Outreach in Community
Mental Health Care

Outreach in Community Mental Health Care
A Manual for Practitioners

SECOND EDITION

Tom Burns
Professor Emeritus of Social Psychiatry, Department of
Psychiatry, University of Oxford, Oxford, UK

Mike Firn
Nurse and Health Care Consultant, South West London
and St George's Mental Health NHS Trust and Springfield
Consultancy, Springfield Hospital, London, UK

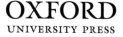

OXFORD
UNIVERSITY PRESS

OXFORD
UNIVERSITY PRESS

Great Clarendon Street, Oxford, OX2 6DP,
United Kingdom

Oxford University Press is a department of the University of Oxford.
It furthers the University's objective of excellence in research, scholarship,
and education by publishing worldwide. Oxford is a registered trade mark of
Oxford University Press in the UK and in certain other countries

© Oxford University Press 2017

The moral rights of the authors have been asserted
First Edition published in 2002

Impression: 1

Published in the United States of America by Oxford University Press
198 Madison Avenue, New York, NY 10016, United States of America

British Library Cataloguing in Publication Data
Data available

Library of Congress Control Number: 2016958453

ISBN 978–0–19–875423–7

Printed and bound by
CPI Group (UK) Ltd, Croydon, CR0 4YY

Dedication

This book is dedicated to Reg Burns
who always put the social workers' perspective,
and to Markus 24.01.01.

Preface

This book is written for all staff who work with seriously mentally ill (SMI) individuals. It focuses on what we can do to help these patients get well and stay well outside hospital. Outreach in community mental health has become increasingly widespread across Europe and several regions of the Americas. In most middle- and high-income countries, it is now the backbone of routine mental health care for the most disabled patients. It contrasts with health care systems based almost entirely on hospital and outpatient clinic services. These make scant provision for individuals with low motivation to attend appointments, or whose lives are so marginalized and chaotic as to make this a very low personal priority. Most of these, but not all, suffer from recurrent psychotic illnesses. As services have matured, this focus has widened to include individuals with persisting affective disorders and some serious personality disorders. Adult services are also now confronted with growing numbers of patients coming from Child and Adolescent Services requiring care for disorders such as ADHD and autistic spectrum disorder.

We wrote this book 15 years ago because our team (and that included us) needed it. We had been working as an assertive outreach team for individuals with severe mental illness since the beginning of 1994. Establishing the Wandsworth assertive community treatment (ACT) team in South West London was prompted by a trip to examine some of the model ACT teams in the US. These US teams were as marked by their differences from one another as by their similarities—hardly surprising, as America is a diverse society with dramatic variations in health and social care. If the approach could make a difference there despite all those differences in context, then we reasoned that the model would probably survive translation to the UK.

When the team was set up, it seemed a useful service development, worth trying out for a few years before deciding whether to continue. Its success was far from guaranteed. Much of what our American colleagues considered characteristic of ACT—continuity of care, outreach, integrated multidisciplinary working—was well established, even taken for granted, in our local generic community mental health teams (CMHTs). Would the smaller caseloads and explicitly targeted work practices make such a noticeable difference as to justify the costs?

Since then, the context of mental health care in the UK has changed almost out of all recognition. Practice has become much more explicitly accountable. The upside of this has been a noticeable raising of standards and consistency— but a price has been paid. The price includes a shift to a greater emphasis on risk management and something of a 'blame culture', with negative effects on staff recruitment and morale. We have also witnessed a quite astounding increase in the degree of prescription of service models and structures. Assertive outreach (encompassing ACT) was one of these prescribed teams in the major reorganization initiated in the UK by the 1999 National Service Framework (Department of Health 1999) and legislated for in the NHS plan (Department of Health 2000). What had started out seven years earlier as a local initiative, though not an isolated one, was now national policy.

When we started, our relative obscurity was a benefit. It meant that we were free to develop a viable way of working, trying out different configurations and styles and learning new skills. It was not always an easy time—we made several mistakes and often had to retrace our steps and start again. It took time to discover what sort of staff liked this intensive working (not everybody does). Tolerance and persistence were necessary to establish effective relationships with all the other components of our mental health services. Our team did not develop in a vacuum, and it had its critics.

Evolution or revolution?

In the first edition of the book, we made it clear that we considered ACT or assertive outreach to have more in common with CMHT practice than it had differences. We believed then that overstating the differences was in nobody's best interest. It set up unnecessary and artificial conflicts and undermined some effective strategies that had evolved over time to fit local needs. Our view was that it was best understood as a refining and targeted application of evidence to a part of CMHT practice rather than a new practice.

In the event, research evidence has eroded these differences. While early trials of ACT teams in several countries demonstrated dramatic reductions in hospitalization (Mueser et al. 1998; Marshall and Lockwood 1998), this was not always found. In the UK, where well-functioning CMHTs were the alternative, ACT consistently failed to deliver its promised reduction in admissions (Burns et al. 1999; Burns et al. 2007; Killaspy et al. 2009). The insistence in the UK on separate ACT teams has since been removed, and local services allowed greater flexibility.

Despite this, ACT remains of enormous importance for this book on community outreach, for two reasons. The first is that the careful attention to practice in ACT teams and the research into them was a step-change in our understanding of practice. It clarified procedures and practices, and provided the drive to improve and codify community outreach in established CMHTs. For instance, one core feature of ACT teams—'a defined maximum caseload per worker'—was a new and radical idea for us all those years ago when we set up the Wandsworth team. At that time there was simply no thought about what was a sensible caseload size: people just took on new referrals and probably neglected many of the older ones who eventually 'dropped off' the caseload. A consequence of introducing ACT teams is that we imported the principle into our CMHTs. Now a caseload of 25–30 would be considered the maximum for a full-time member of staff and is actively managed.

The second reason for ACT's continuing importance is that in much of mainland Europe, Australasia, and the US it has been the vehicle for introducing community outreach. Indeed, in much of mainland Europe, the term ACT is interchangeable with CMHT. Almost any team that offers community outreach—even at quite low intensity—is referred to as an ACT team, or in some instances as a FACT (flexible assertive community treatment) team. Being able to describe the intense ACT practice also helps highlight what does and does not make a difference in good community outreach.

Who is this book for?

We have aimed this book at multidisciplinary staff who work in any form of mental health team which moves out beyond the clinic. It takes assertive outreach teams as one perspective, but we believe that most of the book's content will be found relevant to practice within a whole range of teams and to a whole range of professions. The middle section of the book on health and social care practice will be useful to anyone working with community patients suffering from severe mental illnesses.

How did we choose what to leave out?

No book is perfect. We are conscious that some will criticize us for leaving out more detailed information on specific treatments, or for not summarizing all the available scientific and research evidence. Others will criticize us for putting in too much about research; still others will complain that there is no obvious logic in how much space is accorded various topics. (Why so much on schizophrenia and so little on obsessive-compulsive disorder or anorexia nervosa?)

We have tried to reflect the reality of community outreach work, and have not attempted to describe the various highly specialized teams (eating disorders, forensic teams, etc.). This work is overwhelmingly with a well-recognized group of individuals trying to manage their lives in the most rewarding and dignified manner possible despite severe and enduring mental illness. They are individuals for whom the alternative is, too often, repeated and protracted hospital admissions. We have focused on those issues that kept coming up in our team discussions. Those issues that are rare or peripheral are mentioned but not described in detail.

Some readers may be incensed that we have often given our own opinions on contentious or unresolved matters. We have usually made it clear when we are expressing an opinion. However, medicine and psychiatry advance by the accumulation of knowledge of a type often rather disparagingly referred to as 'clinical anecdote'. Much of practice is based on painstakingly accumulated clinical experience. After all, research studies can only be conducted once there is a hypothesis to test, and those hypotheses are derived from clinical experience. There is a risk in this era of evidence-based practice that clinical experience is too easily dismissed. We hope we have honestly presented our opinions and made clear when they represent professional consensus and the very rare occasions when they are not the majority view.

'Patient' or 'client'?

A pressing issue was whether to use the term 'patient' or 'client' throughout the book. Neither of us think this is a big issue, and in our team meetings we used both terms interchangeably. But in a book one needs o be consistent. As explained in Chapter 2, we eventually chose 'patient' because of a series of surveys that have been published showing that this is the term that patients themselves prefer. It is not a political point and does not imply allegiance to some outmoded form of medical model. We hope it does not give offence, and if it does, we apologize.

The second edition

Practice moves on in mental health. Since the publication of the first edition, CMHTs following ACT thinking have become increasingly common across mainland Europe, while ACT teams have been reabsorbed into CMHTs in the UK. Early intervention services, an academic novelty at the time of our first edition, have become accepted mainstream practice internationally. In the UK, crisis resolution/home treatment teams have become widely established, and in the Netherlands, a hybrid between a CMHT and an ACT team—flexible ACT, or FACT—has established itself and is spreading. These teams have more in common than is often acknowledged. In particular, they all rely on multidisciplinary community outreach to achieve their goals. The emphasis varies, as does some of the content, although even here there is more overlap than some of the service specifications would indicate. Oxford University Press received several requests for this book to be updated and reissued, and we are delighted to see it come to fruition. We have adjusted the title to *Outreach in Community Mental Health Care* because we believe this accurately reflects where we are currently in our services. The change is also to avoid perpetuating an early misunderstanding of the narrow remit of assertive outreach teams which we never really shared.

Thanks

This book started from the discussions that the Wandsworth ACT team engaged in every day from 1993 to 2003. During these discussions, we reviewed and planned care and sought solutions to problems. The book took shape from the many questions raised by visitors to the open days we held in 2000 and 2001. The main stimulus to write the book, however, came from the needs expressed by patients and team members, and its contents reflect those preoccupations. Were it not for them sharing their skill, hard work, optimism, and tolerance, we would never have had the energy or time to write it. Since 2003, we have both moved on from the Wandsworth ACT team, but have remained active in community outreach—as practitioners, researchers, and supervisors—for many years.

We would like to thank all those who freely gave up their experience and knowledge to us through collaborative networking in the National Forum for Assertive Outreach and, by extension, our North American and European cousins at the Assertive Community Treatment Association and the European Assertive Outreach Foundation. We also thank Peter Stevenson from Oxford University Press for his encouragement and support in commissioning this second edition.

Tom Burns and Mike Firn
Oxford and London
December 2015

Contents

Part I **Conceptual issues**

1 The evolution of community outreach *3*

2 Current context and aims *13*

3 Who is assertive outreach for? Referrals and discharges *25*

4 Model variance and model fidelity: The lessons from ACT *41*

5 Key working versus the whole-team approach *56*

6 Access: Office hours, shifts, or 24/7 availability? *62*

7 The role of medication *69*

8 Compulsion and freedom *77*

9 Cultural sensitivity *92*

Part II **Health and social care practice**

10 Engagement *111*

11 Medication compliance *121*

12 Hostility *136*

13 Suicidality *150*

14 Self-neglect *160*

15 Schizophrenia and delusional disorders *169*

16 Bipolar affective disorder *182*

17 Personality problems and disorders *196*

18 Depression, anxiety, and situational disorders *208*

19 Substance misuse/dual diagnosis *218*

20 Finance and appointeeship *231*

21 Housing and homelessness *242*

22 Physical health care *250*

23 Employment *260*

24 Daily living skills *270*

25 Psychosocial interventions with families, carers, and patients *279*

Part III **Management and development**

26 Operational and team management *295*

27 Training *313*

28 Service planning *320*

29 Research and development *327*

References *347*
Index *373*

Part I

Conceptual issues

Chapter 1

The evolution of community outreach

Community psychiatry's two eras

Community psychiatry as we know it began to take shape after World War II responding to the challenge of moving care out of mental hospitals. Its development falls into two phases. The first, from the 1950s to the end of the 1970s, consisted of countless small, local improvements—a slow evolution rather than revolution. Changes were clinically led: doctors and nurses responded to the needs of their patients in a pragmatic common-sense way. They came together in relatively simple multidisciplinary teams and carved out manageable areas of responsibility.

The publication of Stein and Test's landmark paper on what became known as assertive community treatment (ACT) in 1980 (Stein and Test 1980) marked the start of the second phase. This is dominated by evidence-based practice and a flowering of mental health services research. Evidence-based practice had been promulgated by the Canadian physician David Sackett who argued that medical practice should be based on evidence and not just on authority or copying what your teachers did. He encouraged staff to learn how to 'critically appraise' research papers and to challenge their seniors if they recommended treatments that were not based on current best evidence. For the following decades, developments and service innovations were no longer just local trial and error promoted by their champions. Of course, new initiatives still originated as the creative products of local enthusiasts, but their impact on wider practice was now through scientific studies and papers. Stein and Test's revolutionary assertive community treatment did not become an international phenomenon simply because it was an excellent model of care but because they showed it was better than routine local practice in a randomized controlled trial. Although small and simple by current standards, Stein and Test's trial was carefully described, with patient characteristics and outcomes well defined. In addition, they described their service model in real detail—you could replicate what they did yourself and test if it worked.

The arrival of evidence-based practice has radically altered how we evaluate and plan mental health services. No longer do we rely on the eloquence and charisma of whoever is proposing some new idea, but we expect to be able to make a more objective, rational assessment before we try it out. The acceptance of this evidence-based approach has undoubtedly improved our understanding of practice and consistency in applying innovations. It has also introduced a new 'internationalism' to thinking. No longer is it a case of 'this is how we do it round here'. Now evidence gathered in the USA or Australia or Sweden or Germany can directly change practice here in the UK, just as evidence derived in the UK can influence practice elsewhere, and has done so. There are some problems with this approach and these are picked up in Chapter 29.

Conclusions have sometimes been too hasty and, given the increasingly centralized planning of services, led to some unnecessary disruption. However, the volume and quality of research evidence has been steadily improving and its application is now generally much more considered. An important, but often overlooked, benefit of this change to evidence-based practice is that we have come more in line with our colleagues in the rest of medicine. As a result, we are more respected than before. We are less likely to be dismissed as unscientific, riven by factions and basing our treatments on ancient anecdotes, and so able to argue on a more equal footing for funding and staff. Certainly this book could not have been written 30 years ago!

Outreach in the UK and Europe

Community outreach is not new in mental health practice in the UK. Some form of outreach has been a feature of UK mental health care since the establishment of the National Health Service and various local initiatives have been recorded intermittently throughout the nineteenth century. The practice of taking services to severely mentally ill patients rather than requiring them to attend hospitals and clinics has been long established in the UK. Several European countries have also described influential initiatives. Querido started a mobile clinic in Amsterdam in the 1930s (Querido 1968). The French developed their 'secteur' approach including limited home visiting in the 1960s (Kovess et al. 1995). In the USA, Pasamanick had described the benefits of home visiting in discharged schizophrenia patients (Pasamanick et al. 1964).

Community psychiatric nurses

In the UK, the community psychiatric nurse (CPN) has been the backbone of outreach in mental health practice. CPNs first made their appearance in 1954 in Warlingham Park Hospital in Croydon (Moore 1961), an example of a pragmatic 'first era' innovation. As with Pasamanick's study, they followed up schizophrenia patients recently discharged from hospital and their main concern was to encourage them to continue their medication.

CPNs have developed exponentially since these first early days in Croydon. Like social workers, they have always considered their brief to be broad, covering both patient and family, and, also in common with social workers, have conducted the greater part of their work in patients' homes. Over three quarters of CPN services were established in the 1970s (White 1991) and the first CPN training course in 1974. By the end of the 1980s, they outnumbered consultant psychiatrists and, between 1990 and 1996, their numbers rose from 4000 to 7000 in England and Wales (White 1999) as they became fully integrated within community mental health teams (CMHTs). Many CPNs consider the title outdated and over-medical and prefer 'community mental health nurses'. However, 'CPN' has become such a well-known term that it is unlikely to change, so we will stick with it in this book.

The 1959 Mental Health Act in England

The 1959 Mental Health Act set the scene for the UK expansion of CPNs and of outreach more broadly. The Act required any mental hospital that accepted compulsorily detained patients to provide an outpatient service. While this may seem unremarkable to us in the UK, it is not the norm internationally, then or now. It played a key role in developing our current form of comprehensive mental health care based on the multidisciplinary team. The same clinicians responsible for inpatient care were also responsible, in collaboration with the patient's general practitioner, for their care after discharge.

The 1959 Act was passed soon after the welfare state was established and encapsulated the need for coordinated health and social care. It established collaboration between health and social care authorities. At the most basic level it established a central role for social workers in compulsory detention but, more broadly, it led to close working relations. Social workers, unlike doctors, had always been extensively community-based, visiting and assessing clients and their families in their homes. The integration of social workers into CMHTs has been a more complex and less consistent story than that of CPNs. Some teams had fully integrated social workers in the late 1960s, some have only achieved this recently and, sadly, many previously integrated teams have had their social workers removed. Even when working in teams, their influence has sometimes been compromised by overly complex parallel management structures.

The joint influence of social workers and CPNs has dominated the style of CMHTs, ensuring that virtually all would provide some form of home visiting or 'outreach'. The benefits of home visiting, not just for follow-up but also for assessment soon became clear to other members of the team including the doctors (Burns et al. 1993; Jones 1982).

Social influences on the course of mental illness

Home visiting in pioneer services such as Dingleton Hospital in the Scottish borders (Jones 1982), and in social work generally, was not simply because many long-term patients did not turn up to outpatient appointments. It was not just because of their lack of motivation, or difficulty in getting to the hospital. Its rationale was primarily to obtain a richer understanding of the context of the patient's problem, to become aware of the family and personal pressures precipitating and influencing the illness and likely to determine engagement with treatment.

The therapeutic community movement at the end of the Second World War focused on how relationships and external pressures could impede or promote recovery from breakdown (Jones 1952). It had been shown very early on that the progress of even very serious illnesses such as schizophrenia were affected by the environment of different long-stay wards (Wing 1968). So if social pressures were to be reduced and social supports strengthened for outpatients, then staff had to know about their situations. The most effective way of doing this was obviously for them to go and see for themselves. The whole mental health team in these early pioneer services invaded the social worker's traditional territory.

Deinstitutionalization

These fledgling developments in social care in mental health received a massive boost from the recognition of the damage caused by long-term mental hospital care. The concept of 'institutional neurosis' (Barton 1959) changed attitudes towards the apathy and self-neglect seen in long-term inpatients. Rather than being understood as an inherent deterioration as a consequence of the illness, it was recognized as a demoralized response to the monotony and disempowerment of hospital existence. This was an oversimplification, but there were many apparently 'deteriorated' patients who had, in fact, recovered but whose recovery went unnoticed in these vast hospitals and who flourished once they were discharged. The remarkable ease with which many of these 'forgotten' patients adapted successfully to life outside hospital led to an enormous optimism, and a conviction that mental hospitals were redundant. This optimism, compounded by further savage critiques of mental hospitals, sparked the drive to close them down entirely, speeding their rundown. By the 1980s and 1990s the patients being discharged were generally much more disabled, and it forced us to take a more realistic view on the need for more comprehensive long-term care.

Erving Goffman's book, *Asylums*, is probably the most influential text on the damaging effects of prolonged mental hospital care (Goffman 1960). He wrote this after several months working as an aide 'undercover' in a large Washington mental hospital. He described such hospitals as 'total institutions', meaning environments where all an individual's needs—food, shelter, recreation, company—were provided from a single source. He concluded they were inherently damaging to humans. They disempowered patients and robbed them of their individuality and self-determination—precisely the qualities they needed to recover from a mental illness. His vivid portrayal of the toxic effects of unvarying routines and procedures, with no accommodation for individual variation, had a worldwide impact, hastening the mental hospital's demise.

A series of damning reports of degrading and cruel conditions within mental hospitals accelerated the public's desire to see them abandoned. In the USA there were several searing exposés from conscientious objectors who had served in state hospitals. In the UK local scandals gave rise to detailed investigations (Committee of Inquiry 1969). Enoch Powell's now famous 'water tower' speech referred to their ominous and looming presence (Powell 1961). Since the 1950s, there has been a reduction of over two thirds in the number of psychiatric beds. This is equivalent to a 90 per cent reduction in real terms when population growth and ageing are accounted for. All the large Victorian mental hospitals are now closed, with just a few of the sites still used to accommodate newer admission units. This is true of most of Western Europe and the USA although mental hospital care is still prominent in Eastern Europe. This rundown in institutional care means that outpatient services are now dealing with increasingly ill and disabled patients. As a consequence, the need for multidisciplinary working and community outreach have become inevitable.

Community mental health teams (CMHTs)

CMHTs are the service model which has evolved in the UK, and much of Europe, to meet this challenge. In the UK, CMHTs were serving over 90 per cent of the population by the 1990s (Johnson and Thornicroft 1993) and at the turn of the century were routine. There is no universally accepted definition of a CMHT but they are fairly easy to recognize. They are multiprofessional groups who work closely together to provide comprehensive care to individuals requiring secondary mental health services, usually for a defined catchment area. The definition of a catchment area is somewhat inconsistent. Sometimes it is used to refer to the whole of an area served by a hospital and then the area served by each team is referred to as a 'sector', and several CMHTs may fall within a hospital's catchment area. Alternatively, each CMHT has its own tightly defined sector. Increasingly, CMHTs in the UK have defined their catchment areas in terms of the groups of general practitioners from whom they take referrals in order to improve liaison and promote shared care (Burns and Bale 1997).

What constitutes a multiprofessional team? The general consensus is that there needs to be a minimum of three professions; nursing, medicine, and social work are the most common. In addition, most CMHTs also include clinical psychologists and occupational therapists, and increasingly mental health support workers, employment specialists, and substance abuse workers.

CMHT culture

CMHTs developed in the UK at the same time as therapeutic communities and adopted several of their characteristics (Burns 2000a; Jones 1952). Jones believed that mental health practice rested on three levels of competence. The first was a general temperamental one—this work required tolerant, positive individuals who liked people. The second was a generic mental health competence— the ability to work with difficult people and form trusting relationships often despite rejection. The third level of competence was the specific professional skills that doctors, nurses, psychologists, etc. gained in their training. Jones argued that we had often exaggerated the role of this third, professional level, and overlooked the importance of the other two. Many mental health interventions can be delivered by any member of the team, drawing on their generic skills. Most do not require specific professional training. This leads to a 'blurring' of roles. So, for example, either a nurse or a social worker could organize accommodation, or a doctor or psychologist provide psychotherapy.

Most CMHTs contain a healthy tension around the balance between 'generic' and 'specific' interventions. This tension is generally productive and creative when well managed, as demonstrated by the evolution of cross-disciplinary responsibilities within the team. A team may identify a member with special skills and responsibilities that it needs that are not traditionally associated with their profession. For example, an occupational therapist may be the team expert in family management, and a nurse the expert in cognitive behaviour therapy.

Most CMHTs restrict themselves to secondary care, taking all their referrals from general practice, social services, and hospitals. However, some allow direct access. In the 1980s direct access was widely encouraged and tried out, but most teams returned to restricting direct access to known patients. As well as leading to an increased and unpredictable rate of referral, open access was used mainly by individuals who were less ill, sometimes not ill at all. These patients were more vocal and demanding than the more seriously mentally ill who were thus further disadvantaged. It was this steering away from the care of the severely mentally ill by self-referred patients that undermined and discredited the 1970s community mental health centre movement in the USA. Such work is also unrewarding for staff, who are unable to fully use their skills. Self-referral also caused confusion about responsibility with primary care and duplication of work.

CMHTs have had to introduce tighter procedures for referral, systematic care programme reviews (Department of Health 1990), and active caseload management to maintain their capacity to care for the severely mentally ill.

CMHTs evolved pragmatically and were well established before the era of evidence-based practice. Consequently, despite their durability and apparent success, surprisingly little was written about them. Very few research studies have been conducted specifically to examine their functioning (Tyrer 2000a; Tyrer et al. 1999). It is much more common that they are used as the control condition in studies of newer, innovative teams (Burns et al. 2007). This absence of research is in sharp contrast to the development of case management and ACT in the US.

Case management in the US

Case management evolved in the US during the 1970s and 1980s for patients discharged from mental hospitals (Intagliata 1982). Community psychiatry in the US was ushered in by President Kennedy's 'new deal for the mentally ill' in 1963. This launched the community mental health centre movement which suffered from over-ambition and problems in staffing (Talbott et al. 1987). Deinstitutionalization started later in the US than in the UK with an extension of Medicare and Medicaid and followed a more rapid course. The lack of social and welfare provision (such as affordable housing, support, and medical care) for previously long-term patients was strikingly obvious. Where in the UK the patient's general practitioner or local social services office would naturally shoulder responsibility for organizing and delivering care, there was no obvious US equivalent. Case managers (originally described as 'service agents') arose to meet this need.

The case manager was charged with the responsibility of organizing, and often purchasing, services for the individual. Initially they had no clinical training, performing a mainly administrative service of 'brokering' care. Coordinating the care of individuals with complex disabilities and needs, discharged into a confusing and unwelcoming world, made obvious sense. For those with stable disabilities such as mental handicap or dementia, the results were encouraging, but unfortunately not so for severe mental illness (Braun et al. 1981). By the time the research into brokerage case management was published, the penny had already dropped and clinical practice had changed.

Clinical case management

Effective care for the severely mentally ill needs to be built on a supportive and trusting relationship. Establishing such relationships is a core skill which mental health professionals develop and refine during their training. Organizing and coordinating the care of the patient remained important, but the case manager was now a trained mental health professional who provided much of that care personally. This approach has been referred to as 'full support' or, more often, 'clinical case management' (Holloway et al. 1995).

Direct patient care by the clinical case manager is efficient. Most patients are well supported and need no input from other staff. With more complex patients this direct care by the care manager cements the therapeutic relationship and the patient is more likely to accept other input. Such close working also generally yields a better-tailored assessment of need.

Case management became well established in the US in the late 1970s and fitted the plurality and complexity of that country's fragmented health and social care provision. However, the arrival of assertive community treatment 'supercharged' the research and policy agendas, generating a veritable industry in community psychiatry research (Mueser et al. 1998).

Assertive community treatment

Stein and Test's 1980 randomized controlled trial of ACT ushered in a new era in the research and practice of community outreach in mental health. Their study originated from the context of a large, isolated mental hospital surrounded by office-based private psychiatrists and family doctors. They were frustrated by the lack of continuity of care and the rapid readmissions of discharged patients over whose treatment they had no control. They took advantage of a ward closure to conduct their now famous experiment. Stein and Test delivered an intensive form of clinical case management in which the case managers worked in teams with small caseloads of ten patients each. They were committed to following up and treating patients in their own homes and neighbourhoods.

Stein and Test called their service 'training in community living' (TCL), with the aim of teaching patients how to cope with their chronic mental illnesses in the community. They randomized 130 patients with established psychotic illness, at the point of potential readmission, to either their TCL service or standard care, which was almost invariably admission (Stein and Test 1980).

TCL care emphasized stabilizing the patient's living situation, monitoring and ensuring medication compliance, crisis resolution (including 24-hour availability to prevent rehospitalization), and training and supporting the patient in activities of daily living *in their own environment*. Each case manager was expected to develop at least a minimal competence across all these areas and to involve other team members routinely in the care and support of their patients. Professional flexibility was essential—the case manager did what was most necessary to keep the patient well and out of hospital even if this lay outside their normal professional priorities. For instance, it may be more immediately necessary to clean up the flat to prevent the patient being evicted than to increase medication to control symptoms. Contact was several times per week and flexible, dependent on need.

This approach resulted in a dramatic reduction in hospital readmission and inpatient care and even in the cost of care (Weisbrod et al. 1980). Patients also demonstrated modest symptomatic and social improvements with more employed or engaged in structured daily activities (Test and Stein 1980). When the funding for the new service ran out after 14 months, Stein and Test found that all the advantages faded completely. The service they had developed was needed as an ongoing support, not simply a training. They consequently abandoned the term 'training in community living' and renamed it the 'programme in assertive community treatment' (PACT).

Replications of ACT

The PACT approach has become the most widely replicated model of case management in mental illness (Marshall and Lockwood 1998; Burns et al. 2007). It became the accepted model for assertive outreach—although not the only one by a long way (Mueser et al. 1998). There is controversy around which aspects of the PACT model are essential. For example, is a 'team approach' or 24-hour availability a requirement for ACT to function? What constitutes 'frequent contact'; what is 'an emphasis on medication'?

Several scales have been developed to measure the 'ACTness' of a team. These are called model fidelity scales and include the Dartmouth ACT scale (Teague et al. 1998) and the Index of Fidelity for ACT (IFACT; McGrew et al. 1994). However, deciding if a team should be classified as ACT still remains contentious. There have been long-running debates about whether different forms of case management are ACT or not (Marshall 1996; Marshall et al. 1999). The change in practice of case management over time (Holloway et al. 1995) and the tendency of Europeans to use the term 'intensive case management' (Burns et al. 1999) whereas ACT is used in the US provide fertile ground for confusion and conflicting interpretation of studies.

Conclusions

The last 60 years have witnessed a revolution in the care of the severely mentally ill. The locus of activity has shifted from large hospitals to care in outpatient departments or in patients' homes. This shift has reaffirmed the importance of relationships in mental health. Whether they are the relationships with family and friends or the therapeutic relationship with staff members, they are the bedrock of successful treatment. Inpatient care remains an essential provision for times of severe disorganization when patients may need constant monitoring and care. However, it is now simply one temporary option among many over the patient's illness career.

For the severely mentally ill, a flexible and broadly constituted approach has evolved in which both health and social care can be delivered and coordinated by trained individuals working within the same team.

From two quite different health care cultures (the US and the UK), two approaches to outreach have evolved and have converged—the CMHT and ACT. Despite historical and organizational differences these two approaches have much in common and both deliver the community outreach which is the subject of this book. Assertive outreach is an area that has been scarred by dogma and vested interest, and we do not intend to continue such empty arguments. Current practice has been informed by both CMHTs and by discrete assertive outreach teams. What follows in this book is equally applicable whatever the team is called.

Chapter 2

Current context and aims

Modernization of mental health services

The rate of change in provision in mental health services has been gathering pace for the last 40 years. As outlined in Chapter 1, this was initially driven by the move from long-term care in mental hospitals to support in the community, with only brief hospital admissions for acute breakdowns. We have witnessed the process of deinstitutionalization and the closure of the large, old mental hospitals, but this picture is, of necessity, an oversimplification.

There remains an important minority of long-term patients who have not been able to transfer to community care. For some this is because their illnesses are so severe, or their behaviour so unacceptable, that the shelter of a psychiatric hospital is the only tolerant and safe environment for them. There is also a tiny dwindling group still in hospital as their mental illness became compounded by age and infirmity, so-called graduate long-stay patients.

More pressing is the group of 'new long-stay' patients who, despite modern care, often remain in hospitals for months and years. These are usually younger patients with severe psychotic illnesses, often complicated by substance abuse and personality difficulties. Failure to allow for their slowly increasing numbers during the early optimistic phase of community care led to serious underestimates of bed needs (Hirsch 1988). The new long-stay population includes many with offending behaviour who may constitute a risk to those around them. The 1990s saw a recognition of the clinical needs of this patient group with the expansion of medium-secure forensic units (Reed 1992) and some longer-term provision. Current mental health care internationally has witnessed a remarkable rise in the number of forensic beds for this group. Priebe, charting their rise across Europe, has questioned whether it represents a more widespread reversal of deinstitutionalization and refers to it as psychiatric *reinstitutionalization* (Priebe et al. 2005). Forensic services are predominantly inpatient and therefore not the subject of this book. However, some have developed outreach provision (Dawson and Burns 2016), and for these the principles and practices described here are relevant, albeit with a higher intensity of contact and even more emphasis on risk.

Changes in mental health care are not solely the result of deinstitutionalization. There have been other important developments. Among these has been the rise of consumerism in health care, the increasing importance of evidence-based medicine, improved treatments, individual professional developments, the rise to prominence of health services research with its international perspective on practice, and a vigorous interventionist approach by governments. It would be impossible to rank these in order of importance. There is considerable overlap between some of them (e.g. consumerism and government intervention), but each will be considered individually in some more detail.

Consumerism in mental health care

Informed patients

The era of 'doctor knows best' is long dead in modern health care. The challenge to professional authority may seem particularly extreme in the field of mental health but is not restricted to it, nor indeed to medicine alone. The Western world has experienced a profound re-evaluation of its opinion of professions and 'experts' alike. Scientists, doctors, lawyers are all questioned in ways that would have seemed unthinkable only 30 years ago. As the population has become better educated, individuals want to know about the possible courses of action open to them. They also want a say in that choice.

When the medical sociologist, David Tuckett, called his book on the doctor-patient consultation *Meetings Between Experts*, he meant that the doctor was the expert on the treatment and the patient the expert on her own experience (Tuckett et al. 1985). Now, the patient, with access to the Internet may arrive at the consultation informed with more up-to-date information about their illness than the doctor or nurse has. Access to case notes and the practice of copying all significant correspondence to the patient, has been quite revolutionary. It has helped emancipate patients and mould their view of the relationship they have with staff—even if many do not read the letters (Kosky and Burns 1995). The management of disorders (especially long-term conditions) is improved when the patient is as fully informed and active in aspects of self-management as possible. Evidence from a wide range of studies—from terminal care (Hinton 1967), through diabetes (White et al. 1996), to discussing the side effects of antipsychotic medication (Chaplin and Kent 1998)—demonstrates that better-informed patients, who are actively involved in their treatment decisions, do better.

Co-production

'Co-production' has become central to improving many public services, including mental health care. Co-production goes some way beyond simple consumerism. It aims for all aspects of the service (design, delivery, evaluation) to be a partnership between 'consumer' and 'provider'. Originating from innovations in policing in the USA, it has generated a new agenda for how professionals should work. Not only should the relationship be more equal and reciprocal, but professionals should think more broadly about how to engage with and benefit their local community and all patients, not just 'this patient'. Clearly, co-production has endless scope for misrepresentation and politicking, but those of us working in community outreach can hardly fail to see the relevance.

'Patient' or 'client'?

The term 'patient' has been rejected by many staff and users, unacceptable because it implies a passive, dependent role in a paternalistic relationship. Social workers and some nurses prefer the term 'client' to emphasize both the breadth of the relationship (extending beyond the purely medical) and also the control that the client should have of the services they receive. Emphasizing the consumerism of the relationship even more, some insist on the term 'service user' (often shortened to 'user' as in 'users and carers'). Some radical groups use the term 'survivor' to express their antipathy to mental health services, although it is not made clear whether they have survived the illness or the treatment. This attention to terminology can sometimes seem tiresome, generating more heat than light. However, it does indicate a real concern with the nature of the modern therapeutic relationship and a wish to see the status of the two players in it altered.

We have chosen to use the term 'patient' throughout this book when the context is referring to care and treatment. For more general contexts, we will use the words individual or person. 'Patient' could possibly have been 'client'. We rejected 'survivor' because we considered it unnecessarily confrontational. It is, however, important to remain alert to the ambivalence many members of the public feel towards mental health in general and psychiatry in particular. 'User' poses special problems. While it expresses the consumerist preference well, it is confused in US writings with drug users and seems clumsily non-specific, even when expressed as the cumbersome 'service user'. 'Carer' also seems wilfully vague in mental health where carers are almost invariably family members. The role of family is so important in community care that we feel it should be properly acknowledged. 'Carer' also confuses informal (family) and formal (professional) carers.

We settled on 'patient' rather than 'client' because it registers that this is, first and foremost, a therapeutic relationship. We actively welcome its specificity and the fact that it is 'state dependent'. An individual is a patient for as long, and only for as long, as they are receiving treatment (just as you are a passenger when on a bus but cease to be one when you get off). It is not a lifelong characteristic of the individual, nor is it stigmatizing. Few of us will not be patients at some time in our lives. Lastly, and perhaps most importantly, we chose 'patient' because that is what patients say they wish to be called! The only systematic studies of 'patient/client' preference (Ritchie et al. 2000) confirms this emphatically, with 77 per cent of those asked preferring 'patient' over 'client'. Even healthy women attending antenatal clinics prefer the term 'patient'.

Our choice of the term 'patient' should not be taken to imply that we deny the increasing importance of consumerism in mental health. Well-informed patients are a powerful force for improvement. They will enquire about, and insist on, the best up-to-date treatments, and demand ease of access and respectful, polite care. Consumerism will, however, inevitably introduce tensions into the traditional relationship when patient and professional disagree. Few of us, after all, like being told what to do! Patients may also be well aware of the best evidence-based treatments but reject them and insist on some alternative (Laugharne 1999). Disagreements arise not only in individual treatment choices, such as in a preference for 'talking treatments' over medication or vice versa. They also feature in considerations about service structures. An obvious example is the debate over 24-hour crisis access. This is strongly advocated by patient and family groups and endorsed by policymakers and commissioners (Department of Health 1999a). Yet there is little evidence of its value (Glover et al. 2006; Burns 2016) and strong evidence of its impracticability (Cooper 1979).

Planning and delivering outreach services are currently strongly influenced by the rise of consumerism. The views of all relevant stakeholders must obviously be carefully considered, and the rationale behind choices fully explained, or even the best of services will come to grief.

Treatment improvements

A paradox of the increasingly critical attitude and general scepticism towards medicine is that it should be occurring now, just when we are delivering more consistent and effective, and less dangerous, treatments. There is now a range of relatively effective pharmacological treatments for virtually all of the more severe mental illnesses other than dementia. For depression there is a choice between several different tricyclic antidepressants and selective serotonin reuptake inhibitors (SSRIs). In addition there are mood stabilizers such as lithium and carbamazepine for resistant patients and for maintenance in bipolar affective disorder. In schizophrenia and delusional disorders the traditional phenothiazines can now be substituted with the newer 'atypical' antipsychotics and, in resistant cases, the superiority of clozapine is conclusively demonstrated (Kane et al. 1988).

Improvements in treatment extend beyond new drugs and include the refining and testing of structured psychotherapies such as cognitive behaviour therapy (CBT), cognitive analytical therapy, mindfulness-based cognitive therapy, and interpersonal therapy, all for depression, anxiety states, and some persistent personality problems. Behavioural therapies for family work with schizophrenia patients and in obsessive-compulsive disorders have also been vastly improved and operationalized, and their effectiveness confirmed repeatedly by research studies.

This increasing therapeutic armamentarium has influenced the context of our practice enormously. Mental health staff are now appreciated for their skills and knowledge rather than just their wisdom and personality. Services delivery has to recognize that patients are increasingly informed. This can be difficult when some treatments are not available locally and it is important to be able to explain this and why it is so. Neither are all the treatments that are fashionable necessarily well established or appropriate. A willingness to engage in an honest discussion of these issues is now part of the job. The media routinely present misleading and exaggerated reports of new treatments. We need to remember that our patients may, quite understandably, be anxious and clutching at straws. The remarkable improvements in our treatments have, unfortunately, been outstripped by inflated public expectations.

Evidence-based practice and clinical governance

Evidence-based practice and clinical governance are now established as the cornerstone of modern public health care. With an exponential increase in research findings, deciding which treatment is appropriate for which patient requires a careful weighing of the evidence. We can no longer simply rely on clinical experience. Not surprisingly, clinicians form preferences for particular interventions. One psychiatrist might favour a more psychological approach for depressed patients while another vigorously tries a whole range of antidepressants first. Evidence-based practice aims to even out such variations. It involves us examining at regular intervals what is currently known about the subject and then basing our treatment decisions on that knowledge.

Levels of proof

Evidence-based practice favours certain forms of 'proof' above others and has established a hierarchy of evidence (Sackett et al. 1997). In particular, it stresses the randomized controlled trial (RCT) and meta-analyses. RCTs are studies to establish the relative effectiveness of treatments; they are essentially the only type of study that can directly test *causality*. They involve randomly allocating half the patients to the treatment being tested and the other half either to no treatment (placebo) or to a current standard treatment ('active comparator'). In drug trials, great efforts are taken to ensure that neither patient nor researcher knows which group the patient is in (double blind), but this is rarely possible in non-drug studies. RCTs are not the only method of researching treatment efficacy but they are undoubtedly the strongest and are subject to fewer problems in interpretation. Other types of studies include *cohort* studies (following a defined group of patients over time) or *case control* studies (cohort studies that match patients who receive the treatment with patients who do not, but are of, for example, similar age and diagnosis).

Meta-analysis involves collecting together a series of RCTs testing the same treatment and treating the collected data as if it was one big study. Meta-analyses depend on good-quality data and similar outcomes being collected. They are very useful in psychiatry because studies often have quite small numbers. With the larger sample in a meta-analysis, random variations between the studies often cancel out and one can place greater confidence in the conclusions. Meta-analyses can sometimes lead to different conclusions when they are repeated as newer studies are added. For example, in behavioural family management in schizophrenia, data from a series of small studies was added together (Mari and Streiner 1994a). This allowed the number of family treatments required to prevent a single relapse to be calculated (the 'number needed to treat'). As is so often found with new treatments which are often conducted by enthusiasts, the number needed to treat was higher in later studies (seven family treatments to prevent one relapse compared to only five in earlier studies). Similar patterns have been shown in CBT for delusions and hallucinations in schizophrenia such that NICE guidance has had to be modified over time. These issues are taken up in more detail in Chapter 29.

A common misunderstanding about evidence-based medicine is that only treatments with good RCT evidence should be given. This is not the case. Many treatments were well established before RCTs or even structured research trials became the norm. There are more ways of accumulating knowledge than formal research. Many things we do are founded on established clinical practice derived from observation and experience. Examples are providing close monitoring for suicidal patients or ECT for severe delusional depression, and few would question their value. However, where there is established, strong evidence in favour of a treatment such as lithium as prophylaxis in bipolar disorder (Cipriani et al. 2013) or clozapine in resistant schizophrenia (Kane et al. 1988), then one would need a good reason for not using it.

Clinical governance and the need for judgement

Clinical governance is the regular monitoring of health care practice to ensure that the best evidence-based practices are being followed and that they are being applied correctly and competently. For outreach staff, evidence-based medicine and clinical governance set the scene for their practice but they pose very special problems. There is generally little ambiguity about the evidence base for individual treatments (e.g. CBT in anxiety, maintenance antipsychotic medication in schizophrenia), but real controversy surrounds the evidence base for how to *deliver* care. Strongly opposing positions are held by researchers on the benefits of service models such as case management (Marshall 1996; Marshall et al. 1999), ACT (Marshall and Lockwood 1998; Tyrer 2000b; UK700 Group: Burns et al. 1999a), and home treatment teams (Burns 2000b; Pelosi and Jackson 2000; Smyth and Hoult 2000).

There is a real discrepancy between the methodological rigour of treatment studies and the rigour of care systems studies. Treatment studies have a long history of well-established methodologies to reduce bias. However, service evaluations are much newer and the subject matter inherently more complex. Despite this, service studies seem to be more influential on practice than the more robust treatment evidence (Burns 1997). As assertive outreach is such a highly politicized issue (see later discussion) it is crucial to develop skills in critical research appraisal. Only then can one have informed opinions about the strength of evidence rather than blindly accepting the statements from politicians or health service managers. This will be returned to in Chapter 29, 'Research and development'.

Health services research and the international perspective

The study of the organization of health care delivery is referred to as health services research. Deinstitutionalization dramatically demonstrated how the form of care delivery impacted on outcome. The treatments offered outside of hospital were broadly similar but the outcomes very different. Early studies of home-based care (Hoult et al. 1984) soon showed a reduction in the need for hospitalization (taken, in all these studies, as a good proxy measure for relapse). Because of the enormous financial savings of reducing hospital care, studies of alternative community-based services have been encouraged and well funded to support hospital downsizing. Chapter 1 traced how the volume of such research expanded enormously after the publication of the cost-benefit analysis of Stein and Test's 1980 study (Weisbrod et al. 1980). Mental health services research is now big business with a confusing range of study types and outcome measures used.

Interpreting health services research

There are a number of special problems in studying mental health services for the severely mentally ill, and these do matter for accurate interpretation. In the first instance, most of the disorders we treat are 'relapsing-remitting' illnesses so are highly variable from month to month. Studies tracking the changes in clinical state before and after the introduction of a new service are therefore notoriously misleading. Patients are commonly recruited into the study when they are most ill and so improvement is not surprising. This improvement is called 'regression to the mean' and it is very risky to attribute it to the intervention. In large RCTs, it is common for both the experimental and control patients to improve—the important issue is whether one improved significantly more than the other. For example, in an RCT of intensive case management, the UK700 study (UK700 Group: Burns et al. 1999b; UK700 Group: Creed et al. 1999), both the experimental *and* the control patients had significantly reduced hospital care in the two years of the study compared to the two years before. Excluding difficult patients, or patients with more than one disorder, can also mislead as these are precisely the patients who soak up most care (Coid 1994). Similarly, studies of newly set-up services can produce misleadingly positive outcomes because they recruit the most able and enthusiastic staff—the so-called pioneer effect.

Importance of context

Perhaps the most complicated aspect of interpreting mental health services research is that of context. Health service research has fostered a healthy internationalism in mental health planning. Most countries are keen to examine practice in other parts of the world and import them if they seem to work. In the 1980s, Italian community psychiatry attracted the limelight for its radical approaches. Currently, research from the English-speaking US and the UK dominates the field, with the US a clear leader. Most of the early studies into case management and ACT stemmed from the US, and these have influenced thinking about community outreach in Europe and elsewhere. However, a problem with importing services research results from one culture to another is that the context may significantly modify their relative advantages.

A striking case was the failure of European studies to replicate the US advantages for case management and ACT. Explaining this failure led to two diametrically opposed interpretations. One was that the implementation differed—essentially, that European services failed to replicate the American ACT, a failure in 'model fidelity' (Marshall et al. 1999). The other was that it was because the control services in Europe are so different to the US, they are more like the experimental case management service or ACT being tested (Tyrer 2000b). Tyrer also suggested that general social welfare provision would modify any potential impact. There was probably some truth in both positions. Practice does differ and routine services in Europe do contain many of the elements of ACT. Clearly what is needed is greater attention to characterizing the context when such studies are reported (Burns and Priebe 1996; Thornicroft and Tansella 1999). In the event, this issue could be resolved using a form of sophisticated meta-analysis (Burns 2007). Which was right is not so important here; the main message is that care is needed in importing conclusions across different health care cultures.

Importance for community outreach practice

These issues are not simply of interest to academics but are of real importance for staff working in community outreach. Early US studies, such as Stein and Test's, were set against a very rudimentary control service indeed, consisting of little more than hospital care and isolated, office-based private psychiatrists, and no multidisciplinary working. These studies, not surprisingly, reported fantastic outcomes with startling reductions in the need for hospital care. Later US studies (Drake et al. 1998; Mueser et al. 1998) and European ones (Holloway et al. 1995; Holloway and Carson 1998) failed to show anything like the same reductions. Despite this, the belief that intensive outreach will empty wards and make hospitals history remains very strong. Teams need a realistic understanding of what is, and what is not, possible. If not, then disappointment and demoralization can follow.

Professional developments

Mental health care is no longer a case of doctors making diagnoses and nurses looking after patients. The range of disciplines involved has broadened to include social workers, clinical psychologists, occupational therapists, vocational specialists, drug and alcohol counsellors, and many more. Not only has the range extended but the training, skills, and expectations of individual staff are barely recognizable from 30 years ago. Occupational therapists, for example, have moved out from the wards to be integral members of teams. They expect to key work patients and provide counselling and psychotherapy as well as their traditional assessments of disabilities and structuring rehabilitation. Similarly, clinical psychologists have all but abandoned their traditional responsibility for psychometric testing and are busy delivering and evaluating more operationalized forms of psychotherapy (sometimes referred to as 'psychological treatments' or 'talking treatments'). They have also developed a profile in staff supervision and training.

Changes in mental health nursing

Nursing has probably experienced the most radical changes. Community psychiatric nurses led the move into the community and now, rightly, view themselves as an independent profession. Graduate entry and the reconfiguration of basic nurse training as a university degree has increased emphasis on academic achievement and profoundly altered expectations and practice. This has been reflected in the widespread development of nurse specialists and nurse consultants.

Community outreach has been a driving force in this development within mental health. Nurses visiting patients at home must, inevitably, take full professional responsibility in the immediate situation. There is no one there to observe or supervise. This sense of independence, allied with their focus on holistic assessment, has forged an enormously strong professional identity around the nurse-patient relationship. This newly acquired self-confidence of the constituent professions has led to a more equal, interactive style of team working. Such levels of professional self-determination require a commitment to lifelong learning as continuing professional education is often cross-disciplinary. Community outreach has only become possible with such increased levels of skill and self-monitoring.

Government intervention

Mental health care, once the proverbial neglected 'Cinderella' service, is now high up the agenda of most Western governments. The severely mentally ill are cared for within state-funded health care programmes throughout the developed world. Despite widespread market approaches to health care, this is one group of patients who don't find their way into private or insurance-based services. Mental health care is very expensive both because of the long-term nature of many of the disorders and also the complexity of patients' needs. Community care has also made mental illness very visible. The public is concerned about perceived failures of such care, such as vagrancy and homicide, despite clear evidence that they are not a consequence of community care (Leff 1993; Taylor and Gunn 1999).

The result is that we operate within a highly politicized arena which often distorts rational service planning. It certainly can make life difficult for staff, and nowhere more so than in community outreach to severely ill patients. Ever the optimists, politicians select and quote the most successful and dramatic study results when setting targets. Politicians' interests are not served by the dusty academic pursuit of weighing up all the available evidence and forming a balanced judgement. They are guided by advisers who know that they want to hear positive messages (they get enough negative ones from the media). As a result, they expect community outreach to improve engagement with services for disenchanted patients (particularly in the homeless and ethnic minorities), reduce inpatient care (thereby generating financial savings), and, last but not least, prevent homicides and suicides by the mentally ill.

Reviewing current practice

This book is a handbook for mental health professionals working predominantly outside hospitals. It is for anyone engaged in community mental health outreach. The emphasis of the book is practical, focusing on procedures that help patients. Inevitably such a practical approach carries a risk of some redundancy, as treatments change and some of the procedures may be overtaken by better ones. It is important to be aware of this when using the handbook and to keep up to date.

This book aims, however, to do more than simply present a description of current treatments. In this rapidly changing field we want to support a critical approach to reviewing current practice and evidence. It really is not enough just to know of a research study and its published results. One needs to know of all the major studies around a topic to establish their relevance (see Box 2.1).

Box 2.1 Assessing a research study

- How robust was the methodology? Was the sample big enough to prove the findings?
- Is the reported difference in outcome *clinically* important? Is it sufficient to justify the potential upheaval of retraining or even restructuring services to achieve it?
- Was the study carried out with patients who are like those you work with? This is not just diagnosis—were offender patients, drug- and alcohol-abusing patients, or homeless patients excluded? If so, how transferable are the results to local needs?
- How similar is the service context to your own? Do the control and support services seem sufficiently similar so you can anticipate similar gains?
- How feasible is the approach? Do you have similar staff and resources or will an attempt at replication just lead to frustration and disarray?

In each of the practical chapters that follow, these questions will inform the discussion. Only by paying serious attention to them can we ensure that services meet our patients' needs and are not simply following political or financial diktats. The intense public attention focused on community mental health outreach can be a nuisance, but it does provide the spur to improve services. For this to be a reality, clinicians (in collaboration with patients and families and health service planners) must take a very active role in the setting of aims, objectives, and practices.

Chapter 3

Who is assertive outreach for? Referrals and discharges

The wrong question!

Which patients should be targeted is the first question usually asked when the decision is made to establish a separate assertive outreach team. Proposals can be based on evidence, wishful thinking, or simple desperation—'revolving-door patients', 'dual diagnosis patients', 'personality disorder patients', 'offender patients', 'the homeless', etc. A local needs assessment can quickly identify the number of such patients and the size of the team calculated.

Whether considering which patients on a community mental health team's (CMHT's) caseload need assertive outreach or when planning the establishment of a specialized team, this is the wrong question to start from. The fundamental question should be, 'What is assertive outreach for?' In other words, 'What treatments and procedures, of proven worth, can we not provide currently that we could with assertive outreach?' This question gives us the answer of 'Who is it for?'.

What is assertive outreach for?

Len Stein, the iconic figure in establishing assertive outreach, was fond of saying that its purpose is to

1. maintain regular and frequent contact in order to
2. monitor the clinical condition in order to
3. provide effective treatment and rehabilitation

There is no special virtue implied for regular contact in its own right—no magical healing properties are attributed to engagement. It is a tool, a basis, for making the competent clinical assessment that is needed in order to offer effective treatments. This is not to devalue the persistence and sheer hard work of engagement often needed to support a patient's precarious social survival outside hospital, which is dealt with in later chapters. What it means is that the purpose of outreach is to provide treatments. If those treatments can be provided equally well in outpatient clinics or day centres, then there is little reason to invest in assertive outreach.

Being clear what a service is needed for is a crucial question that is often overlooked. We have both been consulted by mental health providers both in the UK and abroad who were planning exclusive assertive outreach teams where it was clear that they are either not needed or not viable. These considerations are particularly relevant in several European countries which have no tradition of outreach. Various intensive stand-alone team models have been introduced, slavishly replicating ACT principles without adjusting for how very different their health and social care circumstances are from inner-city USA. In many rural areas, excellent general practice along with low morbidity and well-functioning CMHTs manage fine. Sometimes assertive outreach is hopelessly compromised by local professional rivalries such as entrenched territorial conflicts between health and social care organizations or between inpatient and outpatient services. In these cases complex accountability arrangements may prohibit the joint, flexible working essential for effective assertive outreach.

Surprisingly, targeted assertive outreach teams are sometimes proposed by organizations that do not consider 'mental illnesses' as a meaningful concept. The thinking behind such groups is well rehearsed and beyond the scope of this book. However, we would question the value of such outreach teams. It is not, however, surprising that these issues arise. The focus on the 'whole person' so central to the outreach approach inevitably attracts many professionals who are sceptical about the 'medical model'. The relative prominence of these issues will vary. For teams who are specifically targeting homeless or hard-to-engage individuals, for example, 'treatment' may play second fiddle to 'engagement'. There does, however, need to be some agreement on what will be offered when engagement has been achieved. This will vary according to the patient's needs, but a core of skills and therapeutic aspirations is required if a team is to function.

Some social service teams attempt to make contact with isolated and vulnerable individuals primarily to determine if they have significant unmet needs. This is, after all, a legal obligation laid on social services. They are assertive in repeatedly approaching patients uninvited (and are often colourfully resisted!). However, their aim is for levels of contact more usual in CMHTs. The model is more one of brokerage case management (Holloway et al. 1995) and not addressed in this book.

Clinical opinion or evidence-based?

Clinical experience has gradually identified those patients whose care seems to be most suitable for assertive outreach, and this has been broadly supported by research evidence. Clinical experience and research have also helped identify patients likely to be responsive and those less so.

With the current emphasis on evidence-based practice, clinical impressions and experience can be too readily dismissed. It is important to remember that research findings can only *follow after* clinical experience and opinion. Experimental studies are designed and conducted to test specific questions, 'hypotheses'. These hypotheses arise from clinical experience. Thus, the first major assertive outreach study (Stein and Test 1980) arose from Len Stein's conviction that patients with unstable psychotic illnesses who were taught intensively how to manage their illnesses in the community would experience fewer relapses.

Research trials involve considerable disruption and cost and are not undertaken lightly. There has to be a significant likelihood of proving an important point or of disproving a commonly held belief with which the researchers disagree. A common mistake is to believe that if there is no published research evidence then treatment is not justified. This is not true. The absence of evidence for effect is not evidence of the absence of effect. Absence of evidence does not undermine clinical experience of effectiveness for a treatment. Many long-established treatments have never been formally tested. Although our clinical experience can sometimes mislead us, it is often the only, and perfectly adequate, guide to practice. Where evidence and experience contradict each other, however, then we should follow the evidence. This is not always straightforward. As detailed in Chapter 2, the applicability of research to your local situation needs to be carefully judged.

Which patients benefit from assertive outreach?

Indicators from research studies

The weight of evidence favours the use of assertive outreach with *psychotic* patients and, in particular, those who relapse frequently, requiring hospital admission (Mueser et al. 1998; Burns 2007; Priebe et al. 2003). This conclusion may be somewhat circular, as most of the research into assertive outreach uses hospitalization as its primary outcome measure. Consequently, only patients likely to relapse and be admitted during the trial period are usually studied. There is considerable clinical support for the belief that it is the *unstable*, often somewhat chaotic, younger psychotic patients who have most to gain. Within this psychotic group, patients who are *poorly engaged* with services are also targeted, along with those with established patterns of *poor adherence* with previous treatment. As a consequence of poor adherence and poor engagement, they often have an extensive history of *compulsory admissions*. Although it is hard to operationalize, most teams try to prioritize for patients who have relapses that are 'more severe'. This usually means relapses associated with *high risk*. This always includes those who harm themselves or relatives, but also patients where the risks can be more complex. Examples are bipolar patients whose hypomanic episodes may ruin their reputation and their family's social survival.

These characteristics broadly define the target population for assertive outreach. They are most often young psychotic patients, usually in the first 10 to 15 years of their illness, where relapses and positive symptoms dominate negative symptoms and social disabilities. They are disproportionately male, often poorly engaged and adherent, and they may be impulsive or hostile when relapsing. Not surprisingly, they may have difficult reputations within the wider service.

Ethnic minorities

Disadvantaged ethnic minority patients fit the foregoing description. In the UK, this often centres on black African-Caribbean patients (Singh and Burns 2006; Bhugra et al. 2011). Controversy rages around whether these patients are poorly engaged and poorly compliant because services fail to meet their needs adequately, or as a reflection of more fundamental and widespread multiple disadvantage, marginalization, and cultural forces. Whichever is the case, there is no doubting the difficulties encountered by mentally ill patients in ethnic minorities (Littlewood and Lipsedge 1997; Singh and Burns 2006), and many assertive outreach services explicitly reach out to them.

Bipolar affective disorder

The mania in bipolar affective disorder probably results in more social disruption than almost any other psychotic condition. It also has several other characteristics that fit it for assertive outreach. The mental state is fragile and markedly unstable, often with poor insight and poor medication adherence. The consequences of relapse can be quite disastrous (e.g. overspending or sexual disinhibition in an otherwise devout Muslim wife). This is a group of patients who often only have contact with the services when they are very ill and rapidly absent themselves when recovered. This disengagement from services is driven partly by the fact that the patient does make a significant and abrupt recovery, with little residual deficit. They may also afterwards feel embarrassed and ashamed of what they did. Getting to know these patients in depth, as real people, is often only possible between episodes and can be achieved by persisting outreach.

> ## Box 3.1 Features of patients who benefit from assertive outreach
>
> ### Established characteristics
>
> - psychotic illness
> - fluctuating mental state/social functioning
> - poor adherence with prescribed treatment
> - poor engagement with services/poor relationships
> - severe consequences of relapse
>
> ### Emerging indicators
>
> - ethnic minority patients
> - severe bipolar affective disorder patients
> - borderline intellectual disability

Psychosis and borderline learning disability

Although there have been no published studies of assertive outreach for individuals with learning disabilities, many services have adopted the approach. The model fits well with established practice with this group. Psychosis patients with borderline learning disability responded better than the other patients in one large trial (UK700 Group: Tyrer et al. 1999). This emphasizes its value for individuals with multiple or complex needs (see Box 3.1).

Which patients do not benefit from assertive outreach?

Starting up an assertive outreach team was often associated with an understandable surge of optimism. Now it will be possible to really help all those patients when, up to now, we had too little time! This may be true for many of the patients outlined earlier, but there are some who, despite real commitment, do not seem to benefit from the extra input.

Personality disorder patients

The selection of psychotic patients for assertive outreach focuses heavily on those who comply poorly with treatment and are difficult to engage. Not surprisingly, they are often patients who have been labelled as having difficult personalities or even diagnosed as personality disordered in addition to their psychosis. Assertive outreach works well with individuals who have difficulty in forming and trusting relationships. This thinking has led to some teams just for individuals with a diagnosis of personality disorder. There are no scientific studies published, but the clinical experience is not encouraging. Little success has been reported beyond initial engagement.

This should not come as too much of a surprise. 'Personality disorder' is a vague term, covering a mixed bag of problems, and there is still no consensus on effective specific treatments (Bateman et al. 2015). Treatments have focused on borderline personality disorder and, to a lesser extent, antisocial personality disorder. Most are institution- rather than community-based (e.g. behavioural dialectical therapy, mentalization day hospitals). Several clinicians report good results in individual cases—mostly reductions in self-harm and emergency admissions in borderline patients provided with intensive supportive outreach. This is, however, a notoriously difficult issue and, while we should remain open-minded, the weight of opinion is that intensive outreach is not a worthwhile investment of resources. Some even argue that persisting engagement with these patients might be damaging for them (raising expectations, delaying pragmatic solutions).

Individuals with predominantly negative symptoms

Most CMHTs carry a significant number of individuals with long-term psychotic illnesses who lead a very restricted existence with poor quality of life. They are often burdened by the negative symptoms of their psychosis, less troubled by their hallucinations and delusions. It is very understandable to believe that assertive input will significantly improve the quality of their lives—that it will introduce more structure, activity, and company, leading to increased motivation and improved self-care. Experience has, however, been disappointing.

There are undoubted benefits from structure and activity, but assertive outreach does not seem to be any more successful in engaging such demotivated patients. It is likely that routine monthly CMHT contact reflects what these patients will tolerate more than a lack of resources.

Forensic and offender patients

The clinical profile of patients selected for more intense outreach is likely to contain a number with extensive offending behaviour. Just under 30 per cent of those in the Wandsworth ACT team that we ran through the 1990s had criminal convictions, and a further 15 per cent had significant offences but without convictions. Attempts to target a purely forensic patient population have not been encouraging. One of the few published studies found that forensic patients with intensive outreach spent longer in prison (Solomon and Draine 1995a, 1995b). To some extent this research is self-fulfilling. This patient group is usually selected for assertive outreach because of its rapid recidivism. In addition, clinical decision-making about admission and discharge can be overridden by judges and magistrates (or the Home Office in the UK). The assertive outreach in this group associated with court-ordered restriction orders will be picked up in Chapter 8.

We have had positive experience with offender patients, but this is dependent on the severity of the offences. Serious offences such as arson and dangerous assaults impose severe restraints on community support. Forensic teams have developed outreach enormously since the first edition of this book when they were still focused on running medium-secure units. There may soon be much stronger evidence on the impact of outreach in this group.

Nuisance crimes (such as repeated petty theft) are not uncommon and frequently pose ethical and treatment dilemmas. Police will often not press charges where the patient is known to be in contact with outreach services. Patients may be deprived of a normal, and often necessary, learning opportunity with no legal sanctions to hold them to account and moderate repetition or escalation of behaviour to more serious criminality.

Which patients may benefit from assertive outreach?

Dual diagnosis: psychosis and substance abuse

An inevitable consequence of community care of severely mentally ill individuals is that they are not protected from society's normal problems. The massive increase in drug and alcohol consumption since the Second World War has not spared those with mental illness. Young men acquire the habits of their peers, and many drink and abuse intoxicants to excess. While more of a problem in the US than in the UK, a significant proportion of individuals with psychosis report alcohol and drug abuse.

There is no doubt that in the short term, substance abuse leads to a more chaotic existence for the patient and for his or her carers. It is highly likely that this is due to fluctuations in mental state as a direct consequence of episodic intoxication and, more importantly, of poor compliance with treatment resulting from a chaotic existence (Kamali et al. 2001). Cannabis and alcohol are the two substances most widely used among young psychotic patients (Green et al. 2005). The contribution of early and heavy cannabis use in the *origin* and *precipitation* of schizophrenia has become a subject of considerable research (Henquet et al. 2005). The risks of its recent more potent forms are incontestable (Di Forte et al. 2009).

Opiates and hallucinogen usage appear to be very rare in this patient group in the UK, although heroin is reported as a significant problem in the US.

Assertive outreach has been recommended as a preferred treatment option for dual diagnosis patients with substance abuse in the US (Essock et al. 2006). Their results strongly emphasize an integrated assertive outreach approach with the same team dealing with both mental health and substance abuse problems, and a less forceful, slower style of substance abuse counselling.

First-onset psychosis patients

First-episode patients (often called 'first break' in the US) were not usually included in early assertive outreach services. This was partly because assertive outreach focused on frequently relapsing patients who used lots of inpatient resources. First-episode patients also often make a good clinical recovery, and there was understandable concern about not 'over-medicalizing' what may be a one-off breakdown.

Recent research has confirmed that although there may be a good clinical response in this first episode (hallucinations and delusions recede quickly when medicine is taken), there are other important, though subtle, changes occurring. These cause educational and vocational decline, loss of social supports, family stress, and possibly even cognitive impairment (Pantelis 2003). A longer duration of untreated psychosis is associated with poorer outcome, so early intervention to reduce it has become a key principle of services (Birchwood et al. 2013). One consequence has been to initiate public education programmes to raise awareness in schools and families about psychosis.

Because of the range of health and social care needs identified in this group, and also because of the understandable reluctance of young patients to be involved in institutional care, assertive outreach is the model promoted. Australia has led these developments based on the work of Pat McGorry's EPPIC (early psychosis prevention and intervention centre) service in Melbourne (McGorry et al. 1996). This is a very ambitious service and includes modules for medication management, psycho-education, individual psychotherapy, coping skills training, etc. (Singh and Fisher 2007). Such early intervention services teams are now established throughout the UK and many other countries. In many respects they are the successors to the original, stand-alone ACT team.

The referral process

Assertive outreach is most useful for patients during the stormy, first half of their illness career. In schizophrenia and bipolar disorder, the first 10 to 15 years are often the worst, and then things may settle somewhat. To what extent this is a 'biological' process or an adaptation to the illness is debated. The slogan 'once a patient, always a patient' was popular in the 1980s to emphasize the value of follow-up and continuity of care. This is certainly not the approach now, especially where 'recovery' principles have been adopted, and emancipation from services is a common goal. It was initially a core principle of ACT. Len Stein favoured a 'no discharge' policy, but in reality it has never been practical.

If the expensive resource of assertive outreach is to be efficiently targeted, then it should target patients during the turbulent phase of their illness, when stabilizing social and clinical functioning really requires intensive input. When they have settled, they can, and should, move back to more routine care and eventually GP care. In our experience, patients seem to need intensive work for about five to six years. Obviously this is very much an average—some hardly engage and some may need it for decades. A six-year average means that key workers may expect two or three new patients a year. A well-thought-through process to identify patients who need assertive outreach has been one of the major contributions of ACT teams. While most of these teams have been disbanded (other than in early intervention services), they left two enduring improvements in CMHT practice: first, the necessity for a set caseload for each worker and the whole team; and second, the need to actively choose who should be on it. A further contribution is the recognition that a rational approach must be developed for stepping down patients to routine CMHT care and subsequently to the GP. This 'handing back' has been previously totally ignored in the research and practice literature.

Explicit criteria

It is vital to have basic, explicit criteria for accepting patients for a separate assertive outreach team. In tightly commissioned services, as in insurance-based health systems, this 'eligibility' for service will be highly formalized for financial reasons. There are three other important reasons for being specific. First, if the target patient group is not clear, colleagues will not know whom to propose and practice is likely to 'drift'. We have already listed the characteristics derived from research and our experience. There may be local demographic reasons for modifying this. Some city areas have focused on serving black African and Afro-Caribbean men, while some prioritize the homeless. This needs to be clearly stated and written down in the team's operational policy and in any literature it distributes. It is both unfair on patients and a frustrating waste of time for team members and linked services to argue over conflicting priorities. Clarity about who gets assertive outreach tends to be very explicit for stand-alone teams, but less so for provision within more generic CMHTs.

Second, there is that natural human tendency to accept patients you like and want to work with, but these may not be those most in need of the intensity. At the opposite end of the spectrum, if the definitions are not clear, it is possible to avoid intense engagement with uncomfortable and potentially hostile individuals. Those with stable, restricted lives are often emotionally rewarding to work with, grateful for the contact, and with ostensibly impressive gains (such as better welfare benefits and keeping the flat cleaner), but they hardly need this level of input. Unclear criteria can be used to discriminate against unattractive patients—'too dangerous', 'not motivated', 'a drinker', etc.

Third, without explicit criteria, the performance of your practice cannot be monitored nor can the comparative needs of new candidates for outreach and those approaching discharge be balanced.

Are there patients who might only episodically need an intensive and assertive outreach approach? Chapter 4 will expand on flexible ACT ('FACT') and other models which attempt to integrate the delivery of two levels of care from within one multidisciplinary team. FACT starts to question the binary argument that there are patients who consistently benefit and people who consistently do not.

Who refers?

Even with explicit eligibility criteria, the decision to provide assertive outreach remains a clinical one. If there is a separate team, one needs to meet with the patient and undertake the assessment, either on the ward prior to discharge or in their home along with their current key worker. The assessment should optimally be by the team leader and one of the other clinical case managers (CCMs). The team leader has to have the final say as he or she is responsible for the overall allocation of the team's resources and knows its capacities. Involving another CCM ensures that there is discussion and an important training opportunity. As often as not, that CCM is most likely to take on the patient, and the assessment is an opportunity to start the handover and engagement process.

When it is a matter of deciding within a generic or FACT team to increase the intensity of outreach, then the procedure is basically the same. The current key worker would make the case in the team meeting and the pros and cons considered. If there is disagreement, the team manager would have the final say. Often it comes down to identifying another patient who is ready for 'step-down'. As well as being the best one to understand the team's capacity, the team leader is usually most aware of local considerations bearing on selection and prioritization. Familiarity with individual patients is essential when dealing with pressures from different referring teams or different team members.

Diagnosis is rarely a controversial issue, so the assessment does not necessarily need a medical input, though where there is real uncertainty involving the doctor may help. Patients who only suffer brief psychotic episodes when intoxicated with drink or drugs may need careful diagnosis and are probably best redirected towards addiction services. There are odd cases where patients have been labelled as suffering from a psychosis after some brief disorganized episode although the overall history is one of a personality disorder. It is questionable that they have much to gain from assertive outreach.

Case study

One of the first patients referred to the Wandsworth ACT team suffered from a reclusive schizoid personality (later to be rediagnosed as a mild form of Asperger's syndrome). His notes carried forward a diagnosis of schizophrenia made years previously, when his difficulties in explaining his problems had been taken as evidence of thought disorder. Not surprisingly, he found regular contact unbearable and was successfully settled in a supportive but unobtrusive hostel.

A waiting list?

Should an assertive outreach team have a waiting list? Should patients in a generic team wait for intensive outreach when it has been agreed for them? In separate teams, it is rarely possible to operate without at least some delay in taking on new patients, and this is one real disadvantage caused by specialization. It can also be almost impossible to motivate the discharge of patients back to CMHTs unless there are at least one or two patients known to be waiting for acceptance. Given a turnover of about two to three patients per CCM (equivalent to 15–20 a year for a team, dependent on size), most teams will be accepting up to two new patients a month.

When running the Wandsworth ACT team, we operated a maximum waiting time of three months. There was no science to this but it seems to make sense. Long waiting lists are unwieldy and things can change rapidly. If there are six to eight patients on the waiting list and no hope of a place for at least six months, then teams may stop referring. More needy patients than those on the waiting list may lose out. It is almost impossible to take someone off the waiting list once accepted, so keeping the list short helps to ensure that the assessment process is rigorous.

Where patients are currently in the ward, there is a strong case for being involved in the discharge process and taking over care promptly. This inevitably means some added delay for patients already in the community. These difficult decisions about prioritization must pay due attention to each individual clinical case, and really have to be taken by the team leader.

A minimum period of engagement

How long should you struggle with a patient before accepting that assertive outreach is not working? No system works with every patient, even those who meet its intake criteria. Some patients will simply not engage and it becomes a waste of resource to continue frequent abortive visits. Some show no improvement (either in clinical stability or reduced admissions) despite intensive contact. We suggest offering all patients 12 months of engagement and support before deciding it has failed. Twelve months is probably longer than really necessary to decide, but staff may otherwise begin to 'ease off' too early if the minimum period is only six months.

We had an exception to this for patients accepted directly from the ward. Sometimes difficult patients, with fairly intractable relapses and behavioural difficulties, are discharged from hospital before they are really fit. Heavy medication allows them to tolerate a brief period outside hospital but, following their quick transfer to the assertive outreach team, they may have to return to hospital ultimately for a prolonged admission. We insisted that the referring team accept these patients back if they relapse within two months, and we see no real prospect of engaging them. This does not mean that they *have* to be handed back, but allows the option if the original assessment now seems hopelessly wrong.

Case study

A young African man with a six-year history of schizophrenia was referred to the team. He had recently experienced his longest admission—on the ward for eight months. Affective features, made much worse by heavy cannabis use, dominated his clinical picture. In his brief stable periods, he revealed that he was intelligent, quite charming, and artistically gifted. At the time of his discharge to his flat and acceptance by the assertive outreach team, he was on depot neuroleptics and high doses of benzodiazepines. He immediately increased his cannabis use and was threatening to both the CCMs and his girlfriend. He had to be compulsorily readmitted after only ten days because of a vicious attack on his girlfriend. It then became clear that these attacks had been escalating for the last two years and that a charge for rape was being pursued against him, which had been 'overlooked' in the referral. We agreed we would reassess him when he was really fit for discharge.

Discharge back to CMHTs

The need for throughput

There is considerable variation in the outcome of psychotic illnesses, from a single episode followed by total recovery to chronic, unremitting deterioration (Harrison et al. 2001). Most patients fall somewhere in the middle with an episodic course of periods of illness and longer periods of full or partial recovery. The most turbulent period is in the first 10 to 15 years; most patients settle after that. Assertive outreach is not usually necessary once this period is passed, and it would be an inefficient use of resources (not to mention an unwelcome intrusion into patients' lives) to continue with it. Assertive outreach practice should target its resources on those who need them most. This means that we must actively monitor caseloads and assess when patients might be equally well served by step-down to more routine care. Only by being alert to the need to scale back input when the patient's condition improves will the team maintain a capacity to care intensively for those who need it.

Throughput is also important to refresh staff perspectives. The experiences of the large mental hospitals should alert us to the risks that staff also can become 'institutionalized'. Without the constant challenge of new patients and changing problems, it is easy to develop a narrow, sterile professional approach. It can be very difficult to distinguish recovery (when the illness has receded as a consequence of its natural fluctuations) from symptomatic control from effective treatment. Only when a patient remains well even with reduced clinical input can we be absolutely sure of recovery. We should not assume all improvements are due to our continuing treatment.

In our Wandsworth ACT team, we experienced about 15 per cent turnover per year. This meant that with a caseload of 100, we discharged and accepted just over one new patient per month. For individual CCMs this represented one or two new patients each year and for individual patients it represented a potential time with the team of ten years. These turnover targets were probably too low. On reflection, we believe that caseloads should perhaps have changed by 15–20 per cent and the average time a patient spent with the team about five years. We cannot be dogmatic about this, however, since nothing has been published about it.

Explicit criteria

While much is written about the criteria for acceptance into assertive outreach, very little is published about when to discharge or step down patients. In the Wandsworth team, we decided that any patient whose mental state and social functioning had been stable for two years (i.e. no admissions and no serious near misses) should always be considered for discharge. This consideration took place in the routine weekly reviews meetings, initiated by the team leader. The criterion is for '*review* for discharge', not for 'discharge'. There is an important difference. We knew from past experience that some patients were only stable as long as they got intensive support. Where a previous attempt at withdrawal of support has resulted either in a rapid deterioration or in potentially dangerous situations, then a longer period of stability can be decided upon.

Case study

A 50-year-old Afro-Caribbean woman with a 15-year history of severe bipolar affective disorder had been stabilized by the team using a regime of high-frequency but low-ambition contact—visits varying from daily to three times per week. Visits were short and the emphasis was on medication. All previous relapses had resulted in compulsory admissions, with the police having to break into her apartment. There had also been a serious assault on the GP on one occasion and a policeman on another.

She is a very private woman who only grudgingly accepts our contact and rejects any expansion of our role. After 30 months of stability, an attempt at reducing the frequency of contact was initiated as a precursor to discharge. She immediately refused access and rapidly deteriorated, requiring compulsory admission. She remained stable for a further three years, but we decided to wait for evidence of a qualitative change in the relationship with us or her functioning before considering discharge again.

Where there is a total failure of engagement, a persistent inability to have face-to-face contact at least once a week, we consider discharge. A minimum of 12 months attempted engagement is our usual requirement, although in exceptional circumstances this may be short-circuited. For one patient we had not been able to achieve even a second contact within four months, so decided that there was nothing to be gained by continued fruitless visits to an empty apartment.

Discharge or step-down may be considered if, on balance, outreach appears not to improve the patient's functioning and well-being. We would expect to take one to two years to come to this decision. Such patients may keep contact with us but do not accept treatments, or they continue the same relapse pattern. On rare occasions one has to simply accept that we cannot support a patient out of hospital. The costs of doing so may be too great for the patient or their carers and those living around them. These are the 'new long-stay' or offender patients already referred to. It is important to acknowledge that assertive outreach will not succeed with every patient.

The process of discharge or step-down

Handing patients back to CMHTs from an assertive outreach team is not a simple process. Careful liaison is required, particularly when the assertive outreach has not succeeded. Before the patient can be handed back as 'successfully stabilized', it is essential that the level of support offered by the assertive outreach team has reduced to that which the CMHT can routinely offer. The patient has to have been stable for at least three months on one or two contacts a month. The step-down process of reducing contacts usually takes about three months, so the discharge process will take about six months. During this time, there is ample opportunity to work through issues of dependency and loss. CMHTs are not best pleased to receive patients who feel 'dumped' or who complain loudly about feeling bereft at the loss of their intensive relationship. Discussion and education with the patient (and carers) is required to effect a successful transfer. Although less formalized, the principles are exactly the same for step-down within a generic or FACT team back to primary care.

Where the discharge is because the assertive outreach team has not been successful, the issues are different and often much more difficult. It is essential that the CMHT is not left feeling that they are being expected to achieve, with fewer resources, what the assertive outreach team failed to achieve. Often it is a matter of agreeing that there are some patients who cannot be engaged and may simply have to be admitted and treated when they present in relapse. This can change over time, and sometimes patients have to learn the benefits of continuing care the hard way. This is particularly true of some young manic patients. Paradoxically, being able to share the sense of defeat with the CMHT can sometimes help professional relationships—especially if the assertive outreach team has been viewed as a bit 'precious'.

Conclusions

Assertive outreach in one form or another has been a component of UK mental health practice for several decades. The introduction of assertive outreach teams, however, marked a major step in what has been, until now, a steady evolutionary process. Our view was always that this was evolution rather than revolution, although the pace of change radically altered. Two benefits have resulted from this 'fault line' in development: first, the introduction of explicitly capped caseloads (both individual and team); second, a deliberate attempt to shape the service from the evidence base rather than local consensus. Both these features focus attention much more clearly on selecting the appropriate target patient group than was ever the case before. While accumulating evidence has led to the resorption of assertive outreach back into general teams, these two features have persisted.

The referral and discharge processes are central to establishing the style and effectiveness of a stand-alone team or the choice of patients for assertive outreach in CMHTs or integrated FACT model teams. Evidence drives us towards prioritizing patients with psychotic illnesses and histories of high service use, so-called revolving-door patients. We have emphasized the importance of being clear which *effective treatments* the assertive outreach offers that could not otherwise be delivered. We have followed the evidence and therefore focused on the group of patients with long-standing, unstable psychotic illnesses with prominent symptoms. It should not be forgotten, however, that research can only follow practice, not lead it. It may well be that assertive outreach is effective with other groups (e.g. personality disorders, substance abuse) but we simply do not have the evidence. A healthy respect for evidence-based practice should not lead to a slavish obedience. We have always admitted some patients into our service who do not meet our referral criteria. Only by being open to observation and experience can we learn and advance our practice.

Any division creates border disputes. If assertive outreach is to remain targeted on those who need them most, then it must maintain some boundaries and thresholds. We must not only resist taking on those for whom there is little evidence of added value, but must also discharge or step down those who have improved and no longer need intensive work. The same process occurs between CMHTs and general practitioners in primary care. It is best to anticipate that colleagues will inevitably gripe about this. This will occur when you cannot take on someone ('Typical elitist specialism!') or when you hand back ('Nothing's changed. What's so special about their approach?'). Managing referrals and discharges is, however, probably the most important long-term influence on how well the team works. Ducking issues or, even worse, letting others determine them for you, will please no one ultimately.

Chapter 4

Model variance and model fidelity: The lessons from ACT

The ACT model of assertive outreach

Assertive outreach is one of the most contentious forms of mental health practice. This is because there is a highly prescriptive model of how the best-known form of it, assertive community treatment (ACT), is configured and delivered (Allness and Knoedler 1998). People do not argue about whether or not a day hospital is a 'real' day hospital or not, but they do argue fiercely about whether an ACT team is 'a real ACT team' or not.

ACT, as first described in a series of papers by Stein and Test (1980), has been taken as the model to follow in minute detail. Because it was so successful, it was assumed that every aspect of its innovative approach was 'essential'. This belief was strengthened by the often-quoted study by McHugo and colleagues (1999) in New Hampshire, which showed that 'high-fidelity' assertive outreach teams achieved better outcomes than 'low-fidelity' teams. Fidelity was assessed by measuring the degree to which the teams followed the practice described by Stein and Test, in particular how it matched the ACT standards (e.g. frequency of contact, *in vivo* practice) that were required in the USA to be funded.

It will be clear from the content of this book that we do not accept this interpretation. There are both theoretical and practical reasons for questioning it. Research has undermined the belief that ACT team practice is beyond modification and uniquely and qualitatively different from other assertive outreach services. Later in this chapter we will present this research (Wright et al. 2004; Burns et al. 2007). This confirms the importance of some components, but not all, in successful outreach, and has reduced the insistence on stand-alone ACT teams. In the UK, a consequence of this is to reabsorb the assertive outreach function of ACT teams back into generic CMHTs. This has not been an entirely retrograde step—many lessons have been learnt from ACT which have been preserved in CMHTs. In the Netherlands, a more systematic approach to integrating ACT principles and practice as a component of CMHT practice has been developed—so-called flexible ACT or FACT. We will describe this in more detail later in the chapter.

ACT was initially introduced as a 'package', and no empirical work had been conducted to identify which parts of this package were the effective ingredients. Which of them could be modified or even abandoned without affecting efficacy? The UK700 study (UK700 Group: Creed et al. 1999) was the first designed to address this question by varying only one element of the ACT model (caseload size). We believe that this is the current, scientific, way forward; each of the ingredients should be tested for its contribution (though not necessarily with the rigour of a large multisite RCT).

The instruments used to measure ACT fidelity, such as the Dartmouth ACT scale (DACTS, Teague et al. 1998), have poor psychometric properties. They are the result of 'expert opinion' rather than any testing of the various propositions. This process is rather circular in that experts are chosen from those who agree with the model in the first place. There is nothing wrong in itself with expert opinion—it is often the first step to designing definitive research. However, these conclusions and the measures from which they are derived are often treated as gospel, as if they are based on independent research. They are not. They are opinions—good opinions for the most, but only opinions, and should be treated with appropriate scepticism, especially when applied to the shifting contexts of other nations and the passage of time.

Perhaps it would be better to think more in terms of indicators of good practice in assertive outreach rather than absolute standards. Indicators would include a clearly defined target group of treatment priorities and patients, and a model that emphasized engagement and individualized, intensive, and comprehensive care.

The failure to implement a model of care faithfully may tell us something important about the skills and commitment of the individuals providing that care. Psychotherapy research has shown that what matters most to success is how closely the therapist follows their particular form of therapy, not so much what form of therapy it is. Mindfulness therapists who follow closely the principles of mindfulness therapy do better than mindfulness therapists who do not; interpersonal therapists who stick to the interpersonal therapy rules do better than those who do not (Rounsaville et al. 1988), and so on.

So such comparative studies may tell us as much about the therapists as the treatments. Teams which deviate from their model do less well. We already know that deviation matters, so it may not necessarily prove the superiority of the model. Deviation presumably indicates casual practice or lack of focus, so it is not surprising that the results are poorer. Until individual components of assertive outreach practice have been demonstrated to affect outcome significantly, claims about model fidelity should be taken with a pinch of salt. There are compelling reasons to continue to explore and develop the model. Tyrer

(2013) makes a radical plea to break the bonds that 'ossify' community psychiatry into narrow models and specialisms, with all their resulting fragmentation of care, in favour of the ability to provide continuity of care through flexible multidisciplinary but also multi-function teams. Purists who treat Len Stein's model as holy writ, as if hewn on tablets of stone, are doing neither him nor ACT a service.

Components of assertive outreach

The components of assertive outreach have been described in many ways and at different conceptual levels. One view is that it is primarily a way of thinking (Tyrer et al. 1999), whereas Len Stein has emphasized that it is only a vehicle for delivering effective treatments and that it is these treatments that matter (Chapter 3). Assertive outreach is an effective vehicle for delivering these treatments, so getting it right does matter. Research has modified our views on the relative importance of these features, but describing them is a good starting point to understanding the practice. They are the features used to measure model fidelity in ACT teams, and many are uncontroversial, even if supporting evidence is lacking. We will indicate where there are doubts (see Box 4.1).

In vivo practice

Whatever else it does, assertive outreach requires staff to leave their team bases to visit and treat patients in their homes and local neighbourhoods. It is not an office-based or outpatient, clinic-centred practice. At the very least, three out of every four contacts need to be on the patient's territory to match current CPN practice (Burns et al. 2000). The ACT programme standards (Allness and Knoedler 1998) stipulate 75 per cent or more of the services to be delivered outside the office closely matches this UK practice.

There are several differing reasons for proposing home visiting. Stein and Test originally considered their approach to be a 'training in community living'—learning how to live with the illness. Training in daily living skills such as using a washing machine or cooking in the hospital was of little value if the machine in the patient's local launderette or his cooker had a totally different set of controls. Stein and Test were particularly concerned about difficulties in transfer of learning in patients with psychotic illness. This difficulty, originally labelled 'concrete thinking', has been long recognized. *In vivo* practice enables appropriate skills to be learnt where they will be applied. Whether this is primarily a learning process or a form of support will be addressed in Chapter 24.

Another rationale is that *in vivo* practice ensures that the assessment of a patient's disabilities, needs, and strengths is comprehensive. It is only in their

Box 4.1 Key elements of the PACT model

- A core services team is responsible for helping patients meet all of their needs and provides the bulk of clinical care.

- Improved patient functioning (in employment, social relations, and activities of daily living) is a primary goal.

- The patient is directly assisted in symptom management.

- The ratio of trained staff to patients should be small (no greater than 10–15:1).

- Each patient is assigned a key worker responsible for ensuring comprehensive assessment, care, and review by themselves or by the whole team (see Chapter 5).

- Treatment is individualized between patients and over time.

- Patients are engaged and followed up in an assertive manner.

- Treatment is provided *in vivo*, in community settings—skills learnt in the community can be better applied in the community.

- Care is continuous both over time and across functional areas.

Adapted from Test, M. A, 'Training in community living', in: *Handbook of Psychiatric Rehabilitation*, edited by Liberman, R.P. 1992, Macmillan.

own personal situation that targeted accurate assessments can be made. Seeing them in their home shows the challenges they face and the practicalities of their existence. It is not unusual to find that somebody who appears quite helpless in the hospital has well-developed routines and survival strategies at home, and, on rare occasions, vice versa (Perkins and Burns 2001). In the patient's home and neighbourhood, both stressors and strengths can be fully appreciated.

Outreach is also of great importance for the simple reason that people with severe mental illnesses are poor at attending appointments. They often lead disorganized lives, lose letters, forget the clinic date, or become distracted by other events. They are very unlikely to have a car and the hassle of getting to a clinic by bus or walking may appear insuperable when they are feeling down or particularly unwell. Many may simply not believe they *need* to keep appointments. They may either lack insight that they have an illness at all or have little appreciation of the importance of their treatment. They may also want to avoid treatment because of side effects. For such individuals, outreach, or *in vivo* practice, is the only way of successfully maintaining any contact and developing effective engagement. Without it we have no opportunity to deliver effective treatments. The need to keep patients successfully engaged is one of the most consistent findings of assertive outreach studies (Marshall and Lockwood 1998): there is no controversy about its central importance.

Case study

A middle-aged woman with long-standing paranoid illness was noted at outpatients to be anxious and losing weight. She said that she was lonely but could not get to the shops to buy food, and found her neighbourhood threatening. Initially, her antipsychotics were increased.

On a home visit, however, her CPN tried to take her shopping to 'confront and desensitize her anxiety'. He found that the route from the flat to the shop was past a very rough school where the patient was taunted and harassed by teenage boys. It was this that frightened her. The CPN worked out an alternative (though somewhat longer) route while approaching the headmaster about the boys (in vain).

During his visit, a neighbour approached her and commented that she had known of the patient for several years and would love to help but 'did not want to interfere'. An introduction was arranged and soon the patient was regularly walking the older neighbour's dog and occasionally spending the evening in her flat watching TV together. Both seemed to really enjoy the company (see Box 4.2).

Small caseloads

ACT teams usually insist that caseloads should be small and fixed. In the US, a maximum of ten patients per full-time CCM is usually quoted (Allness and Knoedler 1998), although in clinical practice this often rises to 12–15 when a number of the patients are well settled. Experienced CCMs in established ACT teams warn against too rigorous an insistence on very small caseloads. The work can become monotonous or, even worse, over-intense and emotionally claustrophobic for the patient. A small enough caseload is deemed essential, however, so that staff can maintain regular and frequent contact. It also ensures that they have the time to provide a wide range of inputs, not restricted to simply monitoring medication. Inputs might include encouraging social inclusion by supporting a patient's leisure activities such as going together to a football

Box 4.2 Reasons for *in vivo* practice

- ◆ maintaining contact
- ◆ poor transfer of learning
- ◆ comprehensive assessment

match, or organizing a cinema visit or an outing. None of this is possible without adequate protected time.

Frequent and flexible contacts (see later) do require small caseloads. In the UK, a contact frequency of twice per week for all patients is hardly possible with caseloads of over 12 per full-time worker. In practice, ACT teams maintain a routine contact frequency of 1–2 visits per week (Burns et al. 2000). About three contacts a month seems to be the norm for the more at-risk psychosis patients in CMHTs (Burns et al. 2015). While there is no strong experimental evidence about what is the optimal caseload size in a routine CMHT, it seems to be between 20–30 per full-time worker (Burns et al. 2007).

Frequent and flexible contact/crisis response

An excessive preoccupation with average contact frequency can be misleading. Patients' needs vary enormously over time, and assertive outreach staff need to be able to be flexible about intensity of input. This applies to both the focus of the visit and the frequency. A routine of visiting at a regular time once or twice a week can be reassuring. But changes in mental state, crises in relationships, or other times of stress (such as a flat being decorated or repair works being carried out) may require increased visiting. A hallmark of good teams is that they can easily visit a patient daily for extended periods of time and, similarly, can provide joint visits at a moment's notice if, for instance, the patient has become hostile. Staff must ensure that they have enough spare capacity in their schedules to respond immediately and with good grace. Team leaders have to see that case managers do not overbook their schedules. If they have too many routine visits planned, they can neither respond to their own patients' changing needs or to requests from other team members.

Learning to 'back off' for a time is also an important part of good assertive outreach working. Maintaining contact even when not immediately clinically required is an essential part of engagement (Chapter 10). However, patients may like to have some breathing space when things are going well. In the Wandsworth ACT team, we often dropped to weekly contact when things were going smoothly, and occasionally even less after team discussion. The research evidence supporting the frequency and content of contacts is well summarized by Charles Rapp of the University of Kansas:

> Three conclusions seem warranted: first, frequency of case manager/client contact rather than hours of contact makes a difference; the use of the telephone may be a helpful supplement, not a replacement. Second, frequency of contact and hospital outcomes will never be truly linear since those who are most ill will often receive the most contact but may also have higher rates of hospitalization. The third conclusion is that the quality of contact, not just frequency, may be a mitigating factor. For example,

small caseloads employing ineffective methods or skill-deficit case managers would probably be ineffective.[1]

Crisis work has been a central tenet of assertive outreach from the outset. Organizing the team so that an immediate response can be mobilized is crucial. A period of daily supervised medication if needed is a good indicator of flexibility. It is a crisis response well worth the investment. Such flexibility needs to be at team level, not just a characteristic of individual case managers. Even if crises have been well spotted in advance, situations can arise where a rapid intervention can avert disaster.

Case study

Robert is a patient the team considers we have done well with—admissions down from twice a year to about one every two years and of shorter duration. He has his own flat but refuses any form of structured daily activity. All relapses are characterized by increased cannabis use, withdrawal from services (often sleeping away), and eventual violence. This results in compulsory admission sometimes requiring the police tactical support squad.

He had been out of contact for nearly three weeks and arrived back home aroused, threatening, and psychotic; he attacked his brother. Police and a social worker were rapidly on the scene and admission was both inevitable and welcome. Two team members went to the scene to take part in the admission process. This helped moderate the potential conflict with the police (who had genuine cause to be worried) and, also, one could stay behind and reassure and support his distraught mother.

As teams become longer established, they find that crisis work diminishes. Staff know their patients better, are aware of stressors, and become increasingly attuned to early signs of relapse. The emphasis shifts more to crisis *prevention* than crisis intervention. It is important, however, not to become complacent— crises will occur. The ability of the team to respond rapidly and coherently is an important measure of its effectiveness.

Comprehensive care (health and social)

Assertive outreach teams have a style of working that could be characterized as a form of 'one-stop shopping' in the care of the severely mentally ill. Wherever the team judges that it can meet the patient's need for care, it endeavours to do it without involving other care agencies. In this way it responds to fragmented and discontinuous services. The team offers continuity of care across functional and service boundaries as well as over time (Test 1992).

---

[1] Reproduced from *Community Mental Health Journal*, 34, 4, Rapp, C.A., 'The active ingredients of effective case management: a research synthesis', pp. 363–80. Copyright (1998) with permission from Springer.

Because many of the most disabled patients have difficulties in asking for what they need and in trusting authority figures, the Wandsworth ACT team attempted to provide a broad range of health and social care services. The stabilization of mental state and social supports go hand in hand. It is not possible to contain anxiety if you are facing possible eviction or moving between one temporary accommodation and another.

Costed care and benefits

Care management is the provision of specific social care such as hostels and meals which have to be provided by or paid for specifically by the local authority. It has to be authorized by social workers in the UK, and has to be assessed, justified, and accounted for through district finances. This has traditionally involved highly bureaucratic processes, whereas health care has been left to professional discretion and funded from within budgets which are often constrained or obscured by political influence.

Assertive outreach teams have to learn quickly how to access the most common components of social care. Case managers with backgrounds in nursing or occupational therapy need to familiarize themselves with the complexities of welfare provisions. They become skilled in applying for the range of financial supports for which individuals with severe mental illness are eligible (Chapter 19). Optimally, an assertive outreach team should contain at least one social worker, as this eases enormously any negotiations with the local authority. Failing that, agreements are needed that the local authority, benefits agencies, and housing departments will accept these assessments from health care workers.

Case managers invariably resent the form filling, but quickly learn how much patients appreciate their efforts. Getting a grant for furniture or an increase in benefits for a new patient is often a powerful boost in engagement. It certainly makes clear to the patient that you are on their side. Our team found virtually all the organizations we have had to work with to be receptive to these arrangements. Apart from applications for very expensive, longer-term accommodation, it was very rare for the team to be asked for the social worker's opinion in preference to the key worker's. Those organizations with which there has been little such contact may still require a doctor to fill out an application.

Role of social workers

Initially, the establishment of assertive outreach teams was viewed with some suspicion by social workers. The range of tasks overlapping their traditional professional territory is extensive. How appropriate was it for these to be carried out by non–social workers? This concern has receded—social workers are as hard-pressed as any of us! Inevitably, if social workers are recruited as case managers, the reverse situation will also arise. Social workers find themselves assessing mental states, delivering medicines, and even examining patients for side effects of drugs. In truth, this is not that radical a departure—psychiatric social workers have always done this. In the assertive outreach team, however, it is explicit, condoned, and visible. The recognition of the value of generic work and the repeated crossing of the health and social care divide soon erases such concerns in assertive outreach teams. Indeed, this breaking of stereotypes often strengthens team identity. The social worker insists that the patient needs an increase in his antipsychotics, the nurse points out that the medicines are not going to do much good without some structured daytime activity.

A systematic review of home-based mental health care (Wright et al. 2004) suggested that provision of health and social care from within the same team is a core feature of successful services. Its effect on outcome probably derives from efficient coordination of the essential components of care. It may also be that the shift of focus from predominantly medical assessments to a more holistic appraisal and treatments makes the case manager that much more acceptable to the patient. The patient feels they are being treated as a person—not just a set of symptoms.

Mainstreaming

The emphasis on comprehensive care should not detract from the importance of 'mainstreaming'. Encouraging patients to use non–mental health facilities where possible promotes their social reintegration. Often, as the patient makes progress, the case manager may actively encourage them to seek social services support through such routine channels. This promotes more independence and also reduces the burden on the assertive outreach team. The default approach, of course, is that patients should receive comprehensive input according to their *current* health and social care needs from within the team. Supporting steps where possible to greater self-management and self-determination avoids creating dependency and restricting recovery goals. The decision to seek alternative sources of support should be a clinical one made in consultation with the patient, not one arising from restrictive professional practices or where the patient experiences this as being 'palmed off' onto other less desirable resources.

Multidisciplinary care/team working

Successful assertive outreach requires close multidisciplinary working. Early brokerage studies in the US with non-clinical staff (Curtis et al. 1992; Franklin et al. 1987) and some intensive home-based approaches by exclusively nursing teams (Muijen et al. 1994) quickly demonstrated their limitations. Our patients have complex and varied needs and a range of skills is needed to keep them well. Case managers can learn many of these skills and indeed do so. It is one of the attractions of working in such teams that there is such opportunity for skill sharing and learning from one another. But to share skills there has to be someone available with those skills; hence the need for a multidisciplinary team.

It may be that the breadth of perspective that comes from a multidisciplinary team is as important as the range of skills it contains. Case reviews in such teams usually involve a discussion that touches on several differing points of view and differing ways of conceptualizing the problems. Sometimes these differences are more of language (see Chapter 25), but they remind everyone that there are alternatives—there is more than one way of moving forward. The process of discussion is in itself valuable. Teams composed of simply doctors and nurses can easily become sterile and rigid because they lack these differences in approach or concepts.

How many disciplines constitutes 'multidisciplinary'?

Model fidelity measurement of ACT teams placed great emphasis on the range of staff employed—insisting on the need for employment specialists and substance abuse workers in addition to the core of social workers and some medical and nursing input. It is generally accepted that there needs to be at least three professions represented in a mental health team for it to count as multidisciplinary. Some would argue that CMHTs in the UK should have a minimum of four disciplines, as three of them (medicine, nursing, social work) are statutory 'essentials' in the team. The doctor could be restricted to assessments, prescriptions, and Mental Health Act duties; the nurse to delivering direct care and treatment; and the social worker to care management and Mental Health Act work. Of course, it rarely happens like this, but the addition of one of the non-mandatory professions (e.g. occupational therapy, clinical psychology) radically alters the dynamic. Their role adds value; it improves care. They must, if they are to achieve this, promote wider clinical discussions and broader reviews.

The weight of current opinion (Wright et al. 2004; Burns 2007) is that psychiatrists are an essential part of the assertive outreach team, or indeed of any home-based care team for mental illness. It would be impossible to run such a service without nurses, given the central importance of delivering and monitoring medications for psychotic patients. They are the backbone of any UK team, as they are in Italy. In the US and Germany, social workers tend to dominate, with a nursing input often strictly limited to medication. In the UK, a social worker is desirable. Assertive outreach teams have, however, managed without them, by drawing on duty social workers and CMHT social workers. Most team members quickly acquire a basic competence in social care.

Occupational therapists have proved themselves invaluable members of teams, bringing a more experienced and disciplined approach to the assessment of daily living skills and structuring activity. Their training in the 'use of the self' in mental health work provides an invaluable touchstone for many of the discussions of personal/professional boundaries in assertive outreach.

Few assertive outreach teams have succeeded in the UK in recruiting and retaining full-time clinical psychologists. In part this reflects the job market, but also derives from resistance to the more generic aspects of the role. This is a particular pity as many of the skills appropriate for assertive outreach are highly developed within clinical psychology.

The issues surrounding the 'whole-team approach' versus a key-working role are dealt with in more detail in Chapter 5, and those concerning extended hours and 24-hour availability in Chapter 6.

Medical involvement

Psychiatrists have been integral members of outreach teams (whether they be more traditional CMHTs or ACT teams) from their inception. The Dartmouth ACT scale (Teague et al. 1998) includes an integrated psychiatrist, suggesting one full-time psychiatrist for teams of 100 patients. Stein and Test's original study involved a team with a dedicated psychiatrist who was responsible for maintaining a focus on adequate medication. A systematic review of all forms of home-based care (Wright et al. 2004) confirmed the importance of integrated medical input. This review did not, however, find a strong effect for the level of medical input (the number of hours available). The value of integrated medical input (i.e. a regular member in team meetings and decision-making) was contrasted with the availability of a doctor to consult on specific questions (e.g. psychopharmacology, diagnosis).

Support workers

Most US teams have always employed non-professional 'aides' who carry out both skilled and less skilled tasks in direct patient care. In the UK, support workers have become increasingly common. They do not usually have their own caseload or key worker responsibility. Nevertheless, support workers have clients whom they see regularly and with whom they establish excellent therapeutic relationships. Their ability to engage with clients who may distrust the professionals (who carry more statutory responsibilities or have less 'street credibility') is invaluable. This is enhanced when support workers are also service users or ex–service users who have had direct personal experience of the treatments they are supporting. In the Wandsworth ACT team, the support worker was involved in supervising patients' self-medication, assessing mental state, providing practical assistance with shopping or transportation, and even with venepuncture for clozapine blood monitoring. Our service-user support worker exercised her own discretion about whether or not to disclose her own history to patients. Roles where service users are deliberately employed with a remit to disclose their personal recovery insights are referred to as *intentional* peer support roles. In many settings, not restricted to psychiatric services, individual and group peer support as a part of the care process is highly valued by patients.

Voluntary sector teams

Although the literature on assertive outreach is unambiguous about the need for medical involvement, and indeed the need for persistent and vigorous treatment, not all teams accept this thinking. The UK policy emphasis on assertive outreach as a service targeted on 'hard-to-engage' individuals (National Services Framework 1999) led to the development of some teams with a significantly reduced medical focus. These teams were run by social services or the voluntary sector, and prioritized slow, non-threatening efforts at engagement. They saw their role as encouraging disaffected and marginalized individuals to re-establish contact with health services, but did not provide direct care themselves. They often had a high proportion of non-professional staff, including service-user staff.

These teams usually had specific target groups, such as black African and African-Caribbean psychotic individuals or homeless individuals. They play an important role in large anonymous cities, but their very individuality and variation makes detailed consideration outside the scope of this book. Many, though not all, of the approaches outlined here will be appropriate to most of them. Obviously, not having a medical member, they cannot seamlessly initiate or monitor medication, nor can they admit to hospital.

Alternative methods

ACT teams are at the intensive and more medical end of a spectrum of the range of models of case management for the severely mentally ill. ACT has, because of its medical and scientific bias, been subject to the most research (Mueser et al. 1998; Catty et al. 2002; Burns et al. 2007). It was the model promoted by the UK government in the National Service Framework for Mental Health (Department of Health 1999a), the NHS Plan (Department of Health 2000), and described in detail in *The Mental Health Policy Implementation Guide* (Department of Health 2001). Nevertheless, other models of assertive outreach do exist.

Brokerage case management (Intagliata 1982) is at the opposite end of the spectrum. It is neither intensive nor does it involve *in vivo* direct care provision.

Brokerage links patients to appropriate services after assessment and care planning. Brokers are expected to monitor care but not to provide it; brokerage is the only such model that is not clinical case management.

The 'strengths model' (Rapp and Wintersteen 1989) has a highly developed philosophy based on consumerism and engagement which follows a patient-led recovery agenda. As the name suggests, the focus is on the individual's strengths rather than their problems or diagnosis. It stresses that people with severe and enduring mental illness can learn, grow, and change using the resources of their own communities, and aided by assertive outreach. The strengths model has broadly been displaced by recovery-oriented outreach (Leamy et al. 2011) which shares most of its thinking.

Rehabilitation-oriented case management draws on the principles of structured psychiatric rehabilitation. This approach has been developed and researched in the US where it is often referred to as 'the Boston' method (Farkas and Anthony 2010). This involves working systematically to reduce handicaps and disabilities. The emphasis is biased towards improving the patient's functioning rather than an intensive focus on managing symptoms and protecting community tenure.

In the Netherlands, doubts about whether patients with severe mental illness continuously require the degree of intensity implied in the ACT model resulted in the development of the 'flexible assertive community treatment' or 'FACT' (Van Veldhuizen 2007; Bak et al. 2007; Drukker et al. 2008). In many respects this represents a 'hybrid' model incorporating some ingredients from assertive outreach practice. For a typical team caseload of people with more severe mental illness, 80–90 per cent get recovery-oriented, individual case management via a multidisciplinary sectorized team typically, receiving 2–4 home visits a month. In Flexible ACT, 10–20 per cent of patients receive an intensive ACT level of service according to need from the same team using shared caseload, daily planning and review, and frequent visits. FACT teams use a sophisticated digital white board to help track which 'zone' of care the patient is currently in, and conduct their daily meetings around planning the shared care for these high-intensity patients. In the UK context, patients can be referred up to the crisis team when out of hours and hospital admission becomes a concern, as shown in Fig 4.1.

Patients can and do move easily and frequently onto the FACT board for shared intensive care, and then back to individual care management. The experience of FACT has helped services recognize that time-unlimited offer of intensive ACT is no longer valid or affordable. Caseload per case manager are typical of CMHTs at 20–30, and weekend working and crisis intervention out of hours are drawn from other parts of the service.

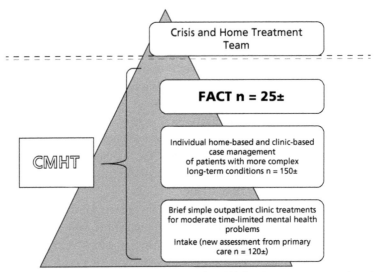

Fig 4.1 Hierarchy of individually case-managed and higher-intensity FACT patients in a typical locality-based CMHT using FACT approaches

We also questioned whether there really was an absolute distinction between the 20 per cent and the 80 per cent group. Are they separate groups, or do patients sometimes belong to one group and sometimes to the other, depending on the thresholds of the system? We suspected that there was a great deal of exchange between the groups. We concluded that the difference between the two groups pertained only to the intensity of care and treatment at a particular point in time and did not have consequences for the composition and attitude of the teams.[2]

FACT has been very successful in the Netherlands, and is spreading as an alternative to ACT in the UK and Norway. The spread of FACT has been aided by its relative affordability, through the availability in several languages of a manualized model description (Van Veldhuizen and Bähler 2013), and more recently by the favourable evaluation of patient outcomes from FACT team care compared to previous periods of ACT team care (Firn et al. 2013, 2016).

Conclusions

Outreach in community mental health benefits from having a clear model. Assertive outreach started with a charismatic service and a strikingly successful

[2] Reproduced from *Community Mental Health Journal*, 43, 4, Van Veldhuizen J.R., 'FACT: A Dutch Version of ACT', pp. 421–33. Copyright © 2007, Springer Science+Business Media, LLC. This is an open-access article distributed under the terms of the Creative Commons Attribution License (http://creativecommons.org/licenses/by/3.0/).

evaluation, and its initial configuration was accepted lock, stock, and barrel. Over 20 years, confirmation of the value of the approach accrued, but also a realization dawned that not all its components are equally important. There has been an understandable tension between the desire to replicate a successful service and the desire or necessity to innovate or vary it according to the relative contributions towards outcomes and the value for money of its constituent parts.

The benefits for reliability and replication of having a clear model with identifiable, essential components are enormous. There is, however, a risk of rigidity, of an ideology, consolidating around what is and is not considered 'real assertive outreach'. Such rigidity can be exaggerated by a focus on measures of model fidelity. Fidelity is not sensitive to changes in the context in which the services are provided. Assertive outreach was the first mental health provision to be subject to such measures. (They are now widely used in individual placement and support, a form of vocational rehabilitation; Bond et al. 2008.) Somewhat ironically, FACT also now has its own fidelity scale and certification process in the Netherlands.

Chapter 5

Key working versus the whole-team approach

Introduction

The central figure in community outreach worldwide is undoubtedly the key worker. Key workers have the strongest and most important relationship with the patient. They provide most of the direct care and are responsible for coordinating those bits they do not deliver. What this person is called—case manager, care coordinator, key worker, clinical advocate—varies between countries and indeed has varied over time. However, the role is intuitively obvious and easily recognizable. In England and Wales, the care programme approach (CPA) (Department of Health 1990) required that all patients cared for by specialist mental health services should be registered on the CPA and that each should have a clearly designated 'key worker'. The legislation and terms used have changed over the years. Now CPA is required only for those with complex and enduring care needs. 'Key worker' became 'care coordinator' to emphasize the specific statutory responsibilities for overseeing and reviewing ('coordinating') care.

Key workers are responsible for ensuring that their patient's care programme is kept up to date, the proposed interventions are carried out, and the various inputs are properly coordinated. They may not be responsible for all aspects of the care patients receive but they are usually responsible for the major part of it. This is a model of care that is well established and fits well with the traditions of multidisciplinary working. Trained professionals work together, but each shoulders appropriate individual responsibility.

The *whole-team approach*, proposed as a key feature of ACT, is in stark contrast to the individual case manager or key worker required by the CPA. Its supporters insist it represents a profoundly different approach. Although no longer the hot issue it once was, it still features in disputes about practice. When European studies failed to find the same advantages for assertive outreach, the absence of a whole-team approach was proposed as one explanation (Marshall 1996; Marshall et al. 1999). In this and the following chapter, we will consider some of the issues which loomed so large in the early debates about orthodox ACT. Although they are now largely historical, they highlight some central concerns that still exercise us, albeit in modified form.

Pathological dependency

In the original Madison team, Stein was particularly concerned to reduce the risk of 'pathological dependency'. He had worked for a considerable period in a state mental hospital and was vividly aware of the risks of institutionalization (Goffman 1960. The more the hospital automatically met patients' needs, the more dependent they became on it—increasingly apathetic and unable to organize their lives. Stein believed this to be the major barrier to patients re-establishing an independent life outside hospital. This is the reason the original initiative was called 'training in community living' (TCL), not 'assertive community treatment' (ACT).

Stein, like most psychiatrists of his era in the US, was also trained in psychodynamic psychotherapy, and he attributed some severe disturbances to a 'pathological dependency' developed in childhood. Pathological dependency had been speculated as a causal factor in schizophrenia. Stein believed it was implicated in the causation of psychoses and that it inhibited personal recovery. He wanted to avoid such relationships being repeated in the patient's relationship with the key worker.

What is the team approach?

In the purest form as proposed by Stein, the team approach meant that patients did not have an individual key worker or care manager. It requires the patient to relate to all members of the team, not just one special worker. The aim was to prevent the relationship becoming too intense, with the patient becoming dependent on a key worker who provided almost all of the patient's care. The result of such a dependent relationship is that the patient then comes to idealize the case manager as supremely competent, and themselves as childlike and helpless. To avoid this, the team organized its work so that no patient could become over-dependent on any one staff member.

A team approach also lifts some of the burden from the staff member—it is not all their fault if things go wrong. Sharing the load across the whole team can also prevent therapeutic pessimism, and avoids resentments arising in the relationship. Such tensions do occur and they can go both ways. A team needs to recognize that staff members can become exasperated with individual patients as well as vice versa. Being professional does not mean being a saint. Intensive, long-term work invariably engages the community outreach worker as a whole person. Such whole-person engagement brings stresses into the therapeutic relationship which need to be acknowledged.

The development of any special or exclusive relationship is prevented by actively ensuring that different parts of the care package are delivered by different team members. Usually this distribution flows logically from the distribution of skill sets. In the most extreme form of a team-based approach, the same intervention is deliberately rotated between different team members (Bond et al. 1990). The patient may not even know who is coming to visit them, just the agreed time and purpose. The Dartmouth ACT scale (Teague et al. 1998) quantifies 'teamness' by asking how many patients have contact with more than one case manager in a given month, but no published studies have reported such data. This did not stop it being fiercely debated.

The US emphasis on the whole-team approach also needs to be understood in the context of their mental health practice of 30 years ago. This was very individualistic, often relying on office-based psychiatrists with little, if any, teamwork. The situation in the UK and much of Europe was quite the reverse. Sometimes referred to as 'shared care', the team approach is also regarded as a feature of flexible ACT (FACT) teams as described in Chapter 4. Developed in the Netherlands as a practical solution to the limitations of individual case management, shared care became part of FACT practice in order to manage the intensity of periods of care without the need to refer outside the team. In the UK, teamwork has been the norm, spearheaded by social workers and CPNs in the community. The risks of unsupervised pathological relationships have always been less, although obviously still possible.

Current position

We have rejected the orthodoxy of the team approach for a number of reasons. First, it simply does not square up with our experience of how people with long-term severe mental illnesses function. As a group, they tend to be shy and have difficulty forming relationships. Certainly those hard-to-engage individuals targeted by community outreach have profound difficulties in establishing a relationship of trust. It takes time, commitment, and consistency to establish such a relationship. Our clinical experience is that for anxious, suspicious individuals, it is best to start with building one relationship and then, gradually, extend the network. Some patients may never accept contact with more than one or two staff.

Second, we are sceptical of the approach because our experience teaches us that independence is only achieved through a period of healthy and supportive dependence. After all, we become adults by slowly gaining our independence from our parents. Attachment theory confirms the crucial importance of a period of secure dependency from which we can then progress. We are convinced that well-trained staff can manage such a therapeutic relationship. Getting this balance right is a common focus in clinical supervision. Meeting legitimate dependency needs supports healthy growth and can avoid an inward-looking and pathological bond.

Third, there are practical drawbacks with a rigorous whole-team approach. Such a 'task-centred' approach adopted by some of the highly orthodox ACT teams has generally been superseded. Even within inpatient nursing teams, the 'primary nurse' system has come to dominate. The hospital setting is much more suitable to a whole-team approach. It allows regular face-to-face contact of the team as well as continuous awareness and monitoring of a limited group of patients; even so, such task-centred practice has been found to be inefficient. It takes too much time and energy to administer and supervise—the continual allocation of tasks which have to be reported back on, the time required to impart and share information and check that everything has been done. Also, quite frankly, patients dislike it. They want the security of knowing that an identified individual has an overview of their needs, remembers about them, and provides continuity. They also want such an individual to turn to when they are worried, one they know knows about them and will take an active interest in their progress.

Finally, we are sceptical because the reality and the rhetoric have never matched up. During a study trip to many of the demonstration ACT teams in the US in the 1990s, one of us (TB) checked it out. While out on visits with case managers, he routinely asked them who else was working with the patient they had just visited. Nearly always the answer was 'Nobody—that's my patient'—despite usually being told by the team leader that the service operated a fully developed 'whole-system team'. Key working seemed to survive even the most clearly articulated theory!

As one report from a US team pointed out:

> The team method of case management is time consuming and manpower intensive. Staff over-saturation with frequently changing information often results in long or incessant meetings, or communication attempts that are sometimes spurious. Staff have a tendency to 'tune out' because of over-arousal or overflow. Additionally, another problem with team case management is accountability in a system where there is no primary care manager except for charting, with resultant ambiguity about who will do the follow-up after treatment planning.[1]

How great is the difference?

In reality, the distinction between the two approaches is less than is portrayed. Community outreach teams usually develop a small network of carers within the team for most patients. At its very least, there needs to be an identified 'secondary' key worker to cover leave or sudden sickness. We found it valuable

---

[1] Reproduced from *Administration and Policy in Mental Health*, 17, 4, Degen K., 'Intensive case management for the seriously mentally ill', p. 268. Copyright (1990) with permission from Springer.

to make joint working a reality, not just an administrative safety net, with a preliminary joint visit undertaken to introduce them in advance of crisis periods. The identity of the secondary worker should be recorded and ideally visible on the boards or charts used for handover. Good handover relies on visual information 'at a glance' showing weekly visit schedules and staff allocated (see Chapter 27). Patients requiring intensive input, such as supervised medication, soon become used to most of the team. Often, certain team members will have special skills which involve them in the treatment of another key worker's patient. For example, a nurse may have to give the depot antipsychotic injections to an OT's patient, or an OT may help in finding employment for a social worker's patient. This is, however, very different from deliberately avoiding special relationships and spreading tasks around the team.

In a team that has run for several years, it is quite possible for all staff to have had direct care experience with virtually all of the patients. Having direct contact makes handovers more meaningful and satisfying and it also improves the contributions made to reviews. This team-level discussion and monitoring of progress also guards against introverted, pathological relationships. The team can comment when they see the key worker becoming over-concerned and preoccupied with detail. They also note when clinical goals have become restricted because of over-familiarity or staleness in the relationship.

Case study

A case manager reported at the second routine six-monthly review in a row that his patient had remained gratifyingly stable; there had been no crises. His colleagues congratulated him on how well things had settled (she had been a very volatile patient). However, they reminded him that a goal of pushing for structured daytime activity had been proposed at the last review but rejected as premature. Now it should be the goal. The key worker had, understandably, focused on stabilizing the patient's medication compliance, almost to the exclusion of all else. His colleagues helped him raise his sights.

The team can also take over the load for a period if a relationship is particularly trying. By familiarity with the patient from direct contact, they can give advice and help without needing the key worker to report concerns.

Case study

The team had been shaken by an unexpected suicide when a young man, who had been doing well, had jumped from a balcony. He had recently got a part-time voluntary job after years of a chaotic and semi-vagrant life. He had also, thanks to dogged detective work by his key worker, re-established contact with his mother, apparently to both their delight. The suicide was debriefed within the team in the usual manner (see Chapter 25).

In the months after this suicide, it became clear that the key worker had upped his level of monitoring across all his patients, especially one who had attempted suicide by jumping in the past. This close monitoring seemed to be raising, rather than reducing, his anxiety.

His colleagues were able to discuss how they also usually found themselves worrying when patients became stable after long periods of psychosis and then started to talk about their 'wasted years'. We all recognized this as a risky period. As well as pursuing this, both in the team and in the individual key worker's supervision, one case manager simply suggested that he would give the key worker a 'break' and do alternate visits for the next month with this worrying patient. In the event, he did most of the visits. The key worker commented afterwards that being 'told' by a colleague what to do had been a great relief—there was no way he was going to ask for such an intervention.

Conclusions

Most patients requiring community outreach teams are likely to have a wide range of needs and may benefit from contact with several team members. Consistency and reliability of care, however, are of paramount importance with highly vulnerable and anxious individuals. It is important that they are not suddenly visited by a complete stranger at a time of crisis or if their key worker is not available. If joint visits are needed, it is preferable that both faces are familiar. Most patients will need to have relationships with more members of the team than just their key worker. The key worker relationship is not meant to be exclusive.

Some might consider this networking and multiple inputs to be a form of 'whole-team' approach, but we think this is confusing. What distinguishes the two approaches is that the responsibility, across time and functions, lies with the key worker. A rigorous whole-team approach deliberately avoids this for clearly stated (though we think, misguided) reasons. Adopting shared care flexibly during periods of intense need and input represents the hybrid position.

While we clearly prefer the key worker and flexible approach, that does not settle the issue. There are still tricky questions to be addressed about the sharing of tasks in community outreach. How should the balance between generic and specialist working be set? What is the role of the secondary key worker? Currently, these decisions are based on local clinical judgement and experience of the patients and team members. Over time, greater clarity and consistency may be achieved.

Chapter 6

Access: Office hours, shifts, or 24/7 availability?

Introduction

Community outreach services in mental health seeks to solve the limitations of reliance on self-presentation to outpatients and to take needed care out to individuals and communities. As consumers of primary care or dentistry, we all now increasingly demand flexible access to services to fit in with our lives. In mental health, the need to improve patient choice and the experience of accessing care is consistent with both the need to engage with people on their terms and also to provide essential safeguards in out-of-hours crisis response. Not least, it ensures that hospital admission is assessed and 'gatekept' properly now that beds are in such short supply. These three aims are widely accepted. What is less accepted is whether out-of-hours accessibility and response should be pooled across services, invested in one team such as a crisis 24/7 team, or held by the team directly responsible for the patient and which knows them best.

Availability seven days a week, round the clock ('24/7'), was one of the rallying cries of ACT purists (Hoult 1986; Marshall and Lockwood 1998; Smyth and Hoult 2000). Like the whole-team approach, it was a central tenet of the ideology and strongly emphasized in early studies. Hoult's service in Sydney is the one where such crisis intervention, round the clock, was promoted in most detail. We do not know how often the original Madison service actually made contact out of hours. The service description (Stein and Test 1978) indicates it was on-call availability from home, more a safety net.

Mature ACT services rarely offered a full service at night. They relied on on-call staff from home who mainly dealt with problems by phone. Some even relied on an answerphone, and most shared duty rotas integrated with local emergency services (Stein and Santos 1998; UK700 Group: Burns et al. 1999a). As with the whole-team approach, the gap between rhetoric and reality was wide for 24-hour services.

Crisis intervention

Crisis intervention has a long history in mental health literature. Caplan (1964) was the first to highlight its potential benefits. Responding to a fire at a dance hall that killed many young people in a small town, he demonstrated the benefits of prompt action in intervening with what nowadays we would probably call post-traumatic stress disorder. Caplan noted how easy it was to engage with traumatic experiences immediately after as compared to the laborious process of overcoming defences and resistance he was used to in traditional psychoanalysis. He saw that crises presented both 'a threat and an opportunity', with real potential for personal growth.

The approach derives more from normal than abnormal psychology; that is, one developed for essentially 'healthy' individuals rather than those with a mental illness. Crisis intervention soon moved from promoting personal growth to intervening quickly to avoid deterioration and damage in established mental health problems. There was a flurry of publications and new services in the 1960s and '70s following Caplan's book (Johnson and Thornicroft 1995), but these services were often short-lived, changing their practice or even disappearing rapidly without fanfare (Cooper 1979).

The 'mobile support team' became the model for community outreach in Australia and parts of Canada, with crisis intervention at its centre. The terms have become confusing and the divisions between 'home treatment' teams, 'crisis resolution' teams, and community outreach teams have blurred. The ability to respond within hours at any time of the day or night to a crisis is central to the remit of home treatment teams (Smyth and Hoult 2000) and to the crisis resolution home treatment (CRHT) teams that became required in the UK National Service Framework (Minghella et al. 1998; National Service Framework 1999; Sainsbury Centre for Mental Health 1998). Although flexibility continues to be an essential component of a community outreach team, crisis resolution is now rarely proposed as a defining characteristic.

24-hour crisis services

The need

For patients with severe and persistent mental health problems, crises and out-of-hours contacts rapidly diminish as patients get to know their teams and teams get to know their patients. The benefits of continuity of care and testing out what works best for each individual within team and key worker relationships are invaluable over the long term.

Separate and specialized 24/7 teams have been implemented nationwide in England since the late 1990s; they have the specific aim and function of providing short-term intensive input as an alternative to admission in crisis. With greater resources than the standard community outreach team, for this purpose they provide an around-the-clock gatekeeping function. They assess the viability of home-based alternative care before anyone is admitted into hospital.

Because this book is aimed at long-term care in the community, we refer you to Johnson et al. (2008) for a detailed textbook on these crisis resolution and home treatment teams as they are known in England.

In long-term relationships, deterioration is anticipated at times of stress and early signs are observed. Training for patients in the recognition of relapse signatures if they have them (Chapter 15) is now a recognized practice in community outreach (Perry et al. 1999). With more intensive contact every few days, it is likely that relapse can be spotted and predicted. This does not mean it can always be prevented, and presentation to the emergency services in the middle of the night will inevitably happen occasionally.

There are two questions to be answered when considering a 24-hour service. First, would an outreach case manager be able to do anything about it that a reasonably well-functioning duty system could not? Second, are the opportunity costs of tying up so much staff time worth it? We audited 24/7 availability for three months in the Wandsworth ACT team when it had been well established and experienced only seven contacts from our 100 patients over the period. Two of these contacts were with the same patient whom we wanted to admit but who had been avoiding us. Eventually, we were able to ensure that the duty psychiatrist admitted him, so that was a plus. The other five were fairly trivial and would have been easily dealt with by the duty psychiatrist. In reality, 24-hour services rarely offer community outreach—it would hardly be safe to be doing home visits at 2:00 in the morning. Even the most ambitious services only offer 'outreach' to emergency departments. So the calculation is about the added benefit of familiarity with the patient rather than outreach as such.

The costs and benefits

The need for 24-hour services will, obviously, depend on local mental health provision. The question is not so much of the possible benefits of a 24-hour service but the cost/benefits of such an investment being made by individual community outreach services rather than relying on a central emergency on-call provision. All mental health services operate from fixed budgets, seeking best value from within them. Outside office hours, there are severe limitations on what can be done. Direct patient and carer contact is possible, but there is little opportunity for any of the complex care planning and liaison which is a core aspect of our job. Nobody else is available out of office hours and certainly not in the middle of the night—social service offices are closed and GPs are only available for emergencies. In early US studies, where the cost of inpatient care was disproportionately greater than non-medical salaries (Weisbrod et al. 1980) and where admission gatekeeping was otherwise absent, then 24-hour cover might have paid for itself.

In a more coordinated local service, however, such as found in Europe and much of the US now, 24-hour availability for small groups of designated patients is prohibitively expensive. It can also deter good staff. The Nacka project in Sweden was one of the earliest comprehensive outreach services in Europe (Stefansson and Cullberg 1986). This service found itself significantly compromised by its early commitment to a 24-hour service that had been written into the service specification. Initially, this 24-hour service was busy and effective. As patients and other services got to know each other and learnt better how to access care during the day, out-of-hours crises rapidly diminished. The 24-hour commitment became effectively redundant but could not be abandoned. Empty night shifts were unattractive to staff, and the cost constituted a massive drain on resources of the whole service and contributed to its eventual closure.

Sustaining the service

In the successful replication of ACT by Hoult et al. (1984) in Sydney, Australia, an on-call system of one person on call between 11 p.m. and 8 a.m. was used. On-call staff had very little to do between these hours during the 12-month study. Patients and carers valued this potential availability of staff but seldom used it. In the UK, several assertive outreach services established 24-hour cover, only later to discontinue it. The reason is usually lack of use other than by a small group of patients who used it inappropriately. Repeated calls from the same individuals complaining of problems with sleep or simply intoxicated have a pretty destructive impact on staff morale.

Staff satisfaction is not a trivial or frivolous issue. Good-quality professionals are not afraid of hard work, indeed most of us find providing good care is our main satisfaction. Being woken in the night to resolve a crisis is fine—surgeons do it all the time—but being woken because someone can't sleep or has had too much to drink soon loses its attraction. Our Wandsworth team members were very clear about this when we evaluated the approach. If the on-call person has to be available to travel to the emergency room at night, this has implications for child care and absolute avoidance of alcohol.

We remain unconvinced that elaborate 24/7 availability adds anything to a well-functioning duty mental health team in the emergency department, and phone triage by inpatient units for patients who are known to the services. The value of experienced mental health nurses being on the emergency on-call system rather than relying entirely on trainee psychiatrists has proved very successful.

Contingency planning with the whole system

Rather than struggling to provide 24/7 cover, community outreach teams are better advised to work with the wider mental health and social care system to provide services in a crisis. Providing the existing 24-hour services, whatever they may be, with a crisis contingency plan for patients is an economical and effective way of ensuring more informed and reliable decisions. NICE guidance (2011) is that patients at risk of crisis are offered a crisis plan. NICE defines a crisis plan as a future statement of preferences and practical arrangements. With the increasing availability of electronic patient records, access to information by appropriate members of the wider care services is readily available at all hours and protected by information governance arrangements. The system must allow access to those likely to come into contact with individuals out of hours in a crisis or to easily contact someone who can.

The NICE guidance (2011) sets out what should be contained in a crisis plan:

- possible early warning signs of a crisis and coping strategies
- support available to help prevent hospitalization
- where the person would like to be admitted in the event of hospitalization
- the practical needs of the service user if they are admitted to hospital (for example, childcare or the care of other dependents, including pets)
- details of advance statements and advance decisions
- whether, and the degree to which, families or carers are involved
- information about 24-hour access to services
- named contacts

Out-of-hours staff must be prepared to follow the future preferences that come out of the collaborative process of generating a crisis plan. The Mental Health Act code of practice (Department of Health 2008) promotes encouraging people to set out their wishes in advance. This will often be a helpful therapeutic tool, promoting collaboration and trust between patients and professionals. It is also a way in which effective use can be made of a person's expertise in the management of crises in their own conditions. Where a formal and valid advance decision exists, it is considered legally binding except when compulsory treatment is considered.

Extended hours

In contrast to controversy over 24-hour services, extended hours are almost universally endorsed by community outreach teams. Early services in the US and Australia were based on a two-shift system providing services for about 12 hours per day, with shifts overlapping in the afternoon. This has been used in the UK (Smyth and Hoult 2000) but has not generally found favour. Although such extended hours are attractive to families and health service managers, there are three major problems with the shift system. The first, and overwhelming, disadvantage is the discontinuity of care it introduces and the amount of time absorbed in handovers. Scheduling regular contacts at the same time each week increases the likelihood that patients will remember them and keep the appointment. If staff work shifts, it is much more difficult to be regular, and often information has to be updated and passed on. Second, there is a serious limit to what can be done 'out of hours' because other agencies are closed. Indeed there is only a restricted range of things that *need* to be done out of hours. For the most part, these involve meetings with carers (who may otherwise be at work) and a range of social activities. Neither of these make much sense if not conducted by the key worker. The third problem is that it makes the job less appealing to staff—not, perhaps, an insurmountable issue if the benefits are significant, but few staff conclude that they are.

An alternative to a shift system is flexible working to cover the activities that have to take place in the evenings. A requirement for some flexible working is not unusual in contracts. In the Wandsworth team, we specified a willingness to work up to one evening a week as flexi-time as a requirement of the job. Too much evening work in lieu of daytime work we found to be disruptive. Staff miss out on too many meetings or are unavailable for joint working during the day. A careful eye has to be kept on this approach to extended hours if the smooth running of the team is not to be compromised.

Seven-day working

Working seven days a week has become a stated national priority for the Health Service in the UK recently. Our Wandsworth team moved to seven days a week many years ago as we increasingly provided daily supervised medication (Chapter 11), and we were a relatively large team in terms of staff and caseload. We had found that patients were more likely to break down or get into trouble at weekends, especially holiday weekends. Medication compliance often faltered or alcohol consumption increased when there was nowhere to go and no visit expected. We had anticipated that an extended service would be most used for dealing with crises, but have found quite the contrary. Weekend working was almost exclusively occupied with planned visits and phone calls.

On the Friday handover, the weekend visits were agreed. These included a significant proportion of patients receiving daily supervised medication (planned routine visits). The next main group was those whose mental state had recently been unstable and who were reassured (as were we) by a booked contact. Being able to see them every day contained this anxiety. For many patients, a phone call to prompt the taking of medicine, ask how they were doing, and to reduce isolation and anxiety was enough.

Weekend work in that team was not rostered but paid for out of a specific overtime budget. This prevented staff from feeling obliged to work weekends when they did not want to, but more importantly avoided absences in the week from time taken off in lieu. Staff readily volunteered for weekend work, usually one per day. The rate of visits was higher than during the week (an average of eight visits compared to five on a weekday), but the traffic is lighter so travelling time less. The visits were also shorter, with simple, explicit goals. Free time was welcomed to catch up with notes and paperwork. The absence of crisis and emergency activity at weekends also confirmed the effectiveness of the routine service.

If there is only one staff member on duty, care is needed about responding to emergencies at the weekend. Many unplanned visits are fine—a patient rings up because they have run out of medicine, or they have a burst pipe and need help in organizing a plumber, etc. If, however, there is a rapid deterioration in mental state and it sounds like there could be safety issues, then community outreach is not a sensible option, and the patient should be encouraged to come to the ward or to A&E for assessment. Safety has always to be considered out of hours, and risks should not be taken. Unscheduled visits could also be undertaken to a day centre if it were open at weekends. In truth, such unscheduled visits should be rare if outreach services are easily available within so-called office hours.

Conclusions

Flexibility and access are key features of good community outreach. A balance needs to be struck between total availability, safety, effective use of limited manpower, and sensible working conditions for staff. Being regularly on call, with little productive work to do, is demoralizing for good staff who want to know that what they do makes a real difference. Well-established teams, in regular contact with their patients, find that what was previously described as a crisis, has, in reality, built up over days or weeks.

Context is important. A 24-hour rapid response service is rarely needed if local services are good. Where local provision is rudimentary, it may be the most effective, perhaps the only, service available. However, the cost-benefit equation for such a discrete service for a small, well-engaged group of patients already offered effective outreach is hard to justify. This does not mean, however, that various stakeholders may not demand it!

Chapter 7

The role of medication

Introduction

Community outreach in mental health has developed mainly for the care of individuals with severe mental illness. The majority of such people suffer from psychoses, essentially schizophrenia, bipolar affective disorder, or other delusional disorder. Together they will affect about 2–3 per cent of the adult population at some time of their life. Patients suffering from these disorders nearly all benefit from medication, and do so for substantial periods. There are, however, also some severe and persistent neurotic disorders (e.g. obsessive-compulsive disorder, eating disorders, a range of anxiety disorders) which require intensive treatment and support, but that usually don't need medication; they represent only a small proportion of the caseload of most services. Effective community outreach services need to be clear about their attitudes towards medication and to establish reliable and effective medication management systems.

This chapter will deal with the place of medication in the overall work and practice of community outreach. Chapter 11 deals specifically with medication compliance enhancement and the chapters devoted to individual disorders pick up the specifics of the relevant medications. There are, however, some general issues that need to be addressed.

It is often forgotten that, in their original description of ACT, Stein and Test stressed the vital importance of patients getting their medicines. This received little attention in their paper, or in many of the subsequent studies, probably because practitioners took it for granted. What they thought was innovative and characteristic of their new services was the broad, flexible, and responsive roles of their case managers. Regular prescription and provision of medication was simply assumed as a core feature. A consequence of this is that outreach staff (particularly those in ACT teams) may be attracted to the work because it is seen as 'anti-drug' or 'anti-medical'. In some ways, this is entirely appropriate and understandable. This is a job with an explicitly holistic approach to patient care, one which values moving beyond traditional professional boundaries.

Effective treatment and rehabilitation of individuals with severe psychotic illnesses, however, does require careful attention to optimal medication. Successful teams need an approach which recognizes the importance of medication and ensures that it is reliably delivered. However, this should not let it erode their broader, more personalized service model. A balanced understanding of what medications can achieve, and what they cannot, is a good place to start. Equally, a recognition of the very real problems that their side effects pose for patients enables the outreach worker to engage in an informed discussion of its pros and cons. Denying or minimizing the burden of side effects is bound to fail as the patient cannot but be aware of them and may conclude that the outreach worker is either not honest or not adequately trained.

The role of maintenance medication in psychoses

Antipsychotic drugs helped drive the revolution in psychiatric care when they were introduced in the mid-1950s. How long one should continue with prescribing was a pragmatic, clinical decision. Initially, antipsychotics were thought to be treatments for acute episodes. Psychiatrists quickly learnt that stopping them as soon as the florid symptoms disappeared was often followed by a rapid relapse. For some psychiatrists, this confirmed a belief in a biological lifelong disorder, where the drugs were simply suppressing the acute manifestations. Many more kept their patients on drugs simply 'for safety's sake'. They were reluctant to stop them, encouraging patients to put up with side effects, to lessen the risk of relapse.

Maintenance antipsychotics

Over the years, custom and practice established that patients with schizophrenia should remain on maintenance antipsychotics as prophylaxis against relapse. This is particularly the case in English-speaking (UK, Australasia, Canada, and US) psychiatry and in Italy and Scandinavia, although much less so in other parts of Europe and elsewhere. Continued prescribing is not just playing safe, however: there is good evidence for the protective benefits of maintenance medication. Early evidence came from random controlled trials with depot medication (Curson et al. 1985; Hirsch et al. 1973). These demonstrated unequivocally that patients receiving the medicines stayed well and remained out of hospital longer. A warning note was sounded, however, by an early study of first-onset schizophrenia patients (Crow et al. 1986). This confirmed that those receiving maintenance medication relapsed and came into hospital less frequently, but they also did slightly less well in terms of their social recovery.

While these early studies demonstrated that more patients without medication relapsed than those with medication, the difference in outcome was *probabilistic*. Not all patients getting the medicines stayed well, and not all those without it relapsed. The attempt to understand these variations illuminated the role of social stressors in precipitating relapse and, in particular, the role of high expressed emotion (Leff and Vaughn 1981) (Chapter 25).

The weight of evidence in favour of maintenance antipsychotics is now so overwhelming that few European ethics committees will permit placebo control trials of new drugs. They will not permit patients with psychotic illnesses such as schizophrenia to be without antipsychotic cover in a trial, even if they give fully informed consent. Unfortunately, much of this evidence is from studies of a year's duration or less; a handful were of two years' duration. We have little solid scientific evidence on which to decide how long we should persist with maintenance medication. A fairly early European consensus statement suggested a minimum of two years after a first episode and five years after a repeat (Kissling et al. 1991). Although now dated, there has been no significant shift from this position (Patel et al. 2003). In practice, most clinicians encourage patients to continue with their antipsychotics as long as they are prepared to, and most continue even after discharge back to their GP (Kendrick et al. 1998). Many patients stop their medication despite such advice, and clinicians dealing with their relapses become confirmed in their view of the need to encourage persistence.

It is highly likely that mental health teams overestimate the duration of continued maintenance medication required. We see the patients who relapse when they stop, while those who do not relapse, stay with their GP and get on with their lives. Hopefully, in time we will develop a more evidence-based strategy for maintenance medication, but for the time being it is likely to rely on clinical consensus.

Atypical antipsychotics and clozapine

The reintroduction of clozaril for the treatment of resistant schizophrenia (Kane et al. 1988; Kane and McGlashan 1995) and the development of the new, 'atypical' antipsychotics has significantly changed prescribing for schizophrenia. This will be dealt with in more detail in Chapter 15. Their introduction has, however, had an effect beyond the pharmacological. The fact of having a range of possible medications, with different profiles of effects and side effects, has meant that negotiation about drugs is no longer simply a token exercise but a meaningful and concrete component in the therapeutic relationship. It is no longer simply a matter of 'taking the medicine' or 'not taking the medicine' but of choosing *which* medicine.

Apart from clozapine, the evidence for an overall significant therapeutic superiority of these atypicals is pretty thin. Even evidence for dropout and side-effect levels, when compared against more appropriate doses of older antipsychotics, is weak (Geddes et al. 2000; Lieberman et al. 2005). However, they 'feel' different, and many patients and relatives seem to prefer the newer drugs. It is important not to underestimate the importance of this sense of choice and empowerment. These are individuals who have often felt themselves passive victims of their disease and powerless recipients of care.

When the first edition of this book was published, none of the atypicals were available in depot preparation. Now there are three in common use and more soon to come. Despite the broad equivalence of outcome between the two classes of antipsychotics (Geddes et al. 2000; Lieberman et al. 2005; Davis et al. 2011), the shift towards the atypicals has been inexorable, mainly based on the differences in their side-effect profiles, especially the avoidance of Parkinsonian motor disturbances.

Monitoring of antipsychotic side effects

When prescribing drugs over long periods for people with severe mental illnesses, it is essential to monitor them carefully for side effects. No effective drugs are entirely free of side effects or of the risk of adverse events. With the older antipsychotic drugs, some of the early side effects were sudden and dramatic (e.g. dystonias, akathisia), while others were more insidious, developing over months or years (e.g. tardive dyskinesia, sluggishness, weight gain).

The severity of these side effects (particularly akathisia and stiffness) substantially compromised the acceptability of the drugs, even if both patient and doctor could see the improvement in mental state. Sometimes the dose required to obtain relief imposed simply intolerable distress and made it impossible to keep taking it. The unpleasantness of the side effects was a driving force in the rapid switch to the newer antipsychotics. Although these also have serious side effects—in particular, weight gain and metabolic syndrome with the risk of developing diabetes—they are not so immediately distressing for patients. The same is true of the new generation of antidepressants, the SSRIs. They do not have the range of anticholinergic disturbances (dry mouth, constipation, blurring of vision) that were so prominent with the original tricyclic antidepressants.

Careful adjustment of dosage is essential with any long-term medication to reduce the risk of side effects. Regular reviews (see Chapter 15) are essential. These are both to ensure effective symptomatic relief and also to avoid troublesome side effects. It is always a balance and it needs to be negotiated and regularly adjusted for each patient.

When the older antipsychotics are still used, appropriate prescribing of anticholinergics for Parkinsonian side effects will reduce distress and enhance compliance with treatment. There is evidence that these were often continued unnecessarily and at high doses. In addition, the 'buzz' they can give led to misuse and street trading. They are more often necessary at the start of treatment (when acute dystonias can be a real risk) but less so over time. Efforts should always be made to find the antipsychotic dose level that is effective without needing long-term concurrent anticholinergics.

Anticholinergics were often mistakenly prescribed incorrectly for akathisia. This is a very distressing sense of restlessness, usually affecting the legs and sometimes the trunk. Akathisia does not respond to anticholinergics, and was originally better treated with either benzodiazepines (Cunningham-Owens 1999) or beta-blockers (Fleischhacker et al. 1990), but now would prompt a change to an atypical antipsychotic.

With the displacement of the older antipsychotics by the newer atypicals, the focus of side-effect monitoring has shifted, but it has also become more sophisticated and important. Careful monitoring for movement disorders is virtually a thing of the past, but sedation still remains an issue. Several of the atypicals, particularly clozapine, can induce terrible lethargy and drowsiness. Loading the dose at night often helps, and many patients do adapt to the drugs. Failure to slowly titrate the dosage, particularly in the early phases of treatment, can lead to persistent refusal.

The main concern with the atypical antipsychotics, however, is weight gain and the development of metabolic syndrome with a much increased risk of Type 2 diabetes. Regular weighing and measurement of triglycerides is now an essential and routine part of an outreach worker's job in managing psychosis patients. Indeed, the whole issue of monitoring the physical health of the long-term mentally ill has now moved centre stage (Chapter 21). Their life expectancy is virtually 20 years less than it should be (Bartels 2015; NICE 2015a). This is for a number of reasons, not just the medication. The current drive for parity of esteem between psychiatric and physical care makes such a difference in life expectation utterly unacceptable. Reducing this gap is unlikely to be achieved easily or quickly. However, careful monitoring of antipsychotic medication and attention to reducing its side effects is an early, essential step.

It is not the place of a book like this to give detailed advice about medication—relevant knowledge evolves far too rapidly. What is important is that outreach workers continually update their knowledge of psychopharmacology and ensure that they obtain regular reviews for their patients. We strongly support the need for reviews to be structured both in time and in content. Nowhere is this more important than in the use of long-term antipsychotics.

The role of mood stabilizers

The evidence is now conclusive that the frequency of relapses in bipolar affective disorders can be lowered by taking regular lithium. Most clinicians consider that the weight of evidence in favour of lithium prophylaxis more than makes up for the need for careful monitoring and the range of side effects (McKnight et al. 2012). In earlier studies, long-term physical damage was associated with lithium. Improved monitoring using regular blood tests and the lowering of the recommended therapeutic levels have dramatically reduced such risks.

Other mood stabilizers have been introduced, such as carbamazepine and sodium valproate. These are much more widely used in the US where lithium, perhaps because it has no commercial value to pharmaceutical companies, has fallen somewhat from favour. None of these mood stabilizers is 100 per cent effective, and often patients find themselves on combinations. There is a view that combining mood stabilizers can improve outcome. Because of their toxicity, maintaining patients on these compounds requires vigilance from the team. This is especially so when the monitoring is shared with the family doctor. When this works it is ideal, but the risk of misunderstanding or a breakdown in communication always remains. This will be dealt with in more detail in Chapter 16.

Antidepressants

Depression in the long-term severely mentally ill is often overlooked. Feeling low, tired, and hopeless can all too easily be attributed either to negative symptoms, to side effects of the drugs, or to an empty and unstimulating life situation. There is strong evidence that depression is common in schizophrenia and other delusional psychoses (Siris 2000; Zisook et al. 1999). It is common in the wake of an acute relapse when there can often be obvious causes of remorse and disappointment. Nonetheless, symptoms can be alleviated and functioning improved by antidepressants as well as by increased support and encouragement.

As with any depressed patient, tablets alone are rarely enough, and attention to problem-solving and support is essential. Visits by the outreach worker need to be increased and the very real risk of suicide considered. It is important not to overlook the potential benefit of antidepressants for patients with long-standing psychoses. They need to be chosen with care, prescribed at therapeutic levels, and continued long after symptom resolution. Antidepressants also need to be monitored for side effects and also to ensure that they are not continued unnecessarily—patients are often loath to come off them if they have experienced a significant lifting of their mood.

Benzodiazepines

A striking and surprising feature of the Italian community mental health services which have attracted such acclaim is that their psychiatrists are much more generous with psychotropic drugs than their UK counterparts. In particular, they prescribe more benzodiazepines, both for sleeping and for the control of daytime anxiety. UK psychiatrists tend to be very puritanical about the use of benzodiazepines given the evidence of their addictive potential. With the atypical antipsychotics, several of which are non-sedating, we have become increasingly aware of the sedative and anxiolytic properties of the drugs we prescribe. It is fairly obvious, in retrospect, that phenothiazines were often used in high doses in acute relapses as much for their sedative as their antipsychotic effects. Now that sedation is a separate element in the management of acute psychosis, we have rediscovered its value in periods of stress in the long-term management of patients.

We have found moderate doses of benzodiazepines (e.g. diazepam 5 mg tds) to be extraordinarily helpful in periods of agitation and stress with psychotic patients in the community. Treatment usually is only for a few days or at most a couple of weeks. We found no evidence of dependency or of a demand for continuation of the medicines in this group. Similarly, we found prompt prescribing of adequate sleeping tablets was often the deciding factor for survival outside hospital. Psychotic patients with troubling delusions and hallucinations need a decent night's sleep to cope. The night can be a particularly difficult time for isolated patients as the support and distraction that treatment can provide is absent. In outpatients with clinically stable schizophrenia, poor sleep is common and associated with an increased severity of positive symptoms (Freeman et al. 2015). Prompt use of hypnotics were a common feature in self-medication contingency plans for our bipolar patients in the Wandsworth ACT team.

Periodic, structured reviews

The mental state and social functioning of patients with long-term problems may change very slowly indeed over long periods. There is plenty of evidence that familiarity with them can lead to our overlooking such changes. In Chapter 27, we highlight the importance of not simply relying on routine clinical judgement but of using regular, structured assessments of clinical functioning. There are a range of such assessments for antipsychotic side effects, and the value of regular, structured screening for them is as important (sometimes more important) as structured assessments of clinical and social functioning. The patient's clinical and social functioning are likely to be uppermost in the mind of the outreach worker when they meet, and drug side effects can easily be overlooked.

Conclusions

The management of medications for specific problems will be dealt with more in the relevant chapters. The thorny problem of how to improve compliance with medicines (or 'adherence' or 'concordance' as it is now called) will be picked up in more detail in Chapter 11. For the severely mentally ill patient, who needs flexible community outreach, medication is likely to be an essential part of their treatment for many years. The last thing such patients need are mixed messages about the value of drugs in their treatment. The purpose of this chapter is to highlight their importance and to stress the need to keep abreast of developments and to devote time and energy to monitoring and fine-tuning their dosage.

This is not to say that medication is the only thing that matters. Far from it. It is simply that medication is an equally important strand in a complex provision. With some patients, it is uncontroversial and simply taken for granted. For others, it is a source of continuous conflict, and, for very few, it may be the only point of contact. It is focused on here separately because it is easily overlooked. This may be because it is thought of as simply the doctor's responsibility or because it fits poorly with the holistic zeitgeist of mental health outreach.

Detailed advice on individual medicines (doses, interactions, etc.) is clearly not appropriate in a book like this. Similarly, the exact arrangements for ensuring regular medical oversight will vary from team to team. What does not vary is the need to take medication seriously. It is a strand in our patients' management that deserves respect and skilled attention.

Chapter 8

Compulsion and freedom

Introduction

Issues of free will and personal autonomy are at the heart of all mental health practice. Although there are overwhelming similarities between psychiatry and the rest of medicine, there are still some fundamental differences. Some sense of 'alienation', either from the normal self or from those around us, is central to the experience of most mental illnesses. In neurotic and depressive disorders, the complaint is often of 'not being my usual self', of being strangely 'anxious, worried, pessimistic, preoccupied', and so on. In psychotic disorders, the perception of the world we live in is changed—the familiar becomes threatening, neutral acquaintances become persecutory and random, irrelevant events become charged with personal meanings.

People with all sorts of physical illnesses may also experience themselves 'changed' and find their environment unbearable. However, they usually link this to the illness and rarely feel that they have changed fundamentally as individuals, or that the world around them is altered. They recognize that their lowered resources or heightened sensitivity account for any altered self-appraisal. In mental illnesses, the patient has to try to restore their normal sense of self, to re-establish a normal relationship with themselves. In more severe psychotic illnesses, the patient also needs to get back to a realistic understanding of the world around them and their relationships with individuals in it. We can capture this difference by saying that mental illnesses manifest themselves in relationships—either relationships with the self or with those around them.

Assessing insight

In the most extreme forms of distortion, we describe the patient as 'lacking insight'. In recent years, several attempts have been made to move psychiatric practice away from reliance on concepts such as insight, which are judged to have 'paternalistic overtones'. Current thinking, particularly when compulsion is involved, prefers terms such as 'capacity' or 'competence'. These issues will be explored in greater detail later in this chapter, but the inescapable reality is that clinicians continue to use their assessment of a patient's insight in key management decisions.

Insight is hard to define but remains an indispensable term that we keep returning to. The more closely one examines it, however, the slipperier it gets. There really is no one clear point of crossover from an accurate world view to an insightless one. Individual world views are endlessly varied. When does a strange view become 'a delusion'; when does a period of pessimism become a 'depressive distortion'? These are, invariably, complex individual judgements. Sometimes it is obvious and nobody would dispute it. Out of the blue, an accountant, father of two and a pillar of the local church, tells everyone that his body has been substituted by aliens and is emitting dangerous radiation. We have little doubt that he is unwell and that his ability to interpret his experiences is flawed. What, however, of the legions of people who are convinced that alien abduction is rife and believe others have been taken away and fundamentally altered before being returned to earth? Few of us would confidently call this view held by several million individuals a delusion.

Clinically, however, insight is essential in day-to-day mental health work, and we have long acknowledged degrees of insight—'he's completely devoid of insight', 'she still has some insight'. In an attempt to bring greater rigour, scales have been developed to measure levels of insight (Birchwood et al. 1994; David et al. 1992; Sanz et al. 1998). A problem with such scales is that they can imply that insight is a fixed quality for each individual. This differs from 'capacity', which is recognized to be context-specific. Individuals can be judged to have capacity for some questions but not others. For example, they can be judged to have the capacity to consent to taking part in research while still being judged to lack the capacity to decide on their treatment. Insight scales have been used mainly in research studies to link functioning with neuropsychosocial tests, but we have not found them routinely useful in our clinical work.

Birchwood et al. (1994) suggested three components of insight:

- awareness of illness
- need for treatment
- attribution of symptoms

In practice, we judge impairment of insight by assessing the strength and pervasiveness of hallucinations and delusions. The assessment requires due attention to cultural norms and the context. We would draw different conclusions from the report of cosmic influences and force fields running through a room when recounted by a young New Age traveller than by an isolated 60-year-old widow. Similarly, the evolution of the ideas and experiences will influence our judgement. 'Bizarre' ideas which come out of the blue are much more suggestive of illness than preoccupations and convictions that have evolved over many years. What both of these contextual issues contain is some form of judgement about how much the person is their 'normal self'. We are not judging the normality of the idea generally, nor how widely it is distributed in the population, but rather its *normality for that individual*. How much are they 'alienated' ('alienist' was an early term for psychiatrist) from their normal understanding of their self and the world? In many ways, it is this very specificity to the individual that can make our judgements seem arbitrary and subjective to outsiders.

Disorder of the brain or disorder of the mind?

Whenever societies are sufficiently wealthy and settled they make the distinction between mental health care and general physical care. While we now very rightly call for 'parity of esteem', it is esteem between two different activities. It is not usually aimed at denying their differences, but eroding the tradition of treating psychiatry as less important. Psychiatry is accepted as a properly established medical discipline but it *is* different from other specialties such as dermatology or neurology. Although some European countries still insist on joint neurology and psychiatry training for psychiatrists, it is because many early symptoms may be the same, but the practice is invariably different. In the 1990s ('the decade of the brain'), the slogan 'mental illnesses are brain illnesses' was adopted. Several eminent academic psychiatrists have also insisted that mental illnesses are just brain illnesses and that it is simply a matter of time before our discipline disappears. The facts speak against this, and the obituary may be premature. The difference lies in the clinical manifestations and how we manage mental illness, not whether it is located in the brain or not. We know that multiple sclerosis and Parkinson's disease are brain disorders, and both display changes in mood and thinking—but we don't think of them as mental illnesses.

What separates mental illnesses and their management from general disorders is the 'alienation' described earlier, and also the central role of the therapeutic relationship in treatment, not just as a vehicle for treatment. The other profound difference that marks out psychiatry as different is the use of compulsion. Issues of compulsion and personal freedom lie at the heart of the practice of mental health care and their use cannot be avoided in any effective and comprehensive system.

Compulsion in community outreach

All the issues about how to balance individual liberty with the need for treatment in the absence of insight affect community outreach practitioners and are often tricky. In more reactive mental health services, without community outreach, disturbance was often very marked before opinions were sought. Patients came with profound delusions and hallucinations, often accompanied by severe distress and self-neglect. That they were in no fit state to decide for themselves was pretty obvious. Now, we often have to make decisions confronted with deterioration that is not immediately intolerable, but we know it is the start of an inevitable decline which will end up that way. How justified are we in intervening early to *prevent* such distress and damage?

Early intervention

Some argue that the early use of compulsion by community outreach workers, and particularly by assertive outreach teams, means that patients are disadvantaged. In effect, increased contact with patients may lower the threshold for overriding their self-determination, and one challenging interpretation of this is that intensive outreach diminishes, rather than increases, patients' autonomy. An alternative view is that waiting until the indications for admission are obvious and unequivocal only serves the needs of staff, not patients. It makes the decision easy for us, but the patient and their family pay the price.

The clinical view of most community outreach staff (including us) is that early intervention may reduce both the severity and duration of the relapse—'nip it in the bud'. It can, however, be legitimately argued that treatment reduces the severity of a relapse, but that its time course is less affected. The evidence is not clear cut. Overall, early studies suggested that assertive outreach seemed to reduce the duration of hospital stays but not the number of admissions (Mueser et al. 1998). In some studies, however, more intensive follow-up was associated with increased admission rates attributed to better identification of clinical need (Tyrer et al. 1995). An Australian study of several thousand patients on compulsory treatment orders found that their rates of admission were increased, presumably because of earlier intervention, but unfortunately there was no reduction in the time spent in hospital (Segal and Burgess 2006). The benefit of early intervention is surely that it avoids the social and personal damage to the patient plus the distress to families caused by the relapse. We need to remind ourselves regularly that it is not the principle goal of high-quality care to reduce costs or hospital stays.

Knowing 'too much'

Another problem with community outreach is that decisions can be made more difficult when you know too much about the patient and their circumstances. Community outreach workers acquire a holistic understanding of their patients. The content of delusions and hallucinations may make a lot of sense, and their symbolism be all too obvious when you know the patient's history well and know what they are struggling with. How do you respond to a young man with schizophrenia who becomes preoccupied with delusions of changes in his abdomen, which you know reflect anxiety about his mother's recently diagnosed cancer of the uterus? Being too close can mean missing the woods for the trees. Identification with a patient you have worked with for a long time can delay accepting the inevitable—hope can sometimes cloud judgement.

Protecting the therapeutic relationship

We have made clear that we consider some use of compulsion to be an inevitable and a justifiable component of good comprehensive mental health care. It is not something to be ashamed of or something to distance ourselves from. Nor is it something to be too worried about. We had ten years of working with over 100 patients in the Wandsworth assertive outreach team of whom many were admitted compulsorily at some time by us. We found that they did forgive us. It is a remarkable fact, but one that we need to remind ourselves of regularly, that only a handful of patients harbour a grudge for any length of time about compulsory admissions. Many remain convinced that we should not have done it, even if, in retrospect, they think it helped (Katsakou and Priebe 2006). Despite this, they are still happy to see us and treat us decently. They often recognize that we have our job to do and that this is part of it. Community outreach teaches us that honest disagreement is perfectly compatible with a respectful and even warm relationship.

Importance of honesty

We would go further and propose that honesty is the most fundamental component of an ethical and successful long-term relationship. Deception should be avoided unless there is real risk of danger. The practice of getting someone else to organize the admission ('to protect the relationship') is short-sighted. Patients will eventually have to be told that you endorsed or even initiated it. They will, quite correctly, interpret your leaving someone else to do the dirty work as weakness and lack of commitment to them.

Just because a compulsory admission is unavoidable does not mean that how it is done will not make a difference. Having a familiar face around during a frightening and distressing experience (as it is highly likely to be, especially if the police have to be involved) makes it more bearable for both patient and family members (see Chapters 5 and 10). The value of some comforting words should not be underestimated:

> 'Don't worry Alice, I'm here, and will make sure that nobody hurts you. The police are here just to make sure nothing goes wrong. I'll come to the ward with you and I'll make it my job to see that you're back home as soon as possible. You know I wouldn't agree to you going in unless I thought you really needed it. Yes, I'll make sure the cat is fed.'

Knowledge of the patient's anxieties and vulnerabilities can ease the process. You know their delusions and fears, so you have a much better chance of being able to reassure them. At the simplest level, it helps to know the layout of the flat and the identities of the people involved.

In several instances, key workers have found their involvement in these dramatic periods (when the patient is often at lowest ebb) can serve as an important shared experience. Later it can be worked through to strengthen the alliance. One of the strengths of mental health nurses as key workers is that their involvement in such emotionally charged encounters, and their ease with direct physical contact, makes the relationship more vivid. The patient experiences it as a 'real relationship', not simply a contract with a disinterested, albeit conscientious, professional.

We find it best to acknowledge disagreement openly and in as matter-of-fact a manner as possible. We explain why we are arranging a compulsory admission, listen whilst the patient 'takes it on board', and explore where we differ. In the end we aim for the patient to understand our actions, not necessarily to agree. We often 'agree to disagree'. There is now good evidence that explaining to the patient why they are being admitted makes a significant difference to how they feel about it afterwards. The same is true of listening to their arguments, even if you are not going to change your mind.

Research into the patients' experience of compulsion and coercion in mental health has taken off in the last 15 or so years. This was stimulated by the recognition that many voluntary patients do not feel themselves free and, more perplexing, that a significant number of involuntary patients do feel free (Kaltialo-Heino 1996). The MacArthur group in the US conducted research into this area for over ten years. They developed a scale for measuring the experience of coercion at admission (MacArthur Admission Experience Survey; AES) (Gardner et al. 1993). One of the three subscales is 'procedural justice', essentially 'Were you listened to and was it explained why this was happening?' If patients rated procedural justice highly, they rated their overall experience of coercion much lower (Lidz et al. 1995). Having a good therapeutic relationship also significantly reduces feelings of coercion (Sheehan and Burns 2011).

Although we strongly advocate honesty and transparency in the process of compulsion, common sense and judgement must prevail. There are occasions when avoiding direct confrontation is prudent. Alone at home with an aroused and hostile patient who asks directly 'Well, are you going to section me?', it may be best to say, 'I've got to think about it, but obviously it's possible if things go on like this', even if the honest answer is 'Yes'. This honest answer may have to be given when you have support and are in a position to achieve it safely. Similarly, there have been times, usually at the start of trying to engage with a new patient with a long history of hostility to case managers, when other members of the team take the responsibility. It should be a rare occurrence and, if it has to be repeated with the same patient, it is probably worth radically rethinking their management.

Balancing the risks and benefits

Decisions on compulsory admission are, as we have discussed, often made more difficult, rather than less, when one knows the patient well. For this reason, community outreach staff need to pay more attention to the balance involved in assessments. Decisions should always involve consultation with the team, unless it is a very extreme emergency. Even then, doctors, social workers, and case managers need time to discuss. Four common issues complicate the decision for community outreach workers, and should always be considered:

1. Familiarity with the patient, fondness for them, or a sense of being their 'advocate' can mean that painful decisions are delayed too long.
2. Admission can mistakenly be considered a 'failure'.
3. The resources exist to sustain ill people out of hospital (even if it is not in their interests).
4. There is a heightened understanding of the risks of deterioration and of the potential benefits of treatment.

Power relationships, persuasion, and leverage

Few significant relationships are absolutely equal or single-stranded. To the extent that any relationship is important to us it will, inevitably, compromise freedom. We will strive to protect that relationship. We do not want to lose it and therefore, by this alone, it exerts a significant power over us. When we refer to relationships as 'the ties that bind us', we are recognizing this restriction, distinguishing them from a casual acquaintanceship. An explicit purpose of establishing supportive and trusting relationships with patients (developing effective engagement) is to be able to influence their decisions later. While the relationship may be open and respectful, there is an expectation that it will have the power to influence.

We need to recognize that when we exert such influence, we may often restrict an individual's personal freedom. Of course, they are ultimately at liberty to break the relationship, but that is easier said than done.

Levels of persuasion

If some degree of informal coercion is a common feature of the therapeutic relationship, we need to increase our awareness of it and our understanding

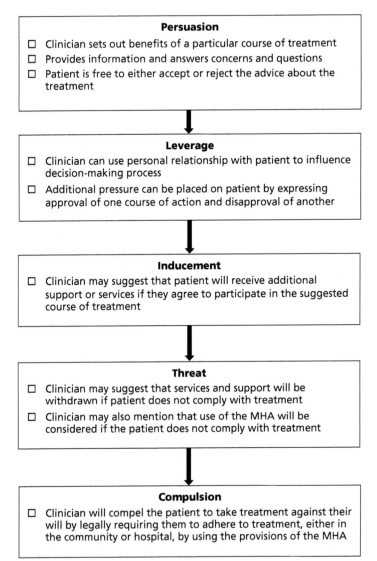

Fig 8.1 Hierarchy of treatment pressures

Reproduced from *Journal of Mental Health*, 17, 3, Szmukler G and Appelbaum PS, 'Treatment pressures, leverage, coercion, and compulsion in mental health care', pp. 233–244. Copyright (2008) with permission from Taylor & Francis Ltd, www.tandfonline.com

of how it is used. A very useful start has been made in a paper by Szmukler and Appelbaum (2008). They identify five types of persuasion, which they rank by increasing degrees of coercion (Fig 8.1). The first level is simple *persuasion* where you explain the benefits of a treatment and encourage the patient to go along with it but do no more than that. The next level involves using the power of your relationship to influence the patient's decision. This is not usually explicit, but relies on your positive and negative responses. It can sometimes be simply your facial expression (looking sad if the patient appears to be rejecting your suggestion or expressing relief or pleasure when they do accept it). Szmukler and Appelbaum call this *leverage*. This is a bit confusing now as leverage has become more widely used as the term to cover the next two steps in the hierarchy—*inducement* and *threat*.

What characterizes leverage as it is now used is that the pressure is *explicit*. You tell the patient that specific outcomes depend on their taking or not taking the treatment. So, for instance, you may say to a patient:

> 'Look, I know you want me to recommend you for a flat in the new development and I would love to see you get a new place of your own. But the truth is that unless I can tell them that you are now taking the medicine regularly, they will not consider you. They tell me that given what happened last time it is too risky.'

This would be considered an *inducement* by Szmukler and Appelbaum, whereas telling the patient that they are likely to lose their tenancy if they don't take the medicine would be a *threat*. They distinguish inducement from threat by whether it increases the options for the patient (inducements add a new potential that was not there before) or reduces them (threats imply taking something away). The more common usage of leverage does not distinguish that much between inducements and threats, but emphasizes the explicit link between what will happen if the patient does, or does not, engage in the treatment.

Szmukler and Appelbaum are committed to the view that the final level of persuasion, *compulsion*, is only acceptable in mental health care when patients lack capacity. Consequently, they draw a very strong ethical distinction between inducements and threats, and are very critical of the use of the latter.

Leverage and financial incentives (contingency management)

Much of the discussion on levels of persuasion is essentially a theoretical one—useful for organizing our thinking on the subject and sharpening our understanding of the therapeutic relationship. Leverage introduces a concrete intervention. A US study of patients with severe mental illness treated in public mental health services in five states (Monahan et al. 2005) found that nearly half of them felt that they had been explicitly pressured into complying with treatment. The use of a CTO was one of these pressures but the others were leverages. The most common was that access to accommodation had been clearly made dependent on complying with treatment. Usually the hostel or apartment lease contained a clause stating that if the patient stopped their medication they would be evicted. The other two leverages were having criminal sanctions (usually prison) waived only on condition that the patient attended their treatment programme and if they failed to do so then they would be jailed. The third was some form of money management such as welfare payments would not be forthcoming unless the patient complied.

Studies in the UK (Burns et al. 2011) and Switzerland (Jaeger and Rössler 2010) found a broadly similar pattern, although there was no CTO available at the time. They found overall lower levels of leverage (about 30 per cent rather than 50 per cent), but the pattern was the same, with housing the commonest, followed by criminal justice leverage and then money management. These lower levels in Europe reflect a difference in the approach to the welfare of disabled individuals to that in the US. Here such benefits are generally considered entitlements, whereas in the US patients often have to earn such benefits by engaging with treatment programmes. Interestingly, in all three studies patients recognized that their autonomy was being compromised, but many considered that the leverages were a good thing and may have helped them. In the UK study, substance abusers were included, and they had much higher levels of leverage; for them access to their children figured prominently. It may be that clinicians feel more comfortable exercising such leverages around substance abuse which they believe is 'more under the patient's control'.

The important thing about these studies is that they revealed just how common such practices are, and also that almost nothing is written about or taught about them in our professional training. None of us have probably been trained in their use or engaged in detailed discussions of when and where they are ethically acceptable.

These ethical and clinical dilemmas are highlighted in a study of what is called 'contingency management'. This means rewarding patients directly for complying with treatment either with money or with some tokens for exchange in shops. Contingency management has been widely trialled in several public health areas—attending antenatal classes, anti-smoking programmes, tuberculosis treatment in homeless individuals. Recently a study tested the impact of paying psychosis patients directly for taking their depot antipsychotics (Priebe et al. 2013).

Paying patients directly to take treatments is obviously not going to become common practice. However, some important things were learnt from this study which had faced considerable objections that it was unethical and undermined the therapeutic relationship. The first finding is that it worked—treatment adherence improved. But more importantly, it seemed, if anything, to *strengthen* the therapeutic relationship. Despite the reservations of the nurses who were doing the administering, it did not appear to devalue the therapeutic relationship to a mechanical commercial transaction. Patients experienced it as evidence that we cared about their outcome and it cast a positive aura over the clinical contact for both patient and nurse. In addition, none of the potential for abuse that was feared at the start of the study—non-study patients refusing to take medication unless paid, stopping the medication as soon as the funding ran out, irresponsible use of the money—materialized.

Clearly, both patients and clinicians recognize that our interactions are complex and involve a range of different types of persuasion. What this research tells us is that we probably need to be more open about incentives and pressures both in our training and with our patients.

Community treatment orders

A major development that has occurred since the first edition of this book has been the introduction of community treatment orders (CTOs). Community compulsion has been discussed for several decades in the UK and several European countries. The Royal College of Psychiatrists proposed a form of CTO in 1993 (Burns and Molodynski 2014). After a long and tortuous passage through legislation, they were introduced in Scotland in 2007 and the rest of the UK in 2008. While they are new to us, they have become widely available in most states in the US since the 1980s, and have become a central feature of community outreach in Australia and New Zealand (Maughan et al. 2014).

Their earliest introduction of CTOs in some US states in the 1970s were pushed by civil rights lawyers as an alternative to long-term incarceration. These were called 'least restrictive' orders and could only be used if the patient was sufficiently ill (usually defined in terms of dangerousness in the US) to warrant current inpatient care. In practice, CTOs are now used for patients who are no longer sufficiently disturbed to warrant inpatient detention, but who are at risk of becoming so, so-called preventive CTOs. CTOs in the UK are preventive (although the legal wording is unclear) and are imposed almost exclusively on 'revolving-door' psychosis patients when there is judged to be a need for regular supervision because of a high risk of rapid relapse.

The UK is unusual internationally in that legal compulsion under the Mental Health Act is imposed directly by clinicians rather than by judges or magistrates based on clinical recommendations. In the UK, the legal input is to the oversight of the order via review by automatic tribunals and managers' hearings, not its imposition. There are arguments for and against this arrangement, and it is often seen as a bit too trusting of professionals, perhaps rather paternalistic. On the other hand, it clearly distinguishes the treatment of the mentally ill from that of criminals and may reduce stigma. This trust also reflects the long-standing absence of commercial incentives in UK health care. CTOs are imposed by both the psychiatrist and an 'approved mental health professional'. This is likely to be the community outreach worker, whether nurse or social worker. Both have to agree.

The community outreach worker is generally responsible for the management of the patient on a CTO, which includes clinical contact and the monitoring of its conditions. When the law was first introduced, there was a lot of discussion about whether CTO conditions should be minimal or extensive. One view was that there should be a very detailed care plan to reflect the seriousness of depriving the patient of their liberty—based on the 'principle of reciprocity' (Eastman 1994). The alternative view was that detailed care plans would be unenforceable and also that the CTO should intrude on the patient as little as possible, commensurate with safety and therapeutic benefit. Overall the minimal care plan approach won out and the conditions imposed are few. These are usually that the patient should live at a specific address, allow access, take prescribed medication, and meet regularly with clinical staff.

About 4000 CTOs are imposed each year in England and Wales, and most last about a year. There is a growing number of patients who have remained on them much longer, and experience from New Zealand and Australia indicates that a significant number may effectively stay on them permanently. The community outreach is almost always by a nurse, and around two thirds or more of the patients are managed on depot antipsychotics.

Whether or not CTOs improve outcome is hotly debated. The evidence has been gathered from case control studies of patient groups before and after imposition of the CTO, and currently from only three randomized controlled trials (RCTs). Most of the studies (including all the RCTs) assess the outcome by the reduction of relapse and readmission over one year follow-up, although most also report duration of hospitalization and time to relapse. The case control studies give conflicting results—in some, CTOs reduce readmission rates; in others, they increase them (Maughan et al. 2014). However, none of the three RCTs find that CTOs reduce the readmission rate (Kisely and Hall 2014). A rigorous application of the general principles of evidence-based medicine would lead us to stop using CTOs, but clearly this is not happening, nor is it likely to do so in the near future. Community outreach workers and teams need to be aware of this lack of an evidence base for their use even if current practice is to continue with them.

A difficult decision facing the clinician is when to stop a CTO. The conditions for imposing one are fairly well described: the patient has to be currently in hospital and soon to be discharged from section but considered to be at high risk of rapid relapse or disengagement if not closely monitored, and such monitoring has to be imposed. However, what to do when the patient has been out for several months and is doing well? Is the fact that they are doing well evidence that they no longer need the CTO, or evidence that it is working and should be continued? This 'lobster-pot' quality of CTOs (easy to get into, impossible to get out of) was one of the strongest arguments levied against introducing the legislation. And how rapid is 'rapid relapse'? It is not sufficient to be at risk of relapse to be placed on a CTO (that would include almost all psychosis patients)—there has to be a significant risk of abrupt and risky relapse.

The risks of abuse of power

If we do not consciously monitor the power within relationships, it is easy to overlook abuses. One of the reasons CTOs were introduced in the UK was to provide formal monitoring of the use of coercion in the community that was already known to occur (such as extended section 17 leave) but which had no judicial oversight. Just because we would say 'No' to someone who tried to encourage (make) us go to a day centre against our inclination, does not mean that our patients feel they can say no. If you are the only person they regularly see, they may be very frightened of losing your support and, consequently, prepared to go along with things you suggest even if they are unwelcome.

The famous Milgram experiment (Milgram 1963) in the 1960s reminds us how powerful hierarchy is in human relationships. In this psychology experiment, ostensibly self-confident subjects administered what they were led to believe were high-voltage shocks to an individual they could see behind a window simply because they were told to do so by someone in authority. Virtually all of them delivered some shocks and 80 per cent delivered shocks labelled 'Strong', even when the individual receiving them (who was, in fact, an actor) exhibited great distress. They simply relied on the authority of the white-coated experimenter. Most of us are unaware of just how much we are influenced by authority. We are the ones with power in clinical relationships and we may be relatively blind to the power we exert.

It is important to recognize the existence of this power if we are to avoid abusing it. How ethical is it to defer a tenancy as an incentive to improve compliance? How ethical even is it to provide lunch at a depot clinic if one of the purposes is to get people to accept medicine they do not really want? How can we be sure that it is a fair trade-off when the patients may not want the injection but have no other source of cooked food? The most stark example is when very poor patients are paid to take treatment (Priebe et al. 2013). Is this incentivization or exploitation?

There are no simple, once-and-for-all answers to such questions. We raise them here to highlight the complexity of even the most benign and empowering therapeutic relationship. We certainly do use leverage to avoid potentially damaging consequences for our patients. The purpose of this discussion is to remind ourselves of our need to constantly consider the ethical dimensions of our work. This mainly plays out balancing individual liberty against therapeutic benefits. However, there are other important ethical principles in medicine—non-maleficence (doing no harm), justice (not letting one patient deprive another by soaking up all your time), risk to others and also dignity (Beauchamp and Childress 2013). Power and compulsion are integral parts of our relationships with patients—they are not simply the concerns of the social worker and the consultant when they arrange an involuntary admission.

Conclusions

This has been a long chapter with few firm conclusions. Debates about balancing effective treatments against personal rights will continue to be at the centre of community mental health outreach. There are no definitive answers, as decisions depend on many factors beyond the illness. Just as society changes, the context of our treatment decisions changes, and the threshold for compulsion is altered. The social acceptability of disorganized behaviour (and hence the stigma and discrimination stemming from such behaviour) depends crucially on the tolerance and expectations of the local community. Risks also depend on where you are. Wandering off the ward was no big deal in a large mental hospital with extensive grounds and many staff about, but can be disastrous in a small district general hospital unit on a busy road. Even climate makes a difference! Wandering out into the winter in Canada or Scandinavia can result in exposure, frostbite, and even death.

Having a caring and involved family and some social stability radically alters the need for compulsion, which may account for much of the cultural variation. Their erosion, along with the scarcity of beds, is likely to explain at least some of the recent remarkable increase in compulsion in the UK (Keown et al. 2011).

The debate about compulsion in each individual case needs to be given space in team discussions, and the unique circumstances around each case should be acknowledged. No team member has a monopoly on wisdom. Although it is codified in law, it is ultimately an ethical decision, and ethical codes derive from all of us.

Team discussions about compulsion are often good starting points to remind us of the power issues in our relationships with patients (and perhaps with each other!). There is no place for a naïve denial of dependency and power in community outreach practice with severely mentally ill people. Psychotherapists have a long tradition of exploring these relationships (in particular, understanding how transference distortions introduce dependency and exaggerate pre-existing power differentials). These are no less relevant because we are dealing with more severe disorders. Even so, we have not found that using external facilitators to explore such issues helpful, although we know other teams do. Our observation is that such facilitated groups often focus excessively on team issues rather than patient issues. We believe that boundaries and autonomy are core issues for routine team meetings and supervision, and that they should not be ignored or reserved for special 'training days'. The scandals of abuse in the old mental hospitals arose because good staff forgot to question their practice with very dependent and difficult patients. We must make sure that something similar does not develop in community outreach.

Chapter 9

Cultural sensitivity

Introduction

It would be true to say that we approached this chapter with more foreboding than any other in this book. Nowhere is there such fierce controversy in modern mental health services than that raging around the care of ethnic minority groups (Singh 2009). In many ways, it mirrors the sound and fury that emanated from the 'nature versus nurture' battles about families and schizophrenia in the 1960s and '70s (see Chapter 15). It is an intensely politicized area. The very strength of feeling on the various sides of the argument (and the passion with which they continue to be advanced) indicates the absence of convincing or conclusive evidence for how to proceed. This is no simple either/or issue—there are almost as many conflicts as there are protagonists!

We do not wish to take sides. We take what comfort we can in data and research and try to avoid value-laden or ideological standpoints. Oversimplifying the complexities of providing mental health care in a multiracial and multicultural society—particularly casting the debate solely in accusations of institutional racism—risks alienating both staff and potential patients. It inhibits the trust and openness necessary for mental health care, and it severely constrains dialogue. Following our clinical habit, we consider it more productive to give all the protagonists in any conflict the benefit of the doubt. We assume that both sides have patients' and families' welfare at heart and aim to relieve distress and safeguard dignity. Conflicts are best understood in terms of differing perceptions and perhaps incomplete information. It rarely helps to write off an opponent's viewpoint as simply mischievous or deliberately malicious. The aim should be to achieve a 'good enough' consensus from which to work.

We have concentrated on ethnicity in this chapter since in our experience it is more pertinent to the day-to-day work in community mental health. That is not to say that the other eight protected characteristics covered by the UK Equality Act (2010) are unimportant. This legislation puts a duty on the public sector, including the National Health Service, to ensure that staff and service users are able to work and access services in a fair manner, free from discrimination. Race is a protected characteristic together with age, sex, disability, pregnancy and maternity, religion and belief, sexual orientation, gender reassignment, and marriage and civil partnership.

However, as Singh (2009) points out:

> Health differences between population groups are not necessarily inequalities; illnesses are neither egalitarian in their occurrence nor equitable in their outcomes. Differences per se neither equate with discrimination nor necessarily result from it.

Ethnic differences in the incidence of diseases less stigmatizing than mental illness raise little controversy. Sickle cell anaemia, diabetes, and cardiovascular disease are just some examples. Socio-economic determinants of health play a large role also. Results reported from the World Health Organisation's Mental Health Survey (Picket et al. 2006) describe a positive correlation between socio-economic inequality and mental health problems across eight developed countries. So economic disadvantage, including unemployment in some ethnic and migrant communities, may be a contributing factor for mental health problems as a whole. In terms of more serious illness, Kirkbride et al. (2008) looked at associations for psychoses, ethnicity, and socio-economic status. Black Caribbean and black African adults were generally twice as likely to experience psychotic disorders compared with their white British counterparts even after controlling for socio-economic status. This study also showed that women of Pakistani and Bangladeshi origin were at higher risk of schizophrenia after adjusting for socio-economic status.

Given the powerful social determination of help-seeking behaviour in all illnesses, it should come as no surprise that there is variation in the perception and acceptance of what mental health services have to offer. Deciding when unusual behaviour is 'illness' is a social process. Social groups will decide what behaviour conforms to their cultural norms—it is a major component in how any group defines itself. When someone's behaviour is thought to be unusual or abnormal, there may then be a whole range of ways of perceiving it. Is it creativity, eccentricity, religious possession, evil, or illness? Transcultural psychiatry reminds us that there can be an equally broad range of responses to a judgement of illness dependent on theories of causation and beliefs about treatment.

Local demographics

Effective community services must know the community that they serve. One of the great strengths of a locality-based service is that it can be adjusted to specific needs. To do so requires knowing about them. Commissioners are required to purchase services to meet the needs of their local population and will publish needs assessments and demographic and socio-economic profiles of the locality together with projections. Local knowledge will also be available informally, built up over time.

Case study

We had struggled for some time to maintain contact with a particularly elusive patient who we knew attended a Pentecostal church just a couple of miles outside our area. Only during his second review did one of the team members identify the particular church, which confirmed that they would be willing to help us maintain contact. When we tried to work out why we had not known this before, it became clear that that team member had been on holiday for the previous review. As a member of the West African community, she was an invaluable resource about these Pentecostal groups and their varying attitudes towards services like ours.

The NHS *Mental Health Policy Implementation Guide* (Department of Health 2001) gives a brief overview of the types of information that a service needs:

* ethnic breakdown of general population
* community languages spoken
* religious diversity
* housing types (including homelessness)
* unemployment
* any vulnerable groups

In the UK, at the end of 2014, refugees, people awaiting asylum decisions, and stateless persons made up 0.24 per cent of the population (UNHCR 2014). Significant proportions of these have psychiatric problems, including post-traumatic stress disorder.

The provision and access to interpreters for patients for whom English is a second or third language is good organizational practice. The use of trained interpreters rather than friends or family is preferable for a full assessment. How many of us would disclose our thoughts, fears, and beliefs via our parents or partners? Concerns about sexuality, religion, persecution, or passivity are most likely to be withheld if mediated through the patient's associate.

Equality and diversity training

Most employing authorities provide equality and diversity training as mandatory for staff. Its purpose is to help us learn more about diverse cultural attitudes, expectations, and assumptions and to allow us to explore any prejudices, misunderstandings, or blocks that we may have.

Scenario-based training is a good way to practice responses to real-life situations. Our team locality has a large Asian population, so our training gives the following scenario with an Urdu-speaking patient newly referred: You ring to make an appointment. Her 14-year old son answers and confirms on behalf of his mum that she can attend. You say that you will arrange for an interpreter to be present. The son then says that his mum prefers for him to act as her interpreter. How do you respond? The correct response is to explain why this would not be appropriate, and to say that you need to book an interpreter.

Staff backgrounds

In a team composed of staff from a wide range of backgrounds (see 'ethnic matching' later), increased cultural awareness is needed so that we can work well with each other, not just with our patients. We do not consider that a 'colour-blind' approach is to be striven for. Quite the contrary. Services should be 'colour sensitive' (La Grenade 1999). Just as our patients are unique individuals with their personal and cultural backgrounds, so our staff also bring the richness of their varied cultures to our day-to-day work. This is a strength which can be utilized in ethnic and cultural matching. It also places an obligation on us to realize that the same event is not always the same experience for each of us involved. Teams need to be able to talk frankly about their experiences, including racism, both from their work and their social lives, so that they can support each other properly.

Case study

Al had been key working John for over two years. It had been demanding but productive work. Both Al and John are African-Caribbean. John has a substantial forensic history, including dangerous violence when psychotic. After over 18 months of stability, John had begun to deteriorate, refusing medicines, smoking cannabis excessively, and avoiding contact. Eventually, Al made contact and ascertained that John was seriously unwell and would need assessment, probably for compulsory admission. Because of John's previous violence, the police insisted on a large squad in protective gear. Along with the consultant and social worker from the team, an extremely unpleasant (but brief and ultimately safe) assessment and transfer to hospital was effected. None of the team thought that anything else would have been possible and we were unanimous that this was the right thing to do. It was John's first admission without injury.

Although we all agreed on it being the right thing and were relieved that it had been achieved, the experience had been different for Al than for the consultant. Both had found it distasteful and menacing. But for Al, the sight of a young black man being subdued by an all-white group of police officers in full riot gear was hard to bear. He talked after of his sense of 'betrayal' of John, mixed with a feeling that the police felt the same way about him. He wanted to demonstrate his solidarity with John (remembering times when he had been stopped and searched by the police), yet equally strongly assert his difference as the responsible professional who had instigated the whole process.

In team feedback, there was relief and praise that Al had organized the admission, but also a recognition that it was not easy for him to do it and no embarrassment in talking about these issues. Fortunately, John did well.

Ethnic representation and matching

Population matching

Much has been written about the pros and cons of ethnic matching. We do not subscribe to a rigid dictate that black patients need black key workers, or that women patients need women key workers, and so on. Such a dictate would, anyway, sit poorly with the notion of shared care and the team approach. On the other hand, it is essential that the overall configuration of the team should roughly represent the population it serves. In inner London, a multiracial team is clearly essential. The same may not be true of, say, rural Ireland.

We subscribe fully to the concept of ethnic representation—both so that the team can be taken seriously by its clientele and, more importantly, so that it can understand the experiences of patients and families and many of the support agencies. At a purely practical level, some gender and ethnic matching is essential. Many Asian families will not contemplate female members being treated by male staff—most of our female patients who need long-acting injectable medication have this administered by female nurses. Some older Asian patients have poor English and it would be perverse not to provide them with an Urdu- or Hindi-speaking key worker if one is available.

Patient matching

Patients who have experienced considerable racial harassment (in the UK, this particularly affects young black men) may have difficulty trusting white staff. They may find it easier to relate to black staff who they know will understand what they have been through. If patients make it clear that they feel this way, it makes sense to try and achieve it. On the other hand, one must be realistic. As the previous example of John's compulsory admission demonstrates, this shared sense of solidarity will be sorely tested. Bitter recriminations will result if too much is made of it. The temptation to over-identify with the patient, against authority, must be carefully balanced with a recognition that the key worker is part of the establishment and, as such, is able to mobilize a full range of care and support for their patient.

When we do have ethnically matched key workers, we are careful, as part of the team approach, to ensure that workers of different cultural backgrounds are introduced. The involvement of other team members will lead to a balanced exposure for the patient. Trust established with the key worker can then (we hope) spread to other staff members as the patient and family experience them working together and see how they treat each other with respect. Dependence on an ethnically closely identified key worker can lead to problems when that key worker is absent on leave or unexpectedly.

Problems with matching

Sometimes, ethnic closeness can be a problem and one needs to recognize this. Patients (though more often families) who have felt discriminated against in the past may also feel discriminated against in this situation. Though very uncommon, we have twice come across families who have talked of 'health care apartheid'. In both instances, things improved when feelings were aired and issues discussed, and in neither case was a change of key worker pursued. For some pitfalls in the key worker/patient relationship from a cultural and psychodynamic perspective, see Box 9.1.

The benefits of improved alliance through identification can be at a price. Many patients (and families) understandably project the restrictions on achievement imposed by the illness on other, more common causes. We will see in Chapter 19 how young men may prefer to attribute their symptoms to alcohol or drugs rather than schizophrenia—it seems somehow more acceptable. Most ethnic minority groups have common experiences of racial discrimination which lend solidarity and social cohesion. For a young black patient, unable to get a job because of his psychotic illness, it can be reassuring to blame racism: it is no longer simply his problem; it is society's unfairness. Working closely with a key worker from a similar background, who has faced similar obstacles, can call into question that defence, or the key worker can identify too closely with this perspective.

Box 9.1 Assumptions and responses by key workers

- Colour blindness: assumption that the minority patient is the same as the majority patient.
- Colour consciousness: all problems result from the minority status.
- Cultural transference: patient's feelings result from the key worker's ethnicity.
- Cultural counter-transference: key worker's feelings towards the patient result from their own ethnicity.
- Cultural identification: the key worker from a minority background defines all problems as racially based.
- Identification with the disadvantaged: the key worker from a minority background denies their status and power.

Adapted from Bhugra, D. and Bhui, K. (2001) *Cross cultural psychiatry: a practical guide*, Edward Arnold, London.

Case study

Anne, a female African-Caribbean patient, formed a good relationship with her female African key worker. This was a considerable achievement as she had always been difficult to engage (particularly because of her complex and stormy relationship with her father who had significant mental health problems to contend with himself). The father initially welcomed the new key worker and supported all her recommendations. He emphasized how much she was on Anne's side and how skilled and conscientious she was. Over time, however, the father's support for the key worker became increasingly idealized. It was clear that he saw her as the daughter he had never had and was holding her up as an example for Anne, undermining her slowly growing self-confidence.

Despite quite intensive work with the pair, nothing seemed to reduce this demoralizing idealization. In the end, Anne herself asked for a change of key worker, and has begun to work well with a white female nurse. Her father occasionally comments that it is easier for white people to get good jobs than for him and his daughter. He is less involved in her care (which has some downsides), but Anne is clearly enormously relieved not to be continually contrasted with her previous key worker.

Racial harassment and abuse

Zero tolerance

Zero tolerance towards racial or sexual harassment or physical threat is a welcome addition to the policies of health and social care organizations. Clear statements to this effect are posted prominently in A&E departments and throughout hospitals. Our local Trust policy on this is stated in a notice at the entrance to all wards and in all outpatient departments. Making a reality of such a policy is not, however, that easy.

It is a good first step that the policy is unequivocal. It is no longer assumed that 'good' or 'experienced' staff will simply take such harassment in their stride as part of the job. This was certainly the attitude 20 or so years ago, when staff were expected to 'toughen up'. Being tolerant to such abuse was considered a professional virtue, almost part of the Hippocratic oath. A commitment to equal treatment for everyone, whatever their political or personal views—which we would agree is a core professional value for health and social care staff—was often confused with a personal tolerance of quite unacceptable behaviour.

It is not by chance that health and social care staff are generally more tolerant of abusive behaviour from patients and clients. We are used to dealing with individuals in crisis. People who are confused or in great pain and distress may say and do things they would never do otherwise, and for which afterwards they are often embarrassed and remorseful. Few of us would hold against them offensive remarks or a glancing blow from an acutely paranoid and scared individual. Being able to rise above unkind remarks is essential when dealing with acutely psychotic individuals. In hypomania particularly (Chapter 16), it is essential not to take to heart what is said (which can often be very accurately personal and pointed). These are symptoms of the illness and to be discounted. Subsequently, one may need to acknowledge and work through their impact when the patient is more recovered.

The central issues relate to dealing with established attitudes and behaviours. It is for managing racial harassment within the day-to-day behaviours of individuals that zero tolerance is needed. Mental health care is much less paternalistic in its practice than before. The benefit for the patient is that the relationship is more respectful and equal. The cost of this equality is that the patient has responsibilities. One of these responsibilities is to treat staff with respect and decency and to act as much as possible as a responsible citizen.

Words and deeds

People can and do think what they like. Our legitimate concern with racial harassment and abuse is what people *do*, not what they think. As children grow up in a more multicultural and varied society, with schools that address issues of racial and cultural tolerance, we can hope over time for more inclusive, less prejudiced attitudes. Working in the community with mentally ill individuals (already the victims of stigma and discrimination), however, the immediate effects of racial harassment and abuse have to be addressed.

When racial harassment and abuse is discussed, it is often assumed that it is always abuse of the (usually ethnic minority) patient by white members of staff or the public. This is, undoubtedly, the most recognized, but not the only, form in which it occurs. Society is highly sensitive to these manifestations and there is a growing consensus about not tolerating them. As suggested in the discussion of zero tolerance, ethnic minority staff must be accorded the same rights as any other in this matter.

There are three forms of racial harassment which are of specific importance in outreach work:

1. harassment of the patient or family by neighbours and the general public
2. harassment of neighbours and public by the patient
3. harassment of staff by patients or their families

Harassment of the patient or family by neighbours and the general public

Protecting patients and their families from racial abuse is clearly one of the roles of an outreach worker. As an advocate for their rights, this means making sure not only that they are not discriminated against either because of their mental illness or their ethnicity. The two are often intertwined, sometimes deliberately. Racial intolerance can be dressed up as a fear of psychotic behaviour when neighbours request an eviction. Resentment against immigrants and asylum seekers can make the position of patients and their families intolerable, with mounting tension leading to relapse. Dealing with these situations requires tact and careful judgement. Simply acceding to hostility and organizing a move may involve enormous upheaval for the family. It can also reveal a loss of vital supports whose existence and importance had been masked by the conflict.

Legal procedures

At its most extreme, it is possible, with the help of the local authority, to instigate proceedings against harassing neighbours, which can result in *them* being evicted and even prosecuted. We have never done this and would be concerned about the degree of risk it would carry for our patients in terms of reprisals and added stress. We have tried to talk to neighbours when patients and families give us permission. Sometimes it has been possible to increase tolerance when neighbours have had a clearer understanding of the situation—why the family has had to flee persecution, why the patient is unable to work, how hard they are trying to get better with treatment.

It is not, however, easy to change attitudes, and our success with such interventions has been pretty minimal. The grim reality is that many severely mentally ill patients in the community will live in deprived areas and be subject, daily, to levels of harassment that most of us would find very difficult to accept. Where such harassment clearly breaks the law, when there are threats or open hostility, then it is our duty to support patients and their families in obtaining justice. Often this means supporting them in contacting the police and keeping up the pressure to get charges pressed.

Harassment of neighbours and public by the patient

It is all too easy to forget that our patients can also harbour and express racist or sexist attitudes. These can be intensified during acute relapses—it is not uncommon for paranoid delusions to involve specific cultural and ethnic groups (black patients feeling persecuted by whites, white patients by the IRA or by Asian groups). On the whole, this is not so difficult to deal with. Both staff and neighbours are able to write off what is said (or sometimes written) in acute episodes. The risk is greater when the patient is not known locally. We have had hypomanic patients assaulted because of uninhibited racist remarks they have made in pubs or in the street.

What to do if the patient or family have racist attitudes that are not related to the illness? We still have a duty to care and cannot simply write off patients because, for example, they come from a far-right nationalist family and are derogatory and insulting about black people, or are from an extremist Hindu family and make disparaging remarks about Muslims. In such circumstances, it is important to maximize the chances of successful engagement. This involves not allocating a key worker who will excite such prejudices. Many of us feel uncomfortable doing this—it is as if we are colluding with the racism. Our approach, however, should be to strengthen the positive rather than focus too much on the negative. Avoiding a match which is likely to be unsuccessful is not essentially that different to meeting a preference for a specific type of key worker (e.g. if a patient specifically asks for a female key worker).

We have found a softening of attitudes over time with some of our very prejudiced patients. As they get to accept their key worker, they become more positive to the team and its members, irrespective of their individual ethnicity. They can form warm relationships with team members and look forward to their visits while we know, from conversations with their key worker, that they still have strong prejudices against that individual's background. We have no hard evidence that the experience of working with a multiracial team does generalize for bigoted patients, but our experience is generally positive.

Distinguishing thoughts from behaviours

At a more practical level, patients and their families may need help in learning not to antagonize their neighbours by racist behaviour. Just as we often work hard to encourage patients not to share their delusional beliefs too widely, we can use the same procedures to help them inhibit racist remarks and behaviour. A pragmatic approach is more likely to succeed than a moral one. The style emphasizes the risks and consequences of such behaviour. Just as cognitive behavioural therapy for hallucinations (Chapter 25) aims to modify the response to them rather than their occurrence, the aim is to help patients keep their racist views to themselves rather than attempt to stop them having them.

This approach makes a very firm distinction between thought and action. We make clear to the patient that, although we do not share his or her beliefs, and indeed disapprove of them, it does not stop us wanting to help. However, we are not going to collude with expressions of such ideas. It is rather like the clergy's obligation to 'love the sinner but hate the sin'. Firm but non-confrontational responses to racist remarks should be used: 'I don't want to hear about that', or even 'I'm not going to listen to any more of this. I'll come back tomorrow when you're able to focus on the task in hand.' Refusing to listen to racist remarks about ethnic minority staff is a very concrete way of demonstrating what is and what is not acceptable: 'Okay, I understand you're upset about Krishna's last visit. I'm happy to hear about what he did that upset you—but not about who he is.'

No matter how hard one tries, patients and their families may persist in racist behaviour towards neighbours or other patients. They will have to suffer the consequences such as exclusion from certain premises. Housing associations and local authorities will evict persistently racist tenants, though obviously only as a last resort if they are mentally ill. We have on several occasions had to rehouse patients because of racist behaviour. Most often this has been to protect them from retaliatory violence from other tenants, but on more than one occasion is was to pre-empt an eviction.

Harassment of staff by patients or their families

Most of us have been roundly racially abused in times of crisis and conflict (e.g. during a compulsory admission). It is unpleasant, but not a big deal. It is much more wearing when it is persistent and in cold blood. Usually such abuse is directed at inpatient staff when patients are detained. In this situation, there is little alternative but to tolerate it.

We can rationalize that the anger stems from the compulsion and the racist content is probably an expression of their sense of helplessness. Staff are well able to distinguish racist abuse that is driven by psychotic experiences from that which is an expression of anger or long-held racial beliefs. Motive clearly does make a difference. The former is strikingly unhurtful whereas remarks that are meant to hurt usually do. Where the abusive remarks arise from the psychosis they will recede; where they are anger at detention, then detention will eventually be lifted as the psychosis is controlled.

Staff need to be protected from racist remarks and, within the ward, reorganizing shifts and nursing patterns may sometimes be necessary. Racist abuse of white and Asian staff is no less common than that of black staff. Black and Asian patients can be equally guilty of such behaviour. Whites making racist remarks about blacks may be getting less, reflecting society's increasing intolerance of them. It may be that zero tolerance policies are often interpreted rather simplistically in terms of old patterns of racism. We need to treat racism equally firmly irrespective of its direction.

Racist remarks by families also need to be treated firmly (after allowing for initial distress). Most services make it explicit that they will not deal with family members who behave in a persistently racist manner. Logical though this is, it is far from easy or simple. Do we withhold schizophrenia family work with a patient who (though not actively racist himself) lives with bigoted and insulting parents?

In all aspects of managing racism within mental health, judgement has to be exercised. This is very much an area where the focus must remain on the patient's welfare. In each individual case, the pros and cons of confronting racism have to be weighed against damage to the therapeutic alliance and the potential of the treatments to make a significant difference over time. A clear and unequivocal policy—which zero tolerance implies—has benefits, but it should be interpreted with clinical judgement and common sense in each individual case.

Community engagement

Active involvement of user and carer groups from the various ethnic minority populations served is one of the most effective ways of improving local cultural sensitivity and acceptability. Such involvement should be encouraged not just on an individual case basis but at all phases of developing and monitoring services. Engaging such groups early and often means that they can give invaluable advice about how best to provide care and support for their members. They can often clarify simple misunderstandings. For instance, when Asian patients in South London requested traditional healing (prayer or dietary advice from a mosque), this did not in fact imply a criticism of our medical approach (Greenwood et al. 2000). We had assumed that requests to take a patient away to a mosque to attend a series of rituals suggested that the family had little faith in Western medicine. Not so, we were informed. They clearly appreciated and wanted the benefits of medication, but they also wanted the added benefits of their familiar interventions. We also learnt from them how hopelessly inadequate terms like 'Asian' are. We now use the country of origin, not the region, in clinical discussions (e.g. 'this Somali man', 'this Bangladeshi family').

The other advantage of close involvement with user and carer groups from ethnic minorities is their spontaneous willingness to help and the offers of support they bring. It is probably not a cliché to propose that many immigrant groups still have stronger and wider support networks than the White British. The variety of such groups makes it difficult to predict where their strengths will lie—hence the simple approach of making sure that they understand as fully as possible exactly what we do so that they themselves can tell us directly how they can contribute.

Political correctness

Concerns about political correctness are particularly acute in the area of ethnic minorities and in mental health generally. It is good that we have realized that casual generalizations can be demeaning to individuals with an experience (whether personal or cultural) of being treated as second-class citizens. Observing that patients in mental hospitals were always referred to by their first names by staff (to whom they replied using staff titles), Maxwell Jones insisted on mutual first names in his therapeutic communities (Jones 1952). He realized the asymmetry of hierarchical relationships. What seems like a friendly familiarity from above may be felt as humiliation from below when you have no choice about it. Long-term unequal relationships are only acceptable if they are entered into freely. Language should be used carefully so that it does not hide unacceptable power relationships. It is now accepted practice throughout medicine to ask patients how they want to be addressed and not make assumptions.

What was central to much of the understanding of the complexity of relationships in therapeutic communities 30 years ago has become commonplace. We are sensitive to how language (often with the appearance of friendliness and humour) can gloss over, or even strengthen, prejudices and practices that, if examined carefully, we could not defend. The success of the women's movement and the fight for genuine equal rights for all members of society has rightly obliged us to examine language more closely and to be careful how we use it.

This has undoubtedly benefited former vulnerable and marginalized members of society. Witness the unacceptability of previously common words (e.g. 'idiot', 'spastic'), along with a heightened awareness that individuals are more than their labels. Changing terms can reduce stigma, though it is naïve to assume it abolishes it. In the field of mental handicap, there has been a deliberate practice of changing the terms for individuals with limited intellectual capacity. This policy is aimed at improving the understanding of the limitation while continually stressing that this is just one aspect of the individual. In exactly the same way, we use the term 'person with schizophrenia' rather than 'schizophrenic patient' or 'schizophrenic' because individuals with this disorder say they feel written off by terms like 'schizophrenic'. There is no consistent logic to this; it depends on the disorder and attitudes towards it. Most people with asthma do not mind being referred to as 'asthmatics' (there is no social stigma attached to that term, as there was to 'schizophrenic' or 'leper', and neither does it imply a complete identity).

Stereotypes

Recognizing a person's individuality means avoiding the shorthand assumptions of stereotypes. Not all young black men will want to attend a community music group; not all white men will be interested in football; nor do all Asian women want to socialize with other Asian women. Racial stereotypes are a form of prejudice. They need not even be negative to be prejudicial—why assume a Jamaican will be a good dancer?

Mental health work can be fun!

The price sometimes paid for such political correctness is that professionals can come to believe that any levity or humour in their work is a sign of disrespect for their patients. This is to throw the baby out with the bathwater. Mental health work is based in honest relationships and these are complex, shifting, and often unequal.

An honest relationship between individuals will allow for humour (as well as for impatience, annoyance, and frustration). As a team we have learnt to be more free with each other as we have learnt to be more supportive and understanding. When we appointed our first peer worker, we were anxious that we would have to stop expressing our frustration with patients in team meetings or making jokes about what we do. She soon disabused us of these anxieties. The last thing that she wanted, she said, was for us to be 'walking on eggshells' around her. She knew that we respected her and her work. She could tolerate and join in the banter but, if it went too far, then she, like any of us, could say so.

We need to complain about patients when things are difficult, just as members of a family complain about each other but remain united. If the relationship slides into dislike or fear, then we are not able to do a useful job. Being able to let off steam prevents, rather than promotes, relationships deteriorating.

A multidisciplinary and multicultural team will also have endless opportunities to find the funny side in difficult situations. There are realistic and healthy tensions between doctors, nurses, social workers, occupational therapists, and psychologists which can be a source of pleasure and enrichment in the work, as well as of conflict. Being able to talk openly about differences is more likely to lead to effective joint working. Similarly with ethnic differences. Pretending these do not exist can only lead to misunderstanding. Being able to enjoy the differences and to gently tease one another seems to promote respect and support. Taking pleasure in the humorous aspects of what at times can be grim work is essential for survival.

Case study

Ed, an African-Caribbean case manager, was reporting on an incident in which he had been assaulted by one of his patients. He had gone to give the patient her routine depot injection and found her in the kitchen baking. Baking was one of the activities that we had been able to interest her in. Unfortunately, on this day she had also been drinking and was very irritable. She shouted at Ed saying that she did not want his injection. She pushed him backwards covering him with flour and breaking his new expensive glasses. Ed withdrew immediately, although the patient had begun already to apologize.

At feedback, Ed was more upset about his new glasses (of which he had been very proud) than of any real worry about being hurt. He was also annoyed that he had flour spilled all over his jacket and face. Andy (a West African case manager) replied that he should not complain that much about his glasses: 'It's not that bad, Ed. After all, you went in black and you came out white. Michael Jackson would have paid a fortune for that.'

The foregoing anecdote may seem tasteless or politically incorrect in some situations. It certainly did not feel that way to those involved. Humour provides a safe area in which differences of experience and expectations can be acknowledged and explored. It allows us to get to know more about each other without being intrusive or pompous.

Apart from explicitly abusive or offensive language, there are no easily imported absolute rules about what can and cannot be said between team members. How it feels will often be the best guide. It will only be a good guide, however, if the team has an open culture where less confident members *really* can indicate if they feel put down or embarrassed by comments. Senior team members must ensure such a culture is sustained (e.g. by ensuring expression from all in team reviews, by putting time aside in team days to allow reflection and criticism, and by being open to criticism themselves). However, being at the top of the pyramid, they are the least well placed to judge the tone. This is not easy to do and there will undoubtedly be mistakes and times when individuals overstep the mark. However, in the long run this is surely better than safety at the cost of rendering the team mechanical and unsupportive.

Conclusions

Cultural sensitivity generally mirrors the core tasks of mental health workers. Our job is to understand each unique individual with whom we work. This involves understanding their history and how they see the world around them. We need to recognize that the same event will be experienced differently by those involved, and that sensitivity and respect must always be used to avoid giving unnecessary offence. Differences may arise because of mental illness, because of a different cultural expectation, or because of the personal history of that individual.

Cultural diversity is a great strength in mental health teams because it deepens our understanding of human experiences by illuminating them from different perspectives. It makes the job more difficult, however, because we need to be aware of a greater range of needs and responses and, perhaps, because consensus is less easy to achieve. It requires us to be more sensitive to how we behave, to be aware that what we do may not be interpreted in the way we mean it. It needs us to be more careful and thoughtful about how we use language, and it runs the risk that, scared of offending others, we become 'wooden' and less accessible as humans. It reminds us, however, that there is no unassailable primacy for any one world view.

Racism has to be confronted in ours, as in any other profession. A balance needs to be struck between carefully monitoring our behaviour to identify prejudices and allowing ourselves to relate as whole individuals. The very complexities of the situations confronting mental health workers in the community prevent any oversimplified or sloganized approach to social inclusion. These situations will continue to present us with incredibly complex ethical challenges where there is no single right answer—another reason why the job is never boring.

Part II

Health and social care practice

Chapter 10

Engagement

Introduction

Engagement is a confusing and under-defined concept in the outreach vocabulary. Definitions range from the ability of teams to retain patients in the service to attempts to describe the qualities required of the patient/worker relationship. We are reminded that in many clinical settings, from paediatrics to psychiatry, 'The importance of organising care in order to support and encourage a good therapeutic relationship is at times as important as the specific treatments offered' (NICE 2011). Perhaps we should allow our patients to tell us how best to approach this challenge. Priebe et al. (2005) interviewed 40 assertive outreach service users who had engaged with the team subsequent to previous disengagement from mainstream services. They valued commitment from staff who were prepared to spend extra time on visits and to address social and practical needs. Engagement came from a genuine relationship where they felt listened to and had a say in decisions about their care. Disengagement was driven by a strong desire to be independent and to avoid the debilitating side effects of medication. Priebe et al. provide some illuminating first-person accounts of these processes:

> When I suggested that I wanted to stop medication for a while, he actually let me and he did actually come across as if he were concerned about me hallucinating again and he wasn't too pushy about things. He warned me I may become delusional again, but he did not come across as though he was trying to prevent me from doing it. He wanted me to be more involved in my own health.[1]

In the UK, the REACT study (Killaspy et al. 2006) found that there was little difference in clinical, social, or service use outcomes between assertive community treatment (ACT) and standard CMHT care, but patients were more satisfied with care and better engaged with ACT. They followed up this randomized controlled trial with a qualitative study, interviewing case managers in each arm of the study about the processes of care, including engagement

---

[1] Reproduced from *The British Journal of Psychiatry*, 187, 5, Priebe S., Watts, J., Chase M., et al. 'Processes of disengagement and engagement in assertive outreach patients: qualitative study', pp. 438–443. Copyright (2005) with permission from The Royal College of Psychiatrists.

techniques (Killaspy et al. 2009). Compared to their CMHT colleagues, staff in assertive outreach teams were more likely to report making patients' interests and building a trusting relationship the central focus of the contact; they were also more flexible in types of support, such as practical help; and they reported fewer missed appointments. In short, 'The majority of ACT staff (16/20) felt they had succeeded in engaging with their clients, whereas half the CMHT staff (10/20) described a continuing struggle to do so' (Killaspy et al. 2009).

Table 10.1 classifies the varied activities and strategies that together can help build regular contact, promote a genuine alliance, and maximize our ability to work together with patients who have come to be known as 'hard to engage'. The selected vignettes and discussion of the strategies in this chapter should equip the reader with a working definition and a toolbox for practice.

It is often the *intention* of the activity that classifies it as 'engagement'. For example, home-based services and interventions are not necessarily related to engagement, but in when they are driven by a desire to make services more acceptable to patients' needs and circumstances, then outreach can indeed enhance the process of engaging.

Housing, welfare benefit payments, and employment activity are all social care interventions in themselves. They appear in our classification because, when they are clearly the patient's priority, their fulfilment will foster a positive attitude towards services. This may then help create the conditions necessary to initiate or change treatment.

Engagement should not be seen only as a means to a treatment end since social contact and recreational activities can have positive effects on quality of life and mood. Successful engagement with a case manager, team, or services will facilitate work with a patient on other difficult issues such as personal hygiene, money, aspirations, relationships, and sexuality. How many of us would discuss these topics with a stranger? They require the establishment of rapport, and trust requires us to be consistent.

Constructive approach

Two quotes encapsulate the need to consider our approach to engagement:

Very few people seek help from mental health services with enthusiasm.

(Onyett 1992)

We often focus on why patients fail to engage with services and less about why services fail to engage with patients.

(Sainsbury Centre for Mental Health 1998)

With any new referral, it is important to spend time working through with the patient why they think they have been referred, and explaining what

Table 10.1 Classification of engagement-related activity and intent

Constructive approach	Monitoring approach	Restrictive approach

◆ Befriending	◆ Assertive outreach; frequent and persistent contact—direct or indirect	◆ Use of legal powers under mental health legislation:
		  • Community treatment order or
		  • guardianship

◆ Collaborative or patient-led agenda	◆ Regular contact with patient's family and carers when no direct contact with patient	◆ Financial leverage through appointeeship or representative payeeship
◆ Strengths-focused interventions	◆ 'Doorstepping': regular attempts at contact despite refusal of access	◆ 'No dropout' policy
◆ Non-judgemental, nurturing approach	◆ Observation of patient's home environment when access denied	
◆ Advocacy and empowering approach	◆ Contact and information gathering through third parties (e.g. neighbours and local community) when necessary	
◆ Home-based care	◆ Contact with housing and welfare payments office	
◆ Preference for 'mainstream' activities	◆ Contact with GP	
◆ Practical assistance and problem-solving		
◆ Social and recreational activity		
◆ Assistance with financial and welfare benefits		
◆ Employment assistance and support		
◆ Support and problem-solving for family and carers		
◆ Obtaining or preserving accommodation		

might be on offer. Such a collaborative approach may not be reciprocated, but it's important to display from the outset an approach that may be perceived as refreshing compared to their experience of hospital restriction or more paternalistic encounters. Many patients will be able to provide their own agenda, given encouragement and some prompts. Where engagement is difficult, patient-led 'wants' should be the starting point, unless the need for an active clinical intervention is critical. When the patients won't tell you their views, it can be useful to put yourself in their position and ask yourself, 'What's in this for me?' At its simplest, this might be the availability and ability of their key worker or team to offer practical help, as illustrated in the following case study.

Case study

Arthur lost his cleaning job ten years previously due to developing paranoid beliefs and increasingly derogatory and disabling auditory hallucinations. Always a loner, he had become extremely withdrawn and neglected. He believed people could read his mind as he heard them castigating him for his heretical or treasonable 'compulsive thoughts'. He had no insight into the psychiatric nature of his condition. He was distressed by his experiences and had a history of barricading himself in his flat for fear of being thrown into prison. As a result, access to his flat was extremely difficult.

At assessment by the outreach team, his flat was spartan and neglected. He had worn the same trousers for three years—they were stiff and waxy. Arthur stated that he did not wish to be visited regularly at home, and if it was more than once a month he would have nothing to say or report since his life was so limited. His only activity was a weekly visit to the local post office, which he described as an ordeal.

We attempted to describe to Arthur how our approach might differ from what he had experienced previously. He would not have to 'report', nor would he be questioned. He was encouraged to think of his key worker's visits more as befriending and supportive. He might, in time, want his key worker to accompany him on his weekly shopping trip, to make it less of an ordeal. Arthur was not much impressed by these proposals and access remained difficult.

On a subsequent visit, his key worker needed to use the toilet and discovered it did not flush. Lifting the cistern, he saw that a piece of plastic had broken in the flush linkage. Arthur had been tipping bowls of water in the bowl to flush it for about five years. A twenty-minute trip to the hardware store, 50 pence, and some rather unpleasant handiwork secured a working flush. This proved to be the turning point in the engagement process. His key worker had proved himself useful, perhaps trustworthy, and the 'what's in it for me' question found a positive response. From this small foundation, other interventions were possible over the years, perhaps the most satisfying being an outing to buy some new trousers.

A powerful and pragmatic engagement tool is knowledge of the state welfare benefit system and related sources of extra finance. Despite attempts to facilitate access to employment, the majority of severely mentally ill patients are wholly dependent on some form of welfare. An ability to help negotiate the complex and shifting benefits system to obtain appropriate disability-related allowances, or sometimes a one-off grant from a local charity, are powerful demonstrations of the alliance in action.

Monitoring approach

Outreach workers may be required to undertake a degree of watchfulness over a patient who has disengaged or is at risk of doing so. This may not always be seen as constructive by the patient, but it is not restrictive. An over-zealous application of monitoring of a deliberately disengaged patient can be experienced as 'therapeutic stalking' (Graham 2006). Unsolicited phone calls or texts, sending unwanted letters, and refusing to stop when told the relationship is over are the hallmarks of assertive outreach, but also of both pathological jealousy and stalking. In English law, at least, an outreach team has a credible defence.

Tensions often exist between the team's duty of care and the patient's desire for self-determination or privacy, or their reluctance to be viewed as mentally ill. Community outreach involves periods of taking responsibility for care. Contact, direct or indirect, provides an early warning system for social or clinical deterioration or crises. This only works if the right enquiries are made and the worker is alert to the signs. Each visit permits assessment of appearance, sleep patterns, mood, irritability, hostility, compliance with medication, unpaid utility bills, eviction notices, damaged furniture, street drugs, drug-taking equipment, alcohol, etc.

If direct contact is refused, then indirect monitoring and information gathering can be a substitute. In the current climate, failure to monitor (and document!) can lead to criticism if an inquiry follows an untoward incident involving the patient. The first step is usually to seek the family's views on the patient's health and need for services. Families may be reluctant to help directly, by giving access, if this risks conflict with the patient. By maintaining contact with the family, feedback on mental state and compliance can be obtained.

Third-party sources of information can also provide knowledge of the patient's routine, places frequented, and friends. Likewise, home visits when the patient is not at home can be a useful opportunity to look through the window, check for piles of unopened mail, and bump into neighbours. Indicators of relapse vary from patient to patient; dirty dishes or mouldy takeaway cartons are not always reliable evidence. Smashed windows, burn marks, and insecure premises are more worrying.

It is generally not advisable to peer through letterboxes as this perhaps crosses the privacy threshold, and stories (probably apocryphal) abound of people being poked at through letterboxes. Entering premises on your own to have a look around, when the door has been left open by a chaotic or preoccupied patient, is also hazardous.

Neighbours will often volunteer information, especially when they are involved. It should not be necessary to endanger confidentiality by declaring your professional identity when making basic enquiries with neighbours. In many cases, a simple 'Have you seen the gentleman downstairs recently?' elicits a history of nocturnal shouting, or other problems only too apparent to the neighbours.

Enquiries with the council can produce other possible indicators of relapse, such as complaints by neighbours or recent rent arrears. Housing and benefits departments will usually take your name and telephone number as a contact and inform you when problems arise to enlist your help in resolving them. Such information gathering can inform the team's risk assessment:

Case study

Olu is a 38-year-old man with a long history of paranoid schizophrenia with. numerous admissions over 25 years, often via the police. His experiences had led to mistrust of services and avoidance of follow-up and treatment.

Olu was withdrawn and always a loner who had no contact with his parents. He had long been labelled 'hard to engage'. He had told social services that his parents had moved back to Nigeria, and attempts to contact them for consultation proved fruitless. Attempts at contact with Olu were met with either his empty council flat or, if he was at home, expletives and the door remaining closed. Even following treatment in hospital, when he became more open, he would barely tolerate a five-minute interaction. Alternative approaches were needed to break this cycle of repeated compulsory admissions, together with the associated risks of rent arrears and distress.

Information on Olu's mental health status could be ascertained indirectly from the reaction to your knock when he was home. He was rarely home during the day, requiring persistent, early morning visits. The ferocity of expletives when grossly unwell would prompt joint visits. With mounting concerns, we eventually decided to talk with immediate neighbours. We had to overcome major doubts, balancing confidentiality with risk. In the end, there were three main reasons for this course of action:

1. Olu's appearance and behaviour were such that the neighbours could be in no doubt about his mental health and social needs.
2. Previous risks existed, both generally and to the neighbours.
3. No relatives were in contact.

Restrictive approach

Restrictive approaches come last, after a long period of attempts at engagement and information gathering. Not all patients who refuse contact will justify this. If someone appears to be coping reasonably well and presents no risks other than future relapse, the team may have to accept minimal direct and indirect contact until such time as the situation may deteriorate. Difficult ethical issues arise in cases where compulsion is prolonged or repeated, and these require team discussion. Liaison with families provides a valuable way of checking out our ethical judgements about whether, or when, to act restrictively.

Case study

Olu was picked up by the police, some distance away, and brought to our local hospital. It was agreed that we would use a restrictive approach.

He was detained compulsorily with treatment consisting of depot medication, as all previous attempts with oral medication had failed. 'Intensive inreach' of three or more visits to the ward weekly by his case manager continued, and Olu's mental state improved quickly, as it always did on the ward. After three long-acting injections, he was given extended leave with the proviso that he attend the ward for his medication every two weeks and meet his case manager in the intervening week. These arrangements were transferred to a community treatment order (CTO) requiring him to attend the ward twice weekly for the purpose of offering treatment and support. He had a better relationship with the ward staff and chose to have his depot from them. It helped that he was also usually given breakfast.

Olu has since been out of hospital for two years and his CTO has been renewed. He defaulted on his injection after six months and, when seen at home, complained of side effects. His injection dosage was reduced and he restarted. The benefits of a protracted period of treatment and contact continue to accrue. He has taken himself for a haircut, removing many years of matted 'locks'. His neighbours are more supportive of him and greet him on passing. He is warmer and less guarded in relationships. He has not been in trouble with the police and has allowed his key worker to accompany him to the housing office to sort out his arrears.

Finally, out of the blue, his mother phoned the team base to enquire after him. Both parents had remained local residents, despite Olu's previous claim! We were able to give glowing feedback on progress to his mother and encourage direct contact. She allowed us to give Olu her phone number and said she would visit her son. They have yet to meet.

Mental health legislation varies both within the UK and internationally, and is discussed in detail in the chapter on compulsion and freedom (Chapter 8). Similarly, the use of financial leverage is addressed both in Chapter 8 and in Chapter 20, on finance and appointeeship.

Failed engagement

NICE (2011) provides a stark quote from the evidence base. reminding us of the challenges particularly with specific groups of patients:

> People with psychosis and coexisting substance misuse are more likely to be non-adherent to prescribed medication, and have poor engagement with treatment programmes, increased risk of suicide, more and longer inpatient stays, increased risk of violence and time spent in the criminal justice system, and poorer overall prognosis.

Indeed, dropout rates from substance misuse treatment services are much higher than we experience in patients with severe mental illness. Our colleagues running diabetes services also experience high levels of missed outpatient appointments and high levels of resulting harm from uncontrolled blood sugars, particularly in adolescents. Imagine the ambivalence and denial that you would experience in accepting that you had a problem with diabetes that restricted your life and diet, and could kill you, or a problem with alcohol that was damaging your relationships and work. Despite the risks posed, neither of these patient groups are offered an equivalent outreach approach to treatment beyond the outpatient clinic. Both, however, offer educational and peer support often through the voluntary sector. In substance misuse, the concept of motivation to change and a stage-wise approach to support for people who are in different psychological stages of readiness for change have developed (Prochaska and DiClemente 1992). This is a useful model to help us consider the stages of engagement and disengagement from the perspective of patient motivation, it is outlined in Chapter 19 on substance misuse.

Ryan and Morgan (2004) list numerous reasons for resistance to mental health services, including fears of having a child taken into care, experiences of prejudicial treatment, dehumanizing care, and holding alternative beliefs about the concept of mental illness. Even though we know these wider psychosocial obstacles are strong, community outreach workers still experience a degree of anguish over failure to engage constructively with a patient. In our experience, staff, particularly new members, find the patient's rejection of the team's considerable efforts difficult. We have to remind ourselves that other services may have tried and failed and that is often why the patient has been referred for outreach. We have certain skills and team resources, but a few patients will still evade all attempts at contact. Individual and team support systems, as described in Chapter 26, help us to depersonalize the problems and not take them too much to heart. Even with the most persistent attempts at care and going the extra mile, one of our patients used the complaints process eloquently, citing harassment. Another patient repeatedly moved out of his flat as soon as he was discharged after each readmission so that even his family did not know where he was, until he appeared in some distant hospital, mute and catatonic.

Measuring engagement and 'dropout'

A simple and routinely collected proxy measure to help teams evaluate their levels of patient engagement is the 'did not attend' rate of missed appointments often shortened to DNA rate. Taken together with patient reported experience of care measures and tracked over time, they can provide basic indicators as to the team's acceptability and customer focus. As with many performance indicators, a degree of caution should be exercised when comparing services with differing patient criteria, populations, demographics, and other confounds.

At a more academic level, Catty et al. (2011) offer a detailed study of the interrelationship between attachment to the clinical team, relationships with their key worker, and the patient's clinical and social functioning. This paper uses several established questionnaires, including measures of attachment in therapeutic relationship with the CMHT key worker, and team attachment. The Team Attachment Questionnaire, for example (Goodwin et al. 2003), has been developed for community services; it records the patient's experience and feelings about the team and key worker they are in contact with. Items include the extent to which they feel they have a partnership, have their needs and problems understood, feel safe with the team, and feel judged or patronized. Interviewing 93 patients mainly diagnosed with psychosis, the authors found that patients' general affability—their disposition for forming personal relationships—did not predict their relationships with clinicians and teams. The authors concluded that higher ratings of therapeutic relationship and service attachment are probably related more to the patients' experience of their care.

The Dartmouth ACT (DACT) scale (Teague et al. 1998) and the Tool for Measurement of Assertive Community Treatment (TMACT) (Monroe-DeVita et al. 2011) offer standards for model fidelity in ACT teams. Both have components that measure the team's application of a 'no dropout' policy, which is measured by how well the service engages and retains patients. The score ranges from low for 50 per cent caseload retention up to a maximum score for 100 per cent retention. The use of 'assertive engagement mechanisms' such as street outreach and legal powers are also measured. These scales recognize that assertive outreach teams use both constructive and restrictive approaches. The TMACT includes measures of more recovery-oriented practices such as person-centred planning, goal setting, and self- management.

The UK700 study (Burns et al. 2000) defined engagement-related activity as any patient contact which fostered a positive attitude to treatment and the service. Only constructive engagement was rated under engagement—appointeeship or payeeship would be rated as 'finance', and Mental Health Act activity as 'mental health'. The proportion of face-to-face activity recorded as engagement (as defined above) was marginally greater in intensive case management (ICM) with caseloads of 10–15 (at 16 per cent) than in standard care with caseloads of 30–35 (at 14 per cent). A greater difference between the two groups was the fourfold increase in the rate of attempted (failed) contacts for ICM compared to standard care: "Case managers with smaller caseloads did strive more vigorously to maintain contact (more telephone calls and failed visits) (Burns et al. 2000).

Conclusions

Engagement is a term used exclusively by professionals and regarded with suspicion by some patients. Patients may not share our positive associations with phrases such as 'preventing people falling through the net'. Is this the sort of net that fish are trapped in or the one that saves the trapeze artist? It is important that we are sensitive to alternative perceptions—our 'conscientious persistence' may be our patients' harassment or 'therapeutic stalking'.

We believe that engagement occurs between the patient and a key worker more effectively than between the patient and the team. The interpersonal skills of the individual worker (such as compassion, empathy, and a nurturing approach) cannot be easily described in writing. The team must foster this approach, having the flexibility to undertake social and practical help when possible. Engagement is not a separate function in itself but permeates everything that we do in community outreach. It is also not restricted to the early part of treatment but persists throughout our contact with patients.

Chapter 11

Medication compliance

Compliance, concordance, or adherence?

When patients are admitted with another relapse of their psychotic illness, there is often discussion about whether they have been taking their medicines regularly. It is common to find that they have either stopped taking their tablets altogether or have been irregular with them in the weeks before admission. The debate then arises about whether they have broken down because they stopped taking the medicine or stopped taking the medicine because they were breaking down. Whichever it is, failure to take medicines as prescribed has been unequivocally demonstrated to increase the risk of relapse (Curson et al. 1985).

Traditionally, this has been referred to as 'compliance'—the degree to which the patient follows the prescribed treatment regimen. Although it is most often discussed in relationship to medicines, compliance or non-compliance can be crucial in all aspects of treatments. For instance, how well patients comply with prescribed diets or exercise regimes is likely to be a factor in outcome variations in some conditions. We will confine ourselves here to issues about medicines (and in particular psychotropic medications). Helping patients comply with the broader treatment package is addressed throughout this book; the chapter on engagement (Chapter 10) is particularly relevant.

Non-compliance can be either covert or overt (Curson et al. 1985). Covert non-compliance is when the patient implies that they are cooperating with the prescribed treatment but, in reality, are not doing so or doing so only partially. This is not at all uncommon. Overt non-compliance is when patients simply refuse to accept the proffered treatment. One of the advantages of depot medication is that although it cannot guarantee 100 per cent compliance, it does ensure that there is no covert non-compliance. If the patient is not taking the injections, then it is clear to all involved.

The last few years has seen a reaction to the term 'compliance' because it is taken to imply an excessively passive role for the patient. We now place greater emphasis on negotiating treatments and ensuring that the patient is, as much as possible, an equal partner in the process. This approach is encapsulated in the policy phrase 'no decision about me without me' from the NHS White Paper on putting the patient first and shared decision-making (Department of Health

2010). At the very least, the patient should be able to express their opinion and have an influence on key decisions. 'Adherence' to the agreed regime became a more acceptable term; even more recently, 'concordance' has been used to drive home the equality of the relationship. Adherence has caught on, whereas concordance has failed to enter common usage, but compliance remains the term most commonly used. We will stick with compliance to avoid confusion, but this should not be taken to imply a passive or submissive role for the patient. Far from it. It is best practice to emphasize negotiation and encourage patients to take as much responsibility for the content and conduct of their treatment as possible.

The extent of non-compliance

There is nothing especially psychiatric about medication non-compliance. Hardly anyone seems able to take tablets regularly over long periods. A simple check of your bathroom cabinet will confirm this! Poor compliance is especially likely if the consequences of forgetting the tablets are not immediate—when you don't experience any immediate change in how you feel. Only about half of patients taking antihypertensives take them absolutely reliably (Johnson et al. 1999); similarly for tuberculosis therapy (Menzies et al. 1993).

Mental health professionals often make the mistake of citing diabetes when encouraging their patients to persist with antipsychotics or antidepressants. This is probably a tactical error. As with antihypertensives, the patient taking antipsychotics or antidepressants will probably feel somewhat better, not worse, in the first few days they forget to take them. The immediate effect is a relief from the side effects. The risks of stopping such medicines (whether of psychiatric relapse or, for the patient with high blood pressure, a stroke) are some time in the future. For the diabetic, the importance of medication is powerfully reinforced by the immediate discomfort associated with any missed insulin injection. Yet even in diabetes, compliance is often quite poor, even though clinicians have the benefit of a routinely used biological marker (HbA1c) which gives an overall picture of what average blood-sugar levels have been over a period of weeks.

Causes of non-compliance

The causes of non-compliance are varied and the situation for each individual will need to be assessed. Not only does it vary between individuals but it can also change over time in the same individual. Although the following sections cover causes of non-compliance, it is generally better to think positively in terms of strategies for improving and supporting compliance. This is not just playing with words. The starting point with our patients should be an acknowl-edgement of the difficulty of sustaining long-term treatment. When we explore the issues, it is to make things easier, not to apportion blame.

Human nature/disorganization

As mentioned previously, there are some general, non-specific factors which interfere with compliance. We are keen to help our patients live as normal a life as possible and minimize the impact of their illness on them. The more success-ful we are with that, paradoxically, the greater the risk of forgetting their medi-cines. We avoid fancy jargon and refer to this simply as 'human nature'. Once they are a bit better and there are more interesting things to concentrate on, it is hardly surprising that attention moves away from their illness.

Many patients with severe mental illnesses lead fairly unstructured, indeed disorganized, lives. A lack of routine makes it even more likely that medicines will be forgotten. A key to success is to take medicines at a regular point in the day (e.g. with breakfast or when returning from work in the evening). This, of course, relies on getting up at a regular time and having breakfast or having a job to go to. In the absence of such personal routines, our interventions need to be directed to introducing some structure.

Side effects

Virtually all effective medicines have some side effects. In the case of the early antipsychotics, mood stabilizers, and antidepressants, these often include dis-tressing motor effects such as stiffness and tremor, gastrointestinal and urinary tract problems including constipation and dry mouth, and also general seda-tion. Weight gain is particularly distressing for many patients.

Undoubtedly, dropout from treatment and poor compliance can be a con-sequence of side effects (Priebe et al. 2005; Lieberman et al. 2005). Out of 40 patients interviewed by Priebe et al. on reasons for previously disengaging from services, the side effects of medication were raised by 28. It is not uncommon to hear statements such as the following transcribed from these interviews:

'I stopped hearing voices but the side effects were so bad I'd prefer to hear voices.'

'I can't do things that I want to do. I want to come off this depot. It makes me put on weight, it stiffens the joints.'

Monitoring regularly for these and ensuring that they are minimized by optimal dosing and, very occasionally, with adjunct medication, is essential if patients are to persist (Chapter 7). Acknowledging the importance of side effects and discussing them frankly can help in itself. A fear that talking about side effects will scare patients off taking their medication is not borne out by experience (Chaplin et al. 1999; Chaplin and Kent 1998). Discussing side effects and the risks for adverse outcomes is such a routine practice in modern medicine that it would now seem odd not to run through them with our patients. It is also important because sometimes patients can misinterpret the side effects as a worsening of their condition and evidence that the treatment is not working. An explanation and honest reassurance can go a long way to preventing discontinuation.

The rapid changeover to the newer antidepressants and atypical antipsychotics has been due more to their benign side-effect profile than to increased effectiveness. However, the challenge posed by excess weight gain and metabolic syndrome is now a major one for community outreach staff.

Insight

So far we have been stressing problems with compliance that are common to all disorders. Lack of insight is often blamed for poor compliance in psychosis patients. Obviously, this is important. A striking feature of psychoses is that the patients are often unaware of the extent of their illness or even deny it altogether, ascribing their discomforts to external agencies (persecutory individuals, direct interference with their thoughts, etc.).

Insight is, however, a complex concept—it is not simply a matter of having it or not. Both Birchwood (Birchwood et al. 1994) and David (David 1990; David et al. 1992) have proposed three components. Insight scales have been developed which recognize that there are degrees of insight (David et al. 1992), but even these have demonstrated only a weak association with compliance. All of us have worked with psychosis patients who are completely devoid of insight and yet happily accept treatment for an illness whose existence they deny. Similarly, most of us have had the frustrating experience of watching patients who have recovered well acknowledge that they were ill and are now better, and yet refuse to take the treatment that would undoubtedly continue to help them.

Increasingly, we conceptualize this area in terms of 'health belief systems'. These vary enormously in our multicultural society. The simple scientific model of illness used by most health care staff is not necessarily shared by our patients, whether psychotic or not. Patients' explanations for illness encountered may range from New Age thinking and the influence of ley lines, a belief in voodoo, or even demonic possession (in some Pentecostal churches).

Different groups within society can have equal information about an illness and come to strikingly differing conclusions about the importance of its consequences. An everyday example of this is how many young people continue to smoke despite the overwhelming evidence about its risks. It is not that they are unaware of the consequences; far from it. However, the balance between immediate gratification versus long-term complications such as strokes and lung disease simply weighs differently with them than with older health care professionals (who regularly observe these consequences). It can be difficult for us to fully comprehend this. For instance, many diabetic patients assess the relative importance of good blood-sugar control totally differently to their doctors (White et al. 1996). Patients are focused on the short-term problems (hypos), and their doctors on the long-term risks (blindness and nerve damage). Recognizing the short-term focus may lead to different strategies for improving compliance (see Box 11.1).

For many of our patients, the risk of a relapse may simply not seem that important compared to the inconvenience of side effects. For the most disabled and socially marginalized, there may not be that much at stake. If you have a job, a family, and some status in your local community, you are likely to put up with almost anything to avoid an acute psychotic episode. If you are living on your own, ostracized by your neighbours, and feel a total failure in life, then the odd period in hospital is not such a price to avoid feeling stiff or sluggish.

In summary, we find the shorthand term 'insight' of limited value in community outreach work. Nor does NICE guidance for psychosis (2014) find sufficient evidence to recommend the use of CBT in the development of insight or in the management of poor compliance. The real issue is almost invariably

---

Box 11.1 Components of insight

David et al. (1992):

+ recognition that one has a mental illness
+ compliance with treatment
+ ability to relabel unusual mental events (delusions and hallucinations) as pathological

Birchwood et al. (1994):

+ awareness of illness
+ need for treatment
+ attribution of symptoms

Data from *The British Journal of Psychiatry*, 161, 5, David A., Buchanan A., Reed A. et al. 'The assessment of insight in psychosis', pp. 599–602, 1992; Data from *Acta Psychiatrica Scandinavica*, 89, 1, Birchwood, J.S., Drury, J., Healy F. et al. 'A self-report Insight Scale for psychosis: reliability, validity and sensitivity to change', pp. 62–67, 2007.

about constructing a space in which to acknowledge and negotiate around complex and, often, conflicting values.

Denial

Denial often contributes to poor compliance and may seem indistinguishable from poor insight. It is, however, different and needs to be worked with. Denial is normal and often very adaptive. Most of us use denial so that we can put aside difficult issues and get on with life. Usually, we then come back to them when we are less stressed. Denial protects us from painful emotions and preoccupations—it has been shown to be beneficial in some circumstances and may be one of the reasons that trauma counselling can be counterproductive (Mayou et al. 2000).

Some years ago, one of our colleagues asked young black men suffering from psychoses and with poor compliance why they did not take their medicines. We had anticipated that the answers would be entirely complaints about side effects or a belief that they were not ill. Several did give such reasons but an equal number told him that they simply wanted to forget about their illness for a time and get on with their lives, feeling they were like everyone else. They had not lost sight of their illness but chose actively to try to ignore it for a period. Denial in psychosis patients requires the same attention that it does in non-psychosis ones; they too need help in coming to terms with the disappointment and loss from having to accept their illness.

The influence of friends and family

It is not just the patients' views about their illness and treatment that matter. Compliance with treatment is powerfully influenced by the opinions of those around the patient, those they depend on and relate to. Family attitudes matter enormously. Do the parents or spouse also accept that the patient is ill and will benefit from the treatment? The improvements found from expressed emotion therapy with families may be due to improved compliance with the medicines, as it helps the family to pull together better (Razali and Yahya 1995).

People whom the patient meets socially are surprisingly likely to be unsupportive, if not actively opposed, to their continuing medication. They will often only meet the patient when relatively well, not seeing them when either in hospital or more withdrawn when ill. It is not surprising, then, if they attribute any residual problems, along with side effects, to the drugs and compare the patient to how they themselves are.

People's attitude towards psychiatric medication is complex but still broadly negative. The strength of society's expressed preference for psychotherapy instead of antidepressants is at variance with both the evidence for relative effectiveness but also with what people do. Educated North European and American populations regularly report very critical opinions about antidepressants while insisting on their prescription and taking them in vast quantities. So, despite the high rates of consumption of psychotropic medicines in our society, patients are likely to be surrounded by sceptical voices.

Scepticism about the value of medication is dramatically demonstrated by a study some time ago of societal attitudes towards the treatment of mental illness (Jorm et al. 1997). In the treatment of schizophrenia, medication came very low on the list, long after the commonest suggestion, 'get out a bit more'.

Many countries, led by Australia and Norway, have established national programmes to improve public understanding of mental health, and there are now several national and international drives to reduce stigma surrounding both depression and schizophrenia as well as mental illness generally. These anti-stigma campaigns often hang their work on evocative titles such as Time to Change (UK), See Me (Scotland), Like Minds, Like Mine (New Zealand), and have strong government backing. The increased willingness of celebrities and politicians to acknowledge their own mental health problems has been one of the most powerful influences. That the prime minister of Norway, Jens Stoltenberg, took two weeks off work because of acknowledged depression would have been unthinkable a decade earlier.

At a more local level, community outreach workers have to devote time to changing attitudes of those individuals whom they identify as key in improving their patients' compliance. There is evidence that educational initiatives for local neighbourhoods may be more effective than large national programmes. A programme to foster acceptance of an aftercare hostel for mentally ill individuals found that inviting the neighbours in to meet the residents was what really worked.

Improving compliance

Just as there are many contributing strands to poor compliance, so there are a number of approaches to try to improve it. Those chosen will reflect the particular circumstances of each patient. The emphasis may vary over time. There is something of a hierarchy in interventions, with patients moving up and down from one to another. In the descriptions that follow, we move from the more general approaches used with all patients to more specific and targeted approaches for patients with severe compliance problems. This is not a rigorous science; nor is it an unvarying sequence. It presents a range that all community outreach staff need to be familiar with. One has to seek alternative strategies when the current one is not working.

The therapeutic relationship

Probably the most important determinant of whether a patient takes their treatment is how well they get on with their case manager. Most of the research in this area has been on compliance with medicines and the relationship with the prescribing doctor, but it is illuminating. Patients who feel their doctors are competent, compassionate, and genuinely interested in them as individuals will take treatment, often despite troublesome side effects (Frank and Gunderson 1990). This seems so central to community outreach that it risks being overlooked. The holistic approach to helping patients that characterizes our work is crucial to sustaining long-term compliance. Time and energy spent on engagement (Chapter 10) is not a luxury but an essential contribution to both the patient's well-being and treatment. Nagging is no substitute for a thoroughly grounded relationship!

There is evidence that a good therapeutic relationship (sometimes called a 'working alliance') predicts outcome in the severely mentally ill (Priebe and Gruyters 1995). Of course, those patients who can form warmer relationships are generally less ill, but the evidence is that it is the later development of a positive therapeutic alliance—rather than how it is at the start of the relationship—that more strongly predicts improved outcomes (Feeley et al. 1999). The improved outcomes also reflect better compliance with the treatment from staff with whom patients engage more and trust more.

Education

Patients need to be well informed about why their drugs are being prescribed. This means detailed (and often repeated) explanations of both their long-term benefits and also their more immediate effects on arousal and symptoms. It will often involve some simple explanation about the relationship between emotional arousal and psychological functioning.

The American social worker Hogarty worked for many years developing psychological strategies to improve outcome in schizophrenia, and concluded that the regulation of mounting anxiety is key (Hogarty et al. 1995). The Yerkes-Dodson law—first described in 1908 (Yerkes and Dodson 1908) and subsequently simplified as a curve (Diamond et al. 2007) (see Fig 11.1)—is helpful for most patients who find it immediately understandable and convincing. It emphasizes how some level of stress and arousal is both normal and beneficial, but how over-arousal rapidly tips over into reduced performance and potential breakdown. The role of medicines to bring arousal back to within the normal range can then be explained.

A full explanation of the therapeutic purpose and effects of the prescribed medicines will involve explaining the side effects and risks. As remarked earlier,

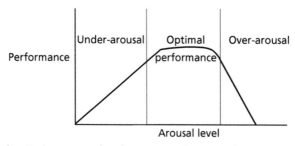

Fig 11.1 Yerkes-Dodson curve of performance against arousal

an honest and frank description of such risks does not reduce compliance. On the contrary, it reassures patients that you know what you are talking about—they will probably already have experienced the side effects.

There now exists an extensive library of professionally produced information leaflets on psychotropic drugs which can be used to supplement personal explanations. While these can be very useful, it is not a good idea to substitute them for an individualized explanation. The more personalized and relevant you can make it, the more likely it will be taken seriously.

Education also must include family members and those who have any significant influence on the patient. This can go beyond simply outlining the rationale for the treatments; they include a careful analysis of the stress points in a patient's life so that they can be anticipated or avoided. Family education is often a part of psychosocial interventions such as 'psycho-education', which has become established in bipolar disorder, as well as expressed emotional work in schizophrenia. These are dealt with more in Chapter 24. Even with patients who live alone, a good understanding of what interferes with compliance can help improve it.

Case study

Barry had been settled on his olanzapine for some years and was happy with it. He had not been admitted for several years, lived with his parents, and had a part-time job in a warehouse with his dad.

Twice in the last year he had become tense and complained of poor sleep and admitted readily, to direct questioning, that he had stopped his medicine for a week on each occasion.

We initially thought that he was experimenting with whether he still needed it, but this proved not to be the case. He explained that on both occasions he had been on a family holiday and, while away, had gone to the pub with his dad and his dad's footballing mates (who knew of his illness). One of them encouraged him to stop taking the medicine, saying that it was making him slow and sluggish and that 'doctors always played safe'. Although he reinstated his tablets on returning home, it was then that his destabilization manifested itself. He discussed this with his father who explained the importance of his medicine to his friend, and there have been no further such incidents.

Prompting and supporting

We have made clear that we consider most of the difficulties in compliance to be best understood as 'normal'. The aim is to help somebody with a difficult task rather than try to find out some pathology for why they cannot cope with an easy task. In practice, this means supporting and prompting them, checking regularly with them about how it is going (see the later section, 'Monitoring and structuring'), and commiserating about the difficulties of complying. We congratulate and encourage them in their success. A positive, committed attitude really works. If the staff member does not really think that the medicines are important, then their support will be compromised. We experienced this in our Wandsworth assertive outreach team. As we gained more experience with clozapine, it became much easier to start and maintain patients on the drug. As team members saw other patients improve, they became more convinced and convincing, being able to point to other patients who were doing well. There is no substitute for the genuine enthusiasm in the support and encouragement offered.

Support and encouragement can be powerfully enhanced by involving other patients, if they are willing. Patients will often listen more willingly to the case made by someone who has experienced the same effects and side effects and who can describe how the medicine has made a real difference to their lives. Asking patients who are doing well if they are prepared to discuss their treatment has to be approached very carefully. However, we have been struck by how many patients are not only willing to but who really value helping someone else. We gained immeasurably in the Wandsworth assertive outreach team by having a user worker who drew on her own experience of how maintenance medication had transformed her life. Seeing her holding down a rewarding and important job despite (or because of?) her medicines strengthened the resolve of many patients to persist. It both demonstrated that the drugs were tolerable and gave a sense of hope and a goal to aim for.

Prompting and supporting are not passive procedures, nor are they particularly 'high status'. They will only happen if they are constantly reasserted on the list of priorities. The importance of medication can easily be overlooked, overshadowed by more fashionable psychosocial developments in outreach work. As outlined in Chapter 7, outreach teams need to explore any resistance to promoting appropriate medications and ensure that it is taken seriously by everyone—it is not just the doctor's job.

Monitoring and structuring

Simply focusing on the medicines (albeit briefly) at each visit really does strengthen compliance. Learning to ask the question 'Have you taken all your tablets?' in a positive way is the first step. Having emphasized how difficult it is to remember to take medicines over long periods, and having stressed how normal that is, the concern can be expressed as a collaboration: 'OK, let's see how you've done with the medicines this week. How's it gone? Did you forget any days or have you remembered them all?'

Such a query can easily be accompanied by a pill count. If compliance is poor, then it is often best to prescribe on a weekly basis. This allows a rapid count of how many tablets are left over and hence how many doses have been missed. The problem can be quickly identified and quantified. It is crucial to be able to do this in a way that is not seen as persecutory or suggests a lack of trust. Many staff we meet think this cannot be achieved and that the therapeutic relationship will be the first casualty of such a manoeuvre. Clumsily done, this may be the case, but our experience is that it is eminently acceptable to most patients. Properly and positively presented, in the spirit of genuine collaboration, it is seen as evidence of professional conscientiousness and concern, not persecution. As with any new technique, particularly if the community outreach worker is doubtful, it is best to get used to it with patients who are already pretty compliant. When you then feel comfortable with it, you can then apply it with the more problematic patients.

As well as asking and checking, many patients can be considerably helped by aids such as dosette boxes. The outreach key worker can fill these up along with the patient, as a joint task, in one of their visits. Alternatively, pharmacists will dispense into them. The advantages are obvious, especially for patients taking a range of medicines for their physical health. It is not unusual for a patient to have to take several tablets. One of our patients with a complex regime for his Parkinson's disease took nearly 20 a day. With lots of tablets, it is very easy to forget or get confused ('Now did I just take that?').

If the patient wants to deceive us, then he can dispose of the pills. This happens sometimes, but simple forgetfulness is by far the commonest reason. When the patient is thought to be deliberately deceiving, daily supervised medicines or depot medication (see later) may be the only alternative.

Supervised medication

One of the major advantages of assertive outreach teams, flexible ACT teams, and crisis resolution home treatment teams is that they can offer periods of intensive supervision of oral medicines. This can involve regular visits—up to twice daily in extreme situations—to make absolutely sure that the prescribed medicines are being taken. In the Wandsworth assertive outreach team this included treatments not only for mental health (antipsychotics, mood stabilizers, antidepressants) but also for physical health (e.g. insulin, antihypertensives). 'Observed meds', as the Americans call it, is a rare, but important and effective, outreach intervention.

In a group of just over 100 patients selected because of poor treatment compliance for the Wandsworth team, 5–10 were on 'observed meds' at any time. For about half of these, it meant a daily visit, sometimes seven days a week, to stay and see they took the pills. For the remainder, visits varied between three and five times a week. For most patients, daily visits are continued until the medication routine is considered established. For this to be a practical option, the medication needs to be effective as a single daily dose.

Because of their sedative side effects, patients prefer to take antipsychotics and some antidepressants as late in the afternoon as possible. Some patients take the bulk of their dose at the delivery and are left to take a further dose themselves either just before retiring or in the morning. This seems illogical (if the patient is reliable enough to take one dose, why not all?), but we have found it works. Patients with limited insight or commitment to the regime will often comply as long as they are kept well with a basic dose. This approach ensures that a substantial dose is taken regularly. The regular visits keep the drugs in the forefront of the patient's mind, so they are less likely to forget the second dose; it is also easy to check at the next visit.

We did an experiment with an evening medicine run, mainly for establishing patients on clozapine, as it is so sedative. Unfortunately, we did not find it sustainable, even with the resources of a dedicated assertive outreach team. It absorbed too much manpower and there were also safety issues. However, evening visits from the home treatment team to patients in crisis are standard practice.

We have emphasized the supportive function of daily supervised medication, but honestly acknowledge the supervisory function. Few patients have any illusions about the importance that we place on their medication, so there is no catastrophic impact on the therapeutic relationship. For the process to succeed, the person delivering the medicines needs to believe in their importance. Training is essential. Most of us feel a bit uncomfortable with this 'controlling' aspect of the job, and teams need time to talk through these issues. Even though experienced members may have been convinced of the value of the approach by previous successes, new members need to be able to explore their ambivalence. The 'user worker' in our Wandsworth team took on a substantial number of daily meds, and her absolute endorsement of the approach ('I wish someone had offered me this years ago, it would have saved me a lot of hard lessons') spoke volumes.

The visits are often short and the patient's case manager should not always conduct them. This is important, because it is when the regular outreach worker is off that one needs most to be able to rely on consistent medication. We did find that patients sometimes accepted regular supervised medicines from 'their' outreach worker but blankly refused them from other team members. It makes sense for the case manager to establish the routine, but second and third members should be introduced as soon as possible.

The delivery of daily medicines should be coordinated for each week at the main team review meeting and the names of those responsible written on a notice board. This ensures that the whole team knows who is on supervised medicines, so that if anyone is away, their visits can be quickly redistributed. This is particularly important in routine CMHTs where daily meds are an infrequent occurrence and could easily be overlooked.

The emphasis on supervised medicines and the change from a five-day to a seven-day service were the two innovations in the Wandsworth outreach team which had the most obvious effect on readmission rates. One needs to regularly remind oneself of this to balance the limited job satisfaction that comes from simply delivering medicines. It may be dull for us, but it makes a real difference to the stability of our patients' lives. As patients became more stable and able to shoulder more responsibility themselves, we can move on to other strategies to improve compliance.

Depot medication

No matter how much work goes into developing a strong, supportive, therapeutic relationship, there will remain some patients who simply will not take their medicines. For such patients, when the consequences of relapse warrant it, depot medication is the only feasible alternative. The UK, Australia, and Scandinavia rely heavily on depots, with up to 50 per cent of patients with schizophrenia maintained on them. This reduced with the advent of the atypicals, but picked up again as atypical depots (referred to as long-acting injectables, LAIs) were developed.

Usually, the case manager administers depots (if they are a nurse) on a visit to the patient's home. While this is the preferred method, there are some patients who are so hard to track down it may be more reliable to get them to come to a ward or clinic for it. Good, fail-safe communication between the ward and the team is essential if this is to work and missed doses spotted.

Compliance therapy

New evidence-based interventions to improve compliance have been developed in recent years. The evidence from randomized controlled trials for compliance therapy is mixed. An early comparison looked very effective despite the number of sessions being small (4–6), rarely taking more than 30 minutes each spread over just 2–3 weeks (Kemp et al. 1996). The authors produced a manual and a video setting out their programme (Kemp et al. 1997). It is based on collaboration, cognitive behavioural approaches in psychosis (Kingdon and Turkington 1994), and the motivational interviewing techniques developed in substance abuse (Rollinick et al. 1992). At 12 sessions divided into three phases, it is longer than the intervention originally trialled. Although a replication study failed to find the same advantage (O'Donnell et al. 2003) and current attention focuses more on CBT to improve compliance (Turkington et al. 2014), most outreach workers still find the thinking behind this approach helpful.

Compliance therapy has three phases. The first is reviewing the illness and attitudes towards therapy. This includes a review of the illness history and previous experience of medication, concentrating on reflective listening and establishing rapport. In addition, the therapist elicits the patient's stance towards treatment, paying attention to their culture and background. At this stage it is important to avoid directly challenging denial of problems (e.g. 'Why does your family think there is a problem?'), to acknowledge negative experiences, and to link medication cessation with relapses.

The second phase is exploring the ambivalence to therapy. It involves exploration of ambivalence towards medication such as side effects, misunderstandings, denial, stigma. The advantages and disadvantages are examined (e.g. 'What bothers you the most about the medication?' 'How has it helped?') and target symptoms are elicited for treatment from patient's feedback. The therapist cautiously explores psychotic symptoms and beliefs that limit compliance and highlights benefits of treatment using metaphors ('Try to see your medicine as a protective layer or an insurance policy').

The third phase is reducing stigma. It encourages self-sufficiency and the recognition of early relapse signs. Normalizing rationales to deal with stigma are provided (e.g. pointing out prevalence, comparisons with physical illness, famous sufferers). The consequences of stopping medication are discussed. Lastly, the therapist encourages maintenance treatment as a freely chosen strategy to enhance long-term quality of life.

Conclusions

Community outreach exists to deliver effective treatments. There is little point in engaging with patients and monitoring their well-being unless there is something to offer them. We have good treatments (pharmacological, psychological, and social), but they cannot work if they are not implemented. With psychological and social treatments, we are often in the driving seat once engagement has been achieved. With drug treatments, we know that these are generally followed only partially and inconsistently by most patients. It is a sobering thought that we could probably achieve almost all the added benefits (in terms of relapse prevention) that can be gained from our range of psychosocial interventions, if only the medicines we prescribe were taken regularly.

We have emphasized in this chapter how vitally important improving compliance is. The paradox is that our experience teaches us that a narrow focus on compliance is counterproductive. If our patients think that we are only interested in them taking the tablets, we can be sure they will not do it. Improving compliance will only work in the long run if our efforts are part of a wider, genuinely patient-focused, approach. Similarly, we would caution against being too 'technical' about compliance, but to stress the normality of the problems and to search for long-term solutions. It is important to provide the compliance therapy, psycho-education, and CBT that help, but it is even more important to convey an understanding that living with a long-term, severe illness is a difficult and demanding exercise and that 'to err is human'. There is no place for moralizing and criticism. The benefits of improved compliance are enormous and worth the effort.

Chapter 12

Hostility

Introduction

We use the term 'hostility' to encompass a range of behaviours that we might encounter in the course of our work in the community. These behaviours are not exclusive to our patients; in daily life we might encounter passive aggression, intimidating behaviour, verbal aggression, and threats—including whilst driving our cars. Actual physical violence, however, remains rare both in our practice and in society. Homicides by people with mental illness are very infrequent, extreme events making them statistically difficult to predict, despite more detailed and sophisticated risk assessment procedures (Munro and Rumgay 2000; Fazel et al. 2012)

This chapter discusses the politics, incidence, assessment, and management of challenging, hostile, and violent behaviour from the perspective of practising community outreach. We seek not to control patients but to work with them collaboratively and safely wherever possible. Patients and patient advocacy groups dislike the public and professional preoccupation with risk because it can lead to a more coercive culture of legislation and practice. It also discourages positive risk taking where individuals may learn from their successes and failures, taking increasing responsibility, supported by a recovery approach to practice.

Incidence and risk factors

Most violent or aggressive incidents in mental health services take place not in the community but in inpatient units. Between 2011 and 2012, there were 60,000 physical assaults reported against National Health Service staff in England: 69 per cent in mental health or learning disability settings, 3 per cent against ambulance staff, 3 per cent involving primary care staff, and 26 per cent involving acute hospital staff. Most acute hospital assaults occur in the emergency department (National Institute for Health and Care Excellence 2015).

The murder of Jonathan Zito by Christopher Clunis in 1992 (Ritchie 1994) triggered investment in mental health community services, and new procedures in the UK, but arguably reinforced the disproportionate public perception of the link between mental illness and extreme violence. Media attention is amplified on at least three occasions for each tragedy—the event, the court sentence, and publication of the inquiry. The social stigma of mental illness and portrayals of psychopathic horror in film and television further distort perceptions for those without personal or professional exposure to mental illness.

The nightmare stereotype of a random act of homicide by someone with a severe mental illness on people unknown to them—so-called stranger homicide—is rare and falling. The National Confidential Inquiry into Suicide and Homicide by People with Mental Illness (2015) provides detailed figures for the UK. This shows that only 7 per cent of stranger homicides are committed by mental health service patients, and the figure has fallen since 2006. However, between 2003 and 2013, an average of 11 stranger homicides a year were committed by people with mental illness, 88 per cent of whom had a history of alcohol and/or drug misuse.

The research evidence to support an association between severe mental illness and violence is mixed. Consensus has emerged that there is a modest but consistent positive association, but researching this area reliably is complex. The MacArthur Violence Risk Assessment Study (Steadman et al. 1998; Monahan et al. 2001) used a combination of data sources collating, for over 1000 individuals discharged from psychiatric care, patient self-reports, information from carers, and criminal records. Once they had factored out those patients with substance misuse, the researchers found no significant difference between the prevalence of violence in patients and others living in the same US neighbourhood. Substance misuse raises rates of violence in people with mental health problems as well as those without, but more so in the former.

Witt et al. (2013) used meta-analysis and meta-regression to try to unpack the strength and direction of some of the detail in associations between violence and psychosis reported across 110 studies. These studies were conducted in both inpatient and community settings and involved over 45,000 individuals, 18.5 per cent of whom were violent. Violence was very strongly associated with a criminal history, especially assault; polysubstance misuse; and being non-adherent to treatments, including psychological therapies. Violence was strongly associated with a history of being violently victimized, moderately associated with homelessness and male gender, and only weakly associated with non-white ethnicity and lower socio-economic status. Table 12.1 summarizes risk factors associated with increased violence.

The best predictor of future violence is previous violence. A risk history from patient and relatives, psychiatric notes, and, where available, criminal records, will provide most of this information. The referral process must include effective written and verbal handover of information on risk as well as clinical state.

Table 12.1 Patient risk factors for violence and aggression

History	Environment	Mental state
◆ Previous violence	◆ Lack of social supports	◆ Persecutory delusions
◆ Offending and prison history		
◆ Substance misuse	◆ Lack or loss of accommodation	◆ Delusions of passivity; e.g. thought insertion
◆ Poor compliance with medication, especially recent discontinuation of medication		◆ Emotions related to violence; e.g. anger, irritability, suspiciousness, hostility
◆ Poorly engaged with services		
◆ Social restlessness and rootlessness		
◆ Recent severe stress		
◆ Evidence of planning such as obtaining weapons		
◆ Specific threats made by patient		

Adapted from *The BMJ*, 312, Jeremy W Coid, 'Dangerous patients with mental illness: increased risks warrant new policies, adequate resources, and appropriate legislation', pp. 965–966. Copyright (1996) with permission from BMJ Publishing Group Ltd.

Further evidence can be deduced from incidents of homicide by patients under the care of mental health services, since they are subject to legal review and reporting. The National Confidential Inquiry into Suicide and Homicide by People with Mental Illness (2015) shows that between 2003 and 2013, a total of 630 patient homicides occurred (57 a year). Of the perpetrators, 51 per cent had been convicted of a previous violent offence (48 per cent had previously been in prison); 6 per cent had a history of admission to a high-, medium-, or regional secure forensic psychiatric unit; 26 per cent had previously been involuntarily detained under mental health legislation; 17 per cent had been non-adherent with prescribed medication in the month before the homicide; and 39 per cent had missed their final service contact before the homicide.

NICE guidance (2015) summarizes the current view in terms of risk to society:

> A mental health problem on its own appears to be only a modest predictive factor for violence while other factors, most significantly substance misuse, are more relevant in predicting risk. Because of the low base rates of mental health problems, its actual contribution to violence in the general population is small and the vast majority of violence is carried out by those without a mental health problem.

Risk assessment

Risk assessments are conducted by unstructured clinical assessment using direct interviews with the service user, carers, and other family members (low reliability mitigated by use by experienced and skilled clinicians), and completing a standardized risk assessment tool, many of which are now incorporated into electronic patient records. NICE guidance (2015b) lists a number of violence-related risk assessment tools currently available, but the evidence is drawn from inpatient settings. The Historical, Clinical and Risk Management Scale (HCR-20) is widely used in forensic outreach and secure settings where risk to the public is highest. As a standardized tool, it has been subjected to testing which indicates its utility as a predictor of both violent and non-violent offending following release from medium-secure units (Gray et al. 2008). Given its length and detail, its use is not proportionate for the risk encountered in the majority of community patients and settings (NICE 2015b): 'Current clinical wisdom is that many of the available risk assessment instruments that predict future violence are broadly similar in their somewhat moderate predictive efficacies'.

Assessment references past events and the clinical history and should occur when a service user first comes into contact with mental health services and under the following circumstances:

- where there has been any significant change, especially following any incidents
- where an individual or family discloses something of concern
- known changes in identified risk factors
- events such as prior to discharge, granting of leave or transfer of care
- transfer between services

Assessment is often categorized into harm to self, harm from others, harm to others, accidents, and other risk behaviours. Each category is typically subsequently graded according to local policy (see Table 12.2).

As we have seen, risk assessment is not an exact science—far from it. Munro and Rumgay's (2000) study of 40 homicide inquiry reports concluded that in 29 the violence could not have been predicted. Twenty-four of the offenders did have a history of violence or high-risk factors for violence, but only eight could have been assessed as high risk at the time of the homicide. In only three cases was the danger predictable, and in these only days prior to the homicide. For community outreach teams, the lessons of being able to easily flex the level of intensity and access to rapid intervention are clear:

> These findings suggest that more homicides could be prevented by improving the response to patients who start to relapse, regardless of their assessed potential for violence, than by trying to identify high-risk patients and targeting resources on them (Munro and Rumgay 2000).

Table 12.2 Local policy risk stratification

Low	No significant indicators of risk. No history or warning signs indicative of risk.
Medium	Current indicators of risk are present, but the risk outcome is unlikely to occur unless additional risk factors intervene. Patient's history and condition indicate the presence of risk and this is considered to be a significant issue at present; a risk management plan and/or contingency plan is required as part of the patient's care plan.
High	Current indicators of risk are present, suggesting that the risk outcome could occur at any time. Continued escalation of risk not reduced by current risk management strategies or previous risk management and/or contingency plan. Any previous risk management and/or contingency plan should be reviewed. The current plan(s) need to be robust, implemented promptly, and frequently reviewed. Highest priority must be given to risk prevention.

Individual management

Risk management planning on an individual level is based on accurate risk histories and knowledge of the current risk and risk factors. This may in practice be very simple: 'If Jason is intoxicated when he answers the door, make your excuses and walk away.'

Some patients need two trigger factors. Beverley has assaulted two key workers and two doctors. On each occasion she has been high, or becoming high, plus she has been demanding antidepressants, which the team has been anxious not to give her. Clearly for Beverley, her ability to accept refusal and her range of coping strategies are severely diminished when she is high. We know that elevated mood reduces most people's inhibitions. We also know that intoxication has the same effect.

These sorts of risk management plans can be easily incorporated into daily practice. Writing them down helps formalize our thinking and allows information to be shared across the team. Care plans and risk management plans (see Tables 12.3 and 12.4) can contain simple statements and instructions and are often most effective when written as concisely as possible, utilizing collaboration with patients and carers when feasible:

> Avoid conflict when high. May make demands that cannot be satisfied e.g. 'Give me some Prozac'. Refusal of demands leads to assault when high. Make excuses and leave; do not wait to rationalize, argue, or discuss.

De-escalation

The ideal is to talk down an aroused patient using psychological de-escalation and problem-solving techniques. This will only be possible and appropriate in the early stages of conflict, before serious escalation occurs. The decision to attempt to resolve the situation through discussion will hinge on your knowledge of the patient, specifically their cognitive abilities and personality. Conflict caused by delusional beliefs about you, or feelings of persecution, are unlikely to respond well if the patient's mental state or level of intoxication are significantly impairing their ability to process information. When psychology and problem-solving are considered unlikely, retreat at this stage is preferable, as in the case of Beverley given previously.

The decision to leave should not be presented as a punishment to the patient and can instead be presented in a neutral, matter-of-fact way: 'I'm sorry if I have upset you, maybe it's better if I leave now and come back another time.' This is a 'face-saving' statement—you accept responsibility for what has happened so that the patient can feel that they have won the argument.

Anger may not lead to aggression in patients with strong internal inhibitions, or when there is no suitable target for the aggression. External inhibitions that help to prevent aggression include fear of consequences or retaliation, material losses, and embarrassment. As professionals, we have a responsibility not to challenge patients inappropriately, hold overly negative views about their motives, or to engage in attempts to dominate. Such staff attitudes can be powerfully transmitted by demeanour and tone.

When problem-solving is possible, then psychological de-escalation techniques can often prevent aggression. We should listen and acknowledge the existence of the problems, show concern and understanding, and attempt to depersonalize the issue. Often disputes occur over medication, either withholding inappropriately requested medication or attempting to implement and improve compliance with current clinically indicated prescription. Explaining to the patient that decisions are made by the team or by seniors can diffuse the personal focus of the grievance: 'I have nothing to gain personally from you taking medication. But with your history, the team's opinion is that you will have more chance of staying well if you stay on the treatment.'

Problem-solving in this instance might include making the treatment more tolerable by adjusting the dose and managing side effects. By personalizing themselves, as distinct from an identity simply as a nurse or doctor, key workers can distance themselves from conflicts that arise from their role. Careful disclosure of personal information about your family, using first names and so on, is a recognized strategy in hostage situations.

Non-verbal techniques are familiar to most of us practising in mental health. Intense eye contact and staring should be avoided, as it is usually perceived as hostile. Intermittent 'normal' eye contact, maintaining a distance that does not threaten the individual's personal space, avoiding 'squaring up' by standing at a slight angle to the patient, and a relaxed posture all help (Davies and Frude 1993). People who are aroused, and those prone to paranoia, have enlarged areas of 'personal space' which, when encroached, make them feel uncomfortable and on edge. Kinzel (1970) demonstrated that violent prisoners identify larger personal spaces than those who are non-violent. Keeping a safe distance and towards the front feels safer for all of us. Similarly, touch may be reassuring for some more sympathetic patients but can be intolerable or misinterpreted by more aggressive and aroused patients.

Remaining calm is the stock response often used when dealing with an aroused person. However, if the patient has a grievance and wants you to sort it out, remaining calm and quiet may give the impression that you are not going to deal with their complaints or demands with the required urgency. 'Mood matching' recognizes this. Davies and Frude (1993) suggest that we match the patient's aggression with a similar degree of arousal directed into concern, involvement, and interest—but not with a similar degree of emotion. This can be difficult to achieve in practice and, together with the use of humour to diffuse situations, is a strategy that requires confidence.

Symptom management

In the community we use medicines to manage symptoms that persist for months and years. Only rarely are we required to administer medication for acute rapid tranquillization. In avoiding hospital admission and the risk of assault on carers and staff, medication can be successfully used to manage symptoms such as arousal, paranoia, and mania in the short term. Frequent contact and a flexible response according to agreed relapse plans can mean the early introduction of antipsychotics or benzodiazepines. Daily team discussion and the availability of medical staff can permit daily titration of medication, for example, with a patient who is becoming manic. Agreeing on these responses (and the threshold at which they are introduced) with the patient at a much earlier stage will minimize conflict and help compliance.

Early attempts at the pharmacological management of a relapsing patient reduce the risk that they become aggressive and may help to avoid the hospital admission which may result from aggressive behaviour. The combination of medication with psychological techniques can help avoid adverse incidents, compulsory admission, and the stigmatizing involvement of the police for severely relapsing patients.

Responding to physical assaults

In the event of a physical assault, it is worth rehearsing a repertoire of responses to minimize injury and maximize the chance of escape. It is also worth realizing that, in the heat of the moment, basic survival instincts may overwhelm any preparation or training. The techniques of breakaway are routinely taught to community workers, and regular refresher courses are advised. Breakaway consists of movements and blocks designed to release or protect a worker from a number of grabbing or striking attacks including strangulation, grasping of hair or clothes, punching, kicking, or attempted sexual assault where the attacker is pressing someone to the ground. All the techniques operate on the principle of reasonable force and the prevention of injury to assailant and assailed. Breakaway movements need to be used in conjunction with techniques such as telling the attacker to stop, assertively and repeatedly if necessary, and shouting for help. Should your attacker have a weapon, rapid escape is preferable to attempts to defend yourself. The main defence would be to place something between you and your attacker (e.g. a door or a chair) and to keep at a distance until escape becomes possible.

Case study

Graham is a 42-year-old man with a diagnosis of paranoid schizophrenia, characterized by suspicion and passivity experiences. He does not drink but smokes cannabis regularly. He was referred because of poor compliance with medication. He was considered hard to engage and hostile, and had had frequent hospital admissions, on several occasions via the courts for violent offences. He lives alone in a block of flats, having recently moved following disputes with previous neighbours.

Graham has a history of a serious assault on a neighbour for which he was convicted. This is the clearest guide to his level of risk. The abuse of cannabis is a further risk factor because of the possibility of it exacerbating his paranoid illness and lowering his inhibitions. A further risk factor is his discontinuation of medication.

Graham is guarded but not yet refusing access to his home, so there is the possibility of early intervention and home-based care. His history and the fact that he is already starting to get paranoid about his neighbours would suggest urgent assessment. He has not made any threats to the new neighbours, and there may be scope to reinstate medication to which he is known to respond quickly. The standard question, 'Have you recently thought about harming anyone such as your neighbours?' is somewhat of a closed question and to a guarded individual is unlikely to be productive. With Graham a better question is to ask him if he feels safe. Without colluding with the delusional fear, enquiries about what the team can do to help him feel safe and what he is currently doing to keep himself feeling safe are more open and inviting questions. If he replies that he is staying up all night so that he can attack them when they come in his house, then the risk is starting to become clearer.

Graham's summary care plan and risk management plan are presented in Tables 12.3–12.4, respectively.

The documentation spells out accountability for interventions and decisions, but does not leave this solely with one person. It will be noted that although the plan is discussed with the patient and attempts are made to agree on a relapse plan, Graham is not given a copy of his care plan. This is because of the possibility, mentioned in the plan, of breach of confidentiality should the neighbours be considered at high risk. Legal precedent is well established that mental health professionals have a 'duty to warn' identifiable third parties and generalized victims, but that breach of this duty renders the professional liable to civil action. Public interest has been found to outweigh the patient's right to confidentiality in such cases where the risk is real and would involve physical harm (Noffsinger and Resnick 1999).

Table 12.3 Summary care plan

Patient's name: Graham K. Address: Flat 3, Ingle House, Archer Street [fictional] Phone: none Date of birth: 09/09/74 GP: Norris Phone: 0208 582 xxxx		CMHT: Wandsworth East Phone: 0208877 xxxx New patient: No If No, date of review: 20/4/20...... Diagnosis: 1. Paranoid schizophrenia ... F 20.0 2. .... F ——. —
Assessed needs or problem	**Intervention**	**Resp. of**
Frequent relapse of paranoid symptoms	◆ Re-establish long-acting injectable medications	JH
	◆ Practical assistance to mediate with potential stressors e.g. housing, finance	
	◆ Continue to educate Graham regarding harmful use of cannabis and link with paranoid relapse	
	◆ Establish collaborative crisis plan to include relapse signature, action to be taken by Graham and the team, and rescue medicine to be used	JH/Graham
Risk of assault when unwell (see risk history and risk management plan)	◆ Frequent contact, 3 to 7 times a week. Joint visits only, **not to be visited alone**	JH
	◆ Low threshold for admission or Mental Health Act assessment	JH/Dr Evans
	◆ Risk assessment on each contact to establish immediacy of any risk; e.g. verbal threats against neighbour	JH
	◆ Consider breach of confidentiality to inform and liaise with neighbour if high assessed risk and delay in admission	Prof Burns

Table 12.4 Risk management plan

Name: Graham K.			
Categories of risk identified:			
Aggression and violence	YES MEDIUM RISK	Severe self-neglect	NO
Exploitation (self or others)	NO	Risk to children and young adults	NO
Suicide and self-harm	NO	Other (please specify).	

Current factors which suggest there is significant apparent risk:

(For example: alcohol or substance misuse; specific threats; suicidal ideation; violent fantasies; anger; suspiciousness; persecutory beliefs; paranoid feelings or ideas about particular people)

History of violent offences (see risk history). Currently has paranoid beliefs about his neighbours who he believes have touched him in intimate places in the past. Believes that the Princess of Wales is touching him. Poorly compliant with medication. Regular consumption of cannabis.

Clear statement of anticipated risk(s):

(Who is at risk; how immediate is that risk; how severe; how ongoing)

Believes that his neighbours have touched him in the past, difficult to assess as is guarded and suspicious. Has not made any specific threats against neighbours but has a history of assaulting neighbours at previous address. Previous assault was severe, with the neighbour suffering a broken jaw. Risk is driven by psychotic experiences.

Action plan:

(Including names of people responsible for each action and steps to be taken if plan breaks down)

Joint visit by key worker (James H) and another member of team, plus team doctor (Dr Evans). Aim to negotiate re-establishing antipsychotic medication immediately in form of long-acting injectable or supervised daily medication. Aim to assess if immediate threat to neighbour or to team members. Does he feel safe presently? If immediate threat he may require hospital admission/referral to Crisis and Home Treatment team with possible compulsory admission under the Mental Health Act. If a delay in admission occurs due to completion of the section discuss with team and consultant (Professor Burns) breaking confidentiality to inform neighbour of risk. If risk considered manageable at home, negotiate frequent joint visits (James H plus place on FACT board for team approach/involve Crisis Team). **Not to be visited alone**. To use safety check system with office prior to visit and establish checking-in time.

Date completed: 20/04/16	Review date: 07/05/16

Team approaches

Inquiries into harm incidents usually highlight failures in coordination, assessment, competency and training and communication. Staff dealing with hostile patients must feel safe and supported within the team and have opportunities to express their anxieties and ask for help freely, such as in frequent handover and systems for sharing complex cases. The focus should be on anticipation through assessment and frequent contact of those at risk. Should a member of staff be threatened or assaulted, then debriefing and support should be available from the team and management to cope with psychological, physical, and legal consequences. Employers have a statutory duty of care for the health and safety of their employees, so far as is reasonably practical, even when their employees have a foreseeable risk of violence at work.

Organizational risk factors that relate to the functioning, policies, and training of the team are:

♦ systematic assessment of risk not carried out

♦ risk indicators denied or minimized by responsible professionals

♦ information not passed from one professional or team to another

♦ clinical responsibility not clearly defined or transferred appropriately

♦ inadequate resources in specialist mental health services and in the community (e.g. hospital beds, housing, forensic services)

♦ management fails to establish, implement, and train staff regarding policies for risk assessment, critical incident analysis, clinical audit, breakaway, and control and restraint[1]

The team leader has a responsibility to ensure that communication, accountability, and training are optimized within the team. We all have a responsibility to raise concerns about patients and systems at the appropriate team meeting. Above all, the team must not be allowed to drift into complacency.

The duty of the employer towards health and safety is partly realized through providing training in de-escalation and breakaway techniques for all staff who come into contact with patients. This should include receptionists and ward clerks. There are several techniques used to prevent, manage, or resolve hostile and potentially violent incidents on an individual basis with community patients. Psychological and pharmaceutical approaches may prevent or ameliorate difficult situations. Physical escape, in the form of breakaway, can minimize injury should an assault take place.

Peer review and support

One of the functions of a good multidisciplinary team is to guard against individual complacency towards risk. The handover, clinical supervision, and individual patient reviews are all opportunities to discuss and problem-solve risk

---

[1] Adapted from *BMJ*, 312, Jeremy W Coid, 'Dangerous patients with mental illness: increased risks warrant new policies, adequate resources, and appropriate legislation', pp. 965–6. Copyright (1996) with permission from BMJ Publishing Group Ltd.

as a team. We may feel that our own relationship with a patient will protect us from assault. However, a relapsing psychotic patient or an intoxicated patient is just as likely to assault a member of their family, so we are not in any way protected by our perceived closeness to them.

Our team operated a low threshold for joint visits and a high degree of flexibility, so that a joint visit could be organized quickly and easily. Many people unfamiliar with community working ask us if we visit patients alone. This question betrays a lack of understanding of the patient group and of community outreach. Most patient contact is one-to-one, in the patient's home. Patients are referred to outreach with a complex pattern of needs, of which intermittent hostility may or may not be a component. Joint visiting has a clear role in periods of concern, but is rarely a prerequisite. At the other extreme, a home visit may not be advisable even with two or more members of staff. For patients showing current signs of hostility or violence, indirect approaches such as telephone contact or contact with carers may be all that is possible until a Mental Health Act assessment, with police in attendance, can be arranged. It is important, however, that such periods of indirect contact are not protracted. If the patient can be persuaded to meet members of the team in a relatively safer environment, such as the team base or ward, this can offer greater backup and protection than in the patient's home.

Safety systems

Teams need to have a clear and reliable safety check system. This can involve both a system for checking in at the end of the day and for checking in before and after visits to individual patients. A safety check system allows the tracking of team members' movements through a daily diary left with the duty worker at the team base. Their role is to receive calls and tick off each member of staff reporting back safe after an individual visit or at the end of the day. The team member's responsibility is to complete the diary and reliably check in.

The duty worker must be confident that if the team member does not check in, is not contactable on their mobile phone, or traceable from diary entries, that they are in trouble and must summon assistance according to agreed protocols. An inconsistent system is almost worse than no system. It must be reliable and continuously reinforced through peer pressure, management supervision, and audit.

The safety value of mobile phones is often exaggerated. They enable team members to check in with the team base and for the person responsible for the safety check to contact staff who have not checked in for whatever reason. They are not, however, effective for summoning assistance during an assault since you will rarely have the time and composure to dial, unless you have managed to escape or lock yourself in a room. Mobile phones also suffer from failed signals or batteries, and should not be thought of as giving protection. Similarly, personal alarms are questionable in their ability to prevent violence and summon assistance. Valuable though these are, they provide perhaps a false sense of security.

Critical incident analysis

Important lessons can be learnt from critical incident analysis. The aftermath of a violent incident has sometimes profound effects on individuals and teams alike. Guilt, loss of confidence, anger, and disillusionment are all common responses. Individual debriefing by the line manager should seek to obtain information, give support, and establish if treatment or time off is required and whether the police should be contacted. Critical incident analysis comes later; it involves the whole team discussing, in a constructive way, the antecedents, predictability, procedures, and both immediate and follow-up responses. Changes to individual and organizational practice, care and contingency plans, resources, and training needs will often be recommended. It is important that these changes are considered carefully and implemented—not just confined to the incident report.

Prosecuting patients for assault

Some organizations operate policies of zero tolerance for assaults on staff (see Chapter 9) and use posters on wards and in clinics to inform patients that prosecutions will be brought against offenders. In practice, it can be difficult to prosecute a patient receiving treatment for severe mental illness, and police responses vary. Often the police will be reluctant to charge a patient unless the assault is severe or involves a weapon, even when a formal request has been made. Some health care staff are also reluctant to press charges against patients, although this convention is changing.

Decision-making needs to take into account the seriousness of the offence, the mental state of the patient at the time, and the effect of prosecution on deterring future violent behaviour towards staff or others. If a patient is regarded at the time of the assault as having the capacity to know the consequences and the morality of the act, then prosecution is usually correct. The formality of a criminal record may protect and alert others should the patient move around the country, and may strengthen the patient's inhibitions and deter a repeat occurrence.

The prosecution service has to consider the impact of proceedings on the defendant's mental health as part of determining if it is in the public interest to prosecute. Should the interests of justice be outweighed by adverse effects on the defendant's health, then proceedings will be discontinued. If the mentally disordered offender is undergoing or about to undergo inpatient treatment, then the police are unlikely to recommend prosecution for minor offences.

Conclusions

For those of us who have worked in both inpatient and community settings, experience suggests that confrontation and hostility are far less frequently encountered with community patients. Collaborative approaches, and the greater sense of personal control that patients feel in their own environments, avoid the situational irritants, constraints, and transgressions that cause frustration and anger in hospital. Of course, patients can still interpret even neutral situations in a paranoid or distorted way, giving rise to conflict, and we still inevitably encounter such conflict in our role as mental health professionals.

Whilst hostility in community outreach may be infrequent, the potential consequences of a violent incident occurring in the relative isolation of the patient's home, without the support of colleagues, are serious. Furthermore, we know that the reliability of risk assessment is low (Munro and Rumgay 2000). We have a responsibility to protect ourselves through training and an understanding of risk factors, by our attitudes and behaviour towards patients, and through the application of risk management plans to everyday practice. The organization in which we work has a responsibility also to provide training, policies, procedures, support, and supervision.

We all have a duty to educate our patients, their carers, the public at large, and policymakers, disabusing them of the perceptions of a rising tide of violent assaults by mentally ill people. Pervasive misconceptions about the level of threat posed by our patients have, undoubtedly, been responsible for making our work more difficult and less rewarding and our patients' lives much more difficult.

Chapter 13

Suicidality

Introduction

In the previous chapter, we considered the risk management of harm to others. This chapter will focus on a behaviour that generates significant risk to self. Suicidality encompasses all of the following behaviours:

Suicide: a deliberately initiated act of self-harm performed in the knowledge of its fatal outcome.

Attempted suicide: a non-fatal act in which a fatal outcome may be expected.

Parasuicide: self-harming behaviour identified by the patient as suicidal but unlikely to actually result in death.

Self-harm: refers to any act of self-poisoning or self-injury carried out by an individual irrespective of motivation. Excludes harm to the self arising from excessive consumption of alcohol or recreational drugs, or from starvation in anorexia nervosa, or accidental harm.

Suicidality may be a result of an individual's recognition of the realities of coping with a life of serious mental illnesses and grief for the losses incurred. It may be that the illness prevents them acquiring the skills needed to cope with such setbacks and disappointments. Poor coping skills and the social and economic marginalization that can accompany serious illness are a common double burden for our patients. For those with positive psychotic symptoms, suicidality can be driven by command hallucinations, acute paranoid delusions of impending doom, or by the dysphoria that accompanies many patients' illness.

This chapter will describe ways of understanding, predicting, and managing suicidality and self-harm in people with severe and enduring mental illness in contact with community outreach teams.

Incidence

There are difficulties with official statistics of suicide, as anyone who has been to a Coroner's Court will know. Currently, the same legal criteria apply to verdicts of suicide as criminal cases—it must be proven 'beyond reasonable doubt'.

Where a suicide note is not left and witnesses' evidence is unavailable or incon-clusive, open verdicts or verdicts of accidental death are often passed, despite a high probability of suicide (O'Donnell and Farmer 1995).

The National Confidential Inquiry into Suicide and Homicide by People with Mental Illness (2015) looks at general population suicides (defined as deaths by intentional self-harm and undetermined intent by individuals aged 10 and over) and the subset of patient suicides (occurring within 12 months of mental health service contact). Between 2003 and 2013 in the UK, the inquiry reports 49,251 deaths in the general population that were registered as suicide or 'unde-termined', an average of 4,477 per year. Most common is hanging and strangula-tion (46 per cent), overdose (22 per cent), and jumping (10 per cent). Drowning (5 per cent), carbon monoxide poisoning (3 per cent), cutting and stabbing (3 per cent), and firearms (2 per cent) make up the less common means.

Some 13,972 (an average of 1,270 per year) of the general population sui-cides during this period were identified as patient suicides (28 per cent of the total). Of these, 17 per cent (2,378) were by patients with a primary diagnosis of schizophrenia or delusional disorders, 9 per cent by patients with a personality disorder, and 54 per cent by patients with a history of drug or alcohol misuse.

Similar rates for means of death in patients are observed as for the popu-lation in general, namely hanging (42 per cent), overdose (26 per cent), and jumping (15 per cent). Opiates were the most common drug used in overdose (24 per cent), followed by tricyclic antidepressants (13 per cent), antipsy-chotic drugs (11 per cent), paracetamol/opiate compounds (9 per cent), and paracetamol (7 per cent).

Gender differences are pronounced, as shown in Fig 13.1.

Risk factors and risk assessment

Risk factors from the inquiry statistics given earlier are clear in terms of gen-der bias towards males in both the patient and general populations. The report further identifies more at risk age groups, identifying a rising trend in men aged 45–54 and psychiatric patients with co-morbid physical illnesses. Some 14 per cent of patient suicides had been non-adherent with drug treatment in the month before death; an average of 158 deaths per year (26 per cent) had missed their final service contact before death (see Table 13.1).

Vulnerable groups include young women (ages 15–24) in the UK from the Indian subcontinent, who are 2.7 times more likely to commit suicide (Soni Raleigh and Balarajan 1992). Single men have suicide rates that are almost as high as for men who are divorced (Charlton et al. 1994). Widowed men have higher rates still. Men who are unemployed run between two and three times

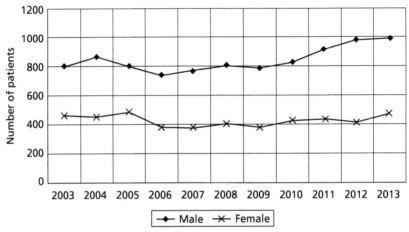

Fig 13.1 Number of patient suicides by gender

Reproduced from *National Confidential Inquiry into Suicide and Homicide by People with Mental Illness Annual Report: England, Northern Ireland, Scotland and Wales*, Fig 7, p. 20. Copyright (2015) Centre for Mental Health and Safety, University of Manchester.

the risk of death by suicide than the average. Clearly, most of these demographic risk factors are not amenable to change, but they serve to raise our awareness of risk in these groups.

Assessment

Individual clinical evaluation—routinely asking our patients difficult questions about the presence of suicidal thoughts, suicidal intent, evidence of planning, command hallucinations, and depression and hopelessness—is the best method of assessment. NICE guidance has not been produced yet for suicide and suicide prevention, but there is guidance on self-harm (NICE 2011). This recommends

Table 13.1 Risk factors for suicide

Illness	Personal factors	Life events	Culture and society
◆ Physical illness	◆ Single marital status	◆ History of parasuicide	◆ Economic depression
◆ Mental illness	◆ Unemployment	◆ Imprisonment	◆ Religious beliefs
◆ Drug or alcohol misuse	◆ Male	◆ Loss of job	◆ Poor social supports
◆ Non-compliance with medication	◆ Younger age	◆ Divorce	◆ Young Asian women
		◆ Family history of suicide	

an integrated and comprehensive psychosocial assessment of needs and risks conducted to engage patients and families in a collaborative relationship. The guidance is dismissive of assessment tools and scales, recommending that they not be used to predict future suicide or repetition of self-harm, or to determine who should and should not be offered treatment. Illustrative of this is the case of a statistical model based on known risk factors, which failed to predict any of the 46 suicides in a large psychiatric hospital (Goldstein et al. 1991). The main problem is the large number of false positives generated by the application of statistical risk factors. Both Appleby (who has been responsible for the national inquiry into homicides and suicides) and Wilkinson argue that prediction is impractical as a goal for health care services:

> The emphasis should be on secondary prevention—concentrating scarce resources on identifying and treating people with mental illness properly. (Wilkinson 1994)

> In the relative absence of specific suicide and homicide prevention measures, the activities that are required—closer supervision, maintenance of treatments, etc.—are in fact aspects of high-quality care. (Appleby et al. 1999)

Clinical evaluation of the severity of underlying psychiatric illness is, however, aided by the use of structured assessment tools. The routine use of the Brief Psychiatric Rating Scale (BPRS) (Overall and Gorham 1962) will help pick up previously unreported depressed mood. Further assessment of depression can be made using the patient self-reporting Beck Depression Inventory (Beck et al. 1961), which includes the statements 'I feel I would be better off dead' or 'I would kill myself if I had the chance'. The presence of hopelessness—'I feel that the future is hopeless and that things cannot improve'—is a particular warning sign for suicidality.

For positive psychotic symptoms (particularly command hallucinations), we should ask our patients the identity of the voices and if they feel that they can resist them. Patients with personality disorder who may have used the expression of suicidal ideation in the past as a method of influencing or controlling situations may require a more considered assessment. Direct clinical evaluations, history of suicide attempt or self-harm, and knowledge of risk factors must all be used to assess the suicide risk for each individual. Recent changes in clinical features such as depression, hostility, distress, and anxiety indicate a higher risk of suicide than a patient who is consistently anxious or distressed.

Individual interventions

Risk management responses

The National Patient Safety Agency's *Preventing Suicide: A Toolkit for Mental Health Services* (revised 2009) focuses on standards, including ensuring that all patients receive the appropriate level of care through assessment, care pathways, and adequate care planning and training of staff. However, the document focuses entirely on inpatient settings.

Treatment responses include offering a psychological intervention that is specifically structured for people who self-harm, with the aim of reducing self-harm. Drug treatment as a specific intervention to reduce self-harm is not recommended (NICE 2011). Increased contact with the patient is an important immediate response in a crisis to reduce suicide risk. Many suicide attempts are predominantly impulsive—a response to an acute or transient stressful circumstance.

If the patient has communicated to you their suicidal thoughts, you can assume that, on one level, they have a desire to stay alive and be helped. Delaying the suicidal impulse becomes the immediate goal together with practical assistance and problem-solving when possible. To delay the impulse, the patient must be able to exercise self-control, otherwise hospitalization is essential. Ask if they feel safe and feel able to resist suicidal or self-harm impulses. An acutely psychotic patient, unable to deny, for example, command hallucinations, will benefit little from negotiation and counselling, whereas, in depressive episodes, counselling techniques of restoring hope are valuable. Working with a patient with bipolar affective disorder, perhaps using mood diaries to track cyclical mood, can reinforce the hope that dark invariably turns to light even when they may be feeling that nothing will ever improve. Remind the patient that as their key worker you will do whatever is necessary to help them through this situation, however complex, finances, housing, relationships, and illnesses can all be tackled, probably one by one, and the patient can be helped to resist being overwhelmed by multiple problems.

Removing the means

Harm reduction strategies include removing the obvious means of self-harm or suicide to reduce the likelihood of an impulsive suicidal act. In wards, great efforts are made to remove ligature points. In the community, these hazards cannot be controlled other than by admitting the patient to hospital. However, supplies of medication to the patient can be limited, hoarded tablets removed and safe alternatives to more toxic medicines prescribed.

Many patients may be tempted to take an overdose given the opportunity, although they would not have the motivation or willpower to take themselves to the railway line. So patients with a history of self-harm in the previous three months should not receive more than two weeks' supply of medication (Appleby et al. 1999). Be aware that illicit drugs and alcohol may be used to increase the effect of an overdose and to reduce inhibitions (provide 'Dutch courage') that would prevent someone from hanging themselves. Team members from different disciplines will need training on relative toxicity, signs of overdose, and the clinical management of overdose. Do not wait for critical incident analysis to identify this need. Team doctors can provide basic training in a team development session.

A patient's key worker, who happens to be a social worker, is informed by the patient that they have taken 20 lithium carbonate tablets, impulsively, half an hour ago. Clearly, the key worker will need advice, but the ability to recognize, assess, and relay information to the team doctor or to the ambulance service can aid intervention and indicate the level of urgency. The patient was able to tell what they had done—so they are conscious. Are they unsteady on their feet? Have they vomited? Is there an empty bottle or packet to verify the amount taken? What strength are the tablets? Did the patient take anything else? Are there signs of other drugs or alcohol? Is lithium dangerous in overdose?

Patients should be encouraged to use the team, not just one individual, for support. If a patient phones feeling suicidal and his key worker is away, other team members should intervene and have access to relapse and contingency plans. Well-established arrangements for shared care, as exemplified by flexible ACT, mean that patients who need intensive or crisis interventions are never denied them because of the absence of a particular staff member.

Restructuring social networks

As a longer-term strategy, patients need to be encouraged to use other supports in the community such as family, friends, drop-in centres, and the church. Helping isolated patients to restructure their social and occupational situation provides a long-term intervention for chronic low self-esteem, depression, and dissatisfaction. Western societies are at long last waking up to the health risks that social isolation and loneliness bring. Many of our patients have lost their social status and supports through illness. Some who developed a psychotic illness early in life have never worked or formed relationships and social groups.

Coping strategy enhancement

Some patients have never learnt the coping skills that help most of us deal with setbacks and failures. The teaching, and reinforcement through rehearsal, of simple strategies and courses of action to take when distressed can help patients avoid getting to the point of crisis and feeling suicidal.

Case study

Julie used to present herself at the A&E department saying she felt suicidal after arguments with her alcoholic partner. On two occasions she had taken a modest overdose of sleeping tablets, believing that her partner would leave her.

Julie was encouraged not to argue with her partner when he was drunk, as this would never produce a satisfactory outcome. Instead, she should walk away to another room, have a cigarette, and listen to some relaxing music. She should remind herself that her partner was drunk, did not necessarily mean what he said, and had not walked out on her in the past ten years. If she was unable to contain her distress herself, she should call her mother. She could also contact the team.

What to do when a suicide occurs

In our experience, a typical urban CMHT or assertive outreach team can expect one or two suicides per year. Given the limitations of suicide prediction described earlier, it is important that suicides should not automatically be considered as a failure. We need a realistic recognition that suicide is part of the job. We must not be complacent about it, but neither should we excoriate ourselves when it happens. The worker most closely involved with the victim is likely to feel crushed, saddened, and often guilty.

The team has two immediate obligations. First, the team as a whole has an obligation to contact and offer support to the family and provide relevant information. Second, it has to support the primary workers, allowing them time to talk it through. It is all too easy for team members to express exaggerated views of what they could have done but failed to do, and equally to exaggerate the impact of things they have done. These concerns need to be heard and taken seriously, not dismissed. Only when they have been talked through in detail can they be weighed and placed in perspective.

The subsequent task facing the service is to conduct a review of the events preceding the suicide to identify anything that may have made it more likely or obscured the detection of warning signs. In England and Wales, the completion of the online returns for the Confidential Inquiry into Homicide and Suicide (2015) is a useful framework for this process. Its detail may help structure the process and reduce the sense of anger and defensiveness that can otherwise inhibit an honest enquiry. Lessons from critical incidents need to be incorporated into routine care. Involving the whole team in a critical incident analysis brings it together at difficult times and identifies strengths and weaknesses.

Gaps in documentation of risks are often identified after critical incidents. Clear team policies, team-based managers able to monitor the application of policy, and standardized documentation assist in consistent risk assessment. The examples presented of our documentation (Tables 13.2–13.3) indicate areas of risk and steps in formulating a clear response.

Outreach teams are resourced and organized to respond as rapidly as possible to patients identified as at risk. Frequent handover, availability of multidisciplinary

Table 13.2 Summary care plan

Patient's name: Richard G. Address: 112 Holden House, Winstanley Estate, Battersea. Phone: 0208 987 xxxx Date of birth: 21/08/77 GP: Jackson Phone: 0208 987 xxxx	CMHT: Wandsworth East Phone: 0208877 xxxx New patient: No If No, date of review: 01/10/16 Diagnosis: 1. Paranoid schizophrenia. F20.0 2. .... F — —.—

Assessed needs or problem	Intervention	Resp. of
Engagement, isolates himself from services, family and friends.	◆ Aim to establish face-to-face contact twice per week. Use of telephone contact as required. ◆ Richard does not tolerate long visits. Explore Richard's wishes; e.g. company, leisure activities. ◆ Liaise with family. Improving level of contact. ◆ Explore local facilities; e.g. library, drop-in-club. Help restructure social network.	BW
Long-term low risk of suicide in response to acute distress driven by psychotic symptoms.	◆ Maintain regular contact. ◆ Increase contact when acutely distressed. ◆ Assess for level of suicide ideation, command hallucinations, paranoia, suicidal intent, depressed mood, and hopelessness. Use team doctor for full mental state assessment.	BW
	◆ Consider admission if extremely distressed and Mental Health Act if refuses informal admission. ◆ Offer medications for symptom relief and arousal. Risperidone long term. Diazepam short term. ◆ Limit supplies of medication to one week. ◆ Try to establish on risperidone. ◆ Psycho-education on illness and origin of distress. ◆ Explore the use of CBT when better.	BW
		Other
		Other
		YES
		YES
		YES

Table 13.3 Risk management plan

Name: Richard G.			
Categories of Risk Identified:			
Aggression and violence	NO	Severe self-neglect	NO
Exploitation (self or others)	NO	Risk to children and young adults	NO
Suicide and self-harm	YES LOW RISK	Other (please specify)	

Current factors which suggest there is significant apparent risk:

(For example: alcohol or substance misuse; specific threats; suicidal ideation; violent fantasies; anger; suspiciousness; persecutory beliefs; paranoid feelings or ideas about particular people)

Non-compliant with medication. Depressed mood. Social isolation. Says he will take the medication when he feels distressed. Current persecutory beliefs around people coming into his flat at night to interfere with his body. Denies suicidal intent.

Clear statement of anticipated risk(s):

(Who is at risk; how immediate is that risk; how severe; how ongoing)

Ongoing low risk of suicide. Risk increased during acute distress driven by psychotic experiences.

Action plan:

(Including names of people responsible for each action and steps to be taken if plan breaks down)

See care plan: Maintain regular contact. Bob Walker and team to increase contact when Richard more acutely distressed.

Assess for level of suicidal ideation, command hallucinations, paranoia, suicidal intent, depressed mood, and hopelessness. Use team doctor for full mental state assessment as level of distress or psychosis increases. Consider admission if Richard extremely distressed and multiple risk factors as above evident. Consider use of Mental Health Act if refuses informal admission. Offer medication for symptom relief and to reduce arousal and distress. Risperidone moderately effective if taken long term. Diazepam effective short term to reduce arousal.

Limit supplies of medication to one week to ensure regular contact and reduce risk of overdose.

Date completed: 01/10/016	Review date: 01/04/17

team members, continuity of care, and regular review of patients all contribute to the safe management of suicidality. Our close knowledge of the patient may alert us to risks through clear contingency and relapse plans. Equally, there is a danger that familiarity leads to tolerance of ongoing risks such as suicidal thoughts and we fail to recognize when this may lead to suicidal behaviour. Clinical supervision and peer discussion of risky patients improves focus.

Case study

Richard is a 39-year-old man whose life has been devastated by psychotic illness. He finds his psychotic experiences (for example, believing that people are coming into his flat and putting pins into his body) extremely distressing. He also has periods of depressed mood when he isolates himself from his family, friends, and services. He does not believe he is ill and does not believe the medicine helps the way he feels. He is highly sensitive to the side effects of medications.

He has had several long admissions to hospital and his symptoms have not reduced significantly with antipsychotic medication. The medication does, however, reduce his arousal and his accusations of others sticking pins into his body.

Several years ago, Richard attempted to hang himself on the ward. He has taken two overdoses of medication. Whilst reluctant to talk about these events, he indicates that they were a response to distressing and painful symptoms at the time, rather than a planned and thought-out assessment of his life.

Conclusions

In brutal epidemiological terms:

> There is little research evidence linking any health service intervention with a fall in suicide rates. (Appleby et al. 2000)

We are not good at predicting suicide; nobody is yet. We must hope that establishing meaningful relationships with our patients, conducting assessments, and our clinical judgement will help identify suicidal intent so that early intervention can follow. A realistic approach to the inevitability of suicide when working with individuals who are often damaged and distressed is needed. We must learn lessons from such tragic events and avoid complacency, while rejecting the pervasive 'blame' culture that equates suicide with a 'sense of failure'. Good mental health practice is based on establishing real relationships between patients and staff, so sadness after suicide is inevitable. It should not, however, develop into persecution or pathological self-doubt.

Outreach teams can vary the level of support utilizing shared care and crisis resolution and home treatment teams according to both the assessed and expressed need. Providing high-quality care and support, together with access to modern treatments and interventions, is the most effective way of serving and protecting patients in the long term.

Chapter 14

Self-neglect

Introduction

Self-neglect often results from the demotivating, negative symptoms of schizophrenia together with the cognitive deficits that strip some patients with psychosis of their ability to manage themselves and the outside world in a normal way. Social factors such as limited social networks, unemployment, and poverty may contribute to a sense of hopelessness or apathy towards self-care and care of the immediate environment. Little is published about self-neglect or its incidence in the general and mentally ill populations. Most accounts are qualitative studies from the nursing and social work literature on clinical observations and ethical decision-making when working with the elderly (O'Brien et al. 2000). Reed and Leonard (1989) describe self-neglect as 'a pattern of intentionally neglecting prescribed self-care activities despite access to available resources and knowledge'.

This chapter will describe ways of managing self-neglect in psychotic patients living in their own homes.

Risk factors and risk assessment

Self-neglect has a low profile as an area of concern for mental health services. As a result, there is no standard measure or method of categorizing self-neglect (Bindman et al. 2000). Patients whose relapse signature includes social withdrawal and psychomotor retardation, to the extent that they fail to eat and drink adequately, must be the main cause of concern to community outreach teams. Patients with a diagnosis of catatonic schizophrenia or with a severe depressive component in either bipolar affective disorder or schizophrenia may self-neglect during relapse and require increased home visits to monitor and assist with self-care and nutrition. Patients at longer-term risk of self-neglect will be those with pronounced cognitive deficits and negative symptoms. These patients will require continued assistance with daily living skills and the monitoring of risk.

Self-neglect is not restricted to patients with psychosis (see Table 14.1). Those with dementia, learning difficulties, and eccentrics can manifest this behaviour. Diogenes' syndrome (named after the Greek philosopher who lived in a barrel) is characterized by gross self-neglect, social withdrawal, and living in squalor (Williams et al. 1998).

Table 14.1 Risk factors for self-neglect

Short-term/acute risk factors	Long-term/chronic risk factors
◆ History of self-neglect during relapse	◆ History of self-neglect
◆ Non-compliance with treatment	◆ Pronounced negative schizophrenia symptoms (social withdrawal, poverty of thought, poor volition)
◆ Psychomotor retardation	◆ Cognitive deficits (schizophrenia or organic disorder)
◆ Severe bipolar affective disorder	◆ Neglect of physical disease (diabetes, hypertension)
◆ Catatonic schizophrenia	◆ Poverty
◆ Financial crisis or problems	◆ Learning disability
◆ Lack of social support	◆ Lack of social support

Assessment

Assessment needs to be sensitive and non-judgemental. Many healthy teenagers may be considered to have problems with personal care. Self-neglecting patients are often not ashamed of their lifestyles and offer good reasons for not going out, mistrusting statutory services, or hoarding. The question of whether patients are putting themselves at significant risk is our overriding concern.

The risk assessment format, which follows the case study in this chapter, can be used to clarify and document assessed risk and to formulate interventions (see Tables 14.2–14.3). Failure to eat and drink due to stupor, depression, or catatonia are the main alerts. It is possible to survive for many weeks without eating, but only a few days without drinking. Assessment should include a history of food and drink intake in recent days, noting evidence of weight loss, pallor, weakness, or fatigue due to starvation.

Gross self-neglect is fairly obvious, but it can come on very gradually and less extreme forms may be underestimated without a visit to the patient in their own home to ascertain the following:

- Is there food in the house?
- What has the patient eaten and drunk today?
- Is there a fridge?
- Is food rotting and dangerous to eat or attracting flies/vermin?
- Is the physical environment of the house safe?

When gross self-neglect is evident, then a full physical examination, using either the resources of the team or by accompanying the patient to the GP, is advisable for new patients.

Assessment of self-neglect presenting less immediate risk needs to focus on activities of daily living such as personal care and household management. The purpose of such assessment is to establish a baseline from which to support the process of change and to gain understanding of the factors that hinder functioning. How often do you bathe and wash? How competent are you with laundry, cleaning of teeth, dress and appearance, shopping, cooking? (See Chapter 24, 'Daily living skills'.)

Formal assessment tools may be off-putting for patients. A patient with a history of reclusiveness and negative symptoms is not going to readily discuss their personal hygiene routine. Scales such as PANSS (Kay et al. 1987) include a subscale to cover the negative symptoms of blunted affect, emotional withdrawal, poor rapport, passive social withdrawal, difficulty in abstract thinking, lack of spontaneity and flow of conversation, and stereotyped thinking. These measures are only regularly used for clinical trials, especially for evaluating the effectiveness of medications. More useful in practice for evaluating progress against baseline are simple scales covering social functioning such as those used by occupational therapists. The Personal and Social Performance Scale (Morosini et al. 2000) rates on four subscales, one being self-care. This clinician-completed scale uses observation and patient and carer interviews to give a rating of absent, mild, manifest, marked, severe, or very severe. For example, a patient or carer can be asked:

◆ In the last [reference period], how often have you taken a shower or a bath? Did you remember to wash or did somebody remind or help you? Have you cleaned your teeth every day?

◆ In the last [reference period], did you always put on clean clothes? Did you ever go out in pyjamas or not properly dressed? Did you ever dress in a way that people might find unusual for the period of the year or the weather?

Common sense needs to be exercised—for example, take into account what resources the patient has available. If they have little or no money, no hot water, and no washing machine or iron, then this will influence your judgement. Equally, a patient with fleas, unintentionally matted hair, and other visual and olfactory clues of self-neglect will not require a scale to measure progress.

Individual interventions

Managing relapse

In some patients, neglect of personal hygiene is part of their relapse signature and not necessarily an ongoing problem. Treatment of the psychosis may be the only intervention needed. Where the self-neglect is life-threatening (e.g. neglect of physical illness, failure to eat and drink), physical treatment takes precedence. Care and risk management plans need to reflect this relapse signature and give clear instructions.

For patients whose mental state changes rapidly, and who are prone to stop eating or drinking, frequent contact with the family is critical for safe community care. Patients with severe bipolar illness can sink to this state in a few days and, for these patients, you must know:

♦ What is their usual pattern?

♦ Will their relative phone you if they do not see them for a day or two?

♦ Have you negotiated a relapse plan with the patient?

♦ Will the patient allow you or their family member to have a key to their home to be used in the event of their being inside, unable to respond?

Neglecting physical health care

The key worker must sometimes also take responsibility for the patient's physical health needs, both identifying problems and registering and accompanying the patient to a GP, and sometimes also treating physical illness (see Chapter 22, 'Physical health care').

We regularly monitor patients' somatic medications, and advocate on behalf of our patients to ensure they get the physical treatments and care they require from services. District nurses and hospital specialists can too often see psychiatric patients as unreliable or low priorities for general health care. Where failure to take life-saving physical treatments such as insulin or antihypertensives is clearly due to psychosis, it is possible to intervene, using the Mental Health Act to treat the psychosis. The use of such legislation with patients who have the capacity to understand the implications and consequences of their self-neglect is much more difficult. For example, a patient without active psychiatric symptoms who is judged to have capacity and who refuses to have life-saving dialysis for renal failure cannot be forced to do so under the Mental Health Act in the UK.

Social linking and networks

Social linking and rebuilding support networks is invaluable for patients who self-neglect. Neglect of personal care is stigmatizing: people avoid contact with malodorous individuals. This initiates a vicious circle as impoverishment of social contacts and occupation reduces incentives for change in the patient's behaviour. Talking to patients about their personal care is not easy. If we have a friend who smells, do we actually come out and tell them? One strategy to avoid offence is to depersonalize the issue by suggesting that if they start attending a resource centre, or if they want to seek paid employment, they will need to tidy themselves up. Otherwise, it is advisable to build up a strong relationship before coming straight to the point!

Daily living skills' training

Teaching self-care and hygiene routines will only be successful once the patient is ready for change and they have expressed realistic goals. Goals must be observable and with achievement dates and intermediate steps constructed. The aim is for goals stated as precisely as possible in the patient's own words. It should be clear when the goal has been achieved or not, so statements like 'dress tidily' are less useful than 'wash seven pairs of underwear every Sunday'. Motivational techniques may include guiding the patient to think about how their appearance or hygiene may negatively influence other people's perception of them. Self-care can be presented as an intermediate step towards further stated goals. Daily living skills' training is discussed in more detail in Chapter 24.

Home care

Practical help with shopping and the provision of a meals service can reduce nutritional risks. Direct assistance with household tasks such as laundry and cleaning, plus the provision of home care, can make the difference between the patient being able to keep their own flat and being in residential care.

So-called deep cleans for grossly neglected flats can be arranged through the social services home care department. Regular home care to keep the flat in a reasonable condition after a deep clean is a worthwhile investment as it can enable the patient to survive in the community for the long term. Such cleaning may need to be paid for from the team or social care budget.

Home carers are not mental health professionals, but domestic staff. With difficult patients, chaotic patients, and hard-to-engage patients, home care arrangements tend to break down. The same applies to home delivery of prepared meals. Regular liaison and problem-solving with the home care agency can keep the service going. Often, however, patients refuse to allow access to the home carer or get into disputes after having possessions moved around or items unwittingly thrown out. In these instances, the only option may be for team members to give direct practical assistance to the patient as part of their regular visits.

Team approaches and responses

Some key workers find the working conditions when patients are living in squalor distasteful, and struggle to hide this in their interactions. They may ask for a reallocation of their caseload. Furthermore, new members of staff may find it hard to resist the immediate temptation to tidy up a messy flat. Imagine a relative stranger coming into your home and being judgemental about your personal and domestic care and insisting they help you tidy up. These situations are best dealt with through clinical and peer supervision. We have had instances of receptionists pointedly spraying air freshener around rooms when malodorous patients have come to the team base. In several services in different countries there have been moves to withdraw domiciliary care for patients who smoke. This is based on the argument that we are all entitled to a smoke-free work environment. This has not yet been insisted on in any mental health services that we know of, but it is bound to be proposed eventually. Withdrawing help from vulnerable patients would seem a draconian step, and one we would find difficult to support. Dignity, respect, and understanding apply equally to patients who self-neglect, and staff may need reminding of this.

The team must respond to more life-threatening self-neglect by assertive efforts to find patients known to stop eating or drinking when they relapse. Well-established relapse and risk management plans and rapid responses to identified risk should be part of the team culture (see Table 14.1). We do have permission from some of our patients to hold their door keys, which allows us to establish quickly if the patient is safe. Entering a patient's house with their keys in the absence of a response to knocking needs to be negotiated, and is usually only undertaken if the team member feels the patient is at immediate risk. Such advanced agreements reduce delay and when written down protect both parties.

Case study

Donald is 60 years' old and developed schizophrenia late in life, when 43. Always a loner, he had spent brief periods sleeping rough, generally working in unskilled and low-stress jobs. He had moved from rural Scotland at 19 to work in Birmingham. He had no friends, had lost touch with his family, and had never had sexual or intimate relationships.

After ten years of declining social function, he was referred following a series of hospital admissions precipitated by gross self-neglect and episodes of barricading himself in his flat due to persecutory delusions and auditory hallucinations. The voices told him he was worthless, should not accept state benefits, and that he would be arrested if he went out.

In Donald's home, his gross self-neglect and spartan living arrangements were most evident:

- He had worn the same clothes for many months.
- He had lost about 15 kg in weight; the majority of his other clothes no longer fit him.

- He did not bathe, but did shave and cut his own hair.
- He ate only dried potato reconstituted with water, and uncooked, tinned fish, biscuits, and cereal with water.
- He had no fridge and tended to hoard packets of food.
- He shopped once a week in the nearest shop when he went out to cash his welfare cheque.
- He avoided going out at any other time for fear of persecution.
- A bed was the only furniture in the flat; Donald had thrown the rest out believing he was going to prison.
- There was no telephone, television, or radio, as Donald believed that 'they' would discuss his personal business over the airwaves.
- He boiled water for tea on a single-ring appliance.

Donald's summary care plan and risk management plan are shown in Tables 14.2 and 14.3, respectively.

Table 14.2 Summary care plan

Patient's name: Donald F. Address: Flat 6, Fraser House, Wandsworth Phone: none Date of birth: 25/10/56 GP: Jones Phone: 0208 675 xxxx		CMHT: Wandsworth West Phone: 0208 877 xxxx New patient: No If No, date of review: 01/6/16 Diagnosis: 1. Paranoid schizophrenia F20.0 2. .... F — —.—
Assessed needs or problem	**Intervention**	**Resp. of**
Engagement	◆ Does not tolerate intensive contact. Frequent short visits. ◆ Offer practical assistance with household tasks as engagement tool.	CP
Self-neglect	◆ Frequent contact to ensure not barricaded in flat and obtaining sufficient food and drink. ◆ Monitor weight. ◆ Negotiate bathing, changing clothes, and bed sheets. ◆ Practical assistance to obtain fridge, clothes, visit launderette, obtain furniture. ◆ Encourage healthy diet by assistance with shopping and meals on wheels three times a week. ◆ Increase variety of social contact and activity in graded way. Visits by different team members. Encourage contact with brother. Accompany to park or café.	CP

Table 14.3 Risk management plan

Name: Donald F.			
Categories of risk identified:			
Aggression and violence	NO	Severe self-neglect	YES
Exploitation (self or others)	NO	Risk to children and young adults	NO
Suicide and self-harm	NO	Other (please specify)	

Current factors which suggest there is significant apparent risk:

(For example: alcohol or substance misuse; specific threats; suicidal ideation; violent fantasies; anger; suspiciousness; persecutory beliefs; paranoid feelings or ideas about particular people)

Two recent admissions due to barricading self in flat and failing to obtain adequate supplies of food and drink. 15 kg weight loss over past six months.

Clear statement of anticipated risk(s):

(Who is at risk; how immediate is that risk; how severe; how ongoing)

Intermittent episodes of self-neglect resulting in starvation. Moderate risk of severe consequences if not discovered quickly.

Action plan:

(Including names of people responsible for each action and steps to be taken if plan breaks down)

Early intervention in the event of withdrawal from services, barricading self in flat, noticeable weight loss, or failure to eat or drink adequately. Early detection through twice-weekly visits.

If barricaded in flat, team member discovering this to initiate Mental Health Act assessment after discussion with medical staff and social worker and to contact council immediately to gain access.

Date completed: 01/06/16   **Review date: 01/12/16**

Conclusions

Self-neglect is under-reported and often overlooked, but is a very important aspect of community outreach. It is not glamorous as a focus for mental health professionals' attention and almost nothing is written in terms of interventions The chronic and insidious nature of some patients' self-neglect can lead to therapeutic pessimism or acceptance of the behaviour. Self-neglect may be profoundly hindering the integration of the patient into their community. Patients with an unstable mental state who self-neglect during relapse are a particular target group for frequent regular contact. Long-term self-neglect can result in premature death, particularly when it involves neglect of chronic physical illnesses such as diabetes.

Community outreach teams must recognize and assess these problems and provide comprehensive support over the longer term. Social linking and rebuilding support networks provide scope for enduring improvements in patients' lives.

Chapter 15

Schizophrenia and delusional disorders

Introduction

Schizophrenia is the archetypal mental illness. It is what most people think of when they talk about 'madness'. It affects all aspects of mental functioning—thinking, feeling, perception, and even movement. More than any other mental disorder, it is the one where the loss of contact with reality is most obvious. It was first described as a specific disorder in 1896 by Kraepelin, who called it 'dementia praecox' (early dementia) to emphasize its long-term, deteriorating course in distinguishing it from manic-depressive disorder (Kraepelin 1919).

The term 'schizophrenia' was coined in 1911 in Zurich by Eugen Bleuler, who based the diagnosis on the patient's current clinical features rather than the course of the disorder (Bleuler 1950). He used the term to draw attention to the disruption (or splitting) of a wide range of mental processes. Bleuler described the core features of schizophrenia as the 'four As'—*autism* (withdrawal from close personal contact), *associations* (disruption in thought processes), *affect* (blunting and disturbances of mood), and *ambivalence* (loss of motivation). He considered that hallucinations and delusions were not the core symptoms of the disease but secondary results of the patient trying to make sense of their disturbing mental experiences.

The focus of diagnosis shifted decisively to these 'secondary symptoms' when Schneider introduced his list of so-called 'first-rank symptoms', those features of the acute illness that could often be identified in a single interview (Schneider 1959). These are essentially hallucinations, delusions, disorders of thinking, and passivity feelings. Schneider's approach has persisted, with subsequent diagnostic systems continuing to emphasize the more 'positive' symptoms of hallucinations, delusions, and thought disorder (American Psychiatric Association 1994, 2015; World Health Organisation 1992). The introduction of antipsychotic medicines (which only really act on the positive symptoms, not the negative ones) consolidated this diagnostic approach, although it is now being challenged for missing the 'essence' of schizophrenia (Parnas 2011).

These early pioneers in schizophrenia research worked in large mental hospitals and tended to see only the patients who did not recover. Not surprisingly, they—especially Kraepelin—developed a very gloomy view of schizophrenia. Follow-up studies of patients discharged from hospital show that a more balanced prognosis has emerged, suggesting that perhaps up to a third of patients make a fairly good recovery, returning to self-sufficiency in their own homes (Ciompi 1988; Harding et al. 1987).

However, these follow-up studies have serious flaws, leading to overestimation of positive outcomes. Ciompi calculated the proportion of good outcomes based on the very reduced sample he could find at 20 years, and the Harding study was of 'patients considered ready for discharge'. Presumably those who died or were lost in Ciompi's study and those who were not considered ready for discharge in Harding's were likely to have had poorer outcomes.

A systematic review of 50 studies by Jääskeläinen et al. (2013) concluded that one in seven people with schizophrenia could be said to recover based on the review criteria. This study has been criticized as an underestimation for including studies which were just too varied in their methods, such as choice of patients (many followed up patients who were admitted to hospital rather than from the general population), and in their definitions of recovery (Slade and Longden 2015). Caution should therefore be taken when commentators are quoting selectively from individual studies or from a statistical figure. Maintaining a balanced and more optimistic view of the disorder remains a problem for community outreach workers, as we also inevitably must concentrate on those who are doing less well.

Classifications

A disorder as complex as schizophrenia (some insist on referring to it as 'the schizophrenias') has been subject to various attempts at subclassification. The primary purpose of classification in medicine is to improve the prediction of prognosis and to target treatments more accurately. It is not an attempt at ultimate truth. It is a pragmatic exercise and there are no logical links between the different classificatory systems; various terms persist from outdated classifications. Of the first classification (into paranoid, catatonic, hebephrenic, and simple), 'paranoid' (where the picture is dominated by persecutory delusions) is still in regular use. The method of diagnosing schizophrenia based on criteria introduced in DSM-III in 1980 and persisting into DSM-V and ICD-10 so emphasizes hallucinations and delusions, that paranoid schizophrenia has effectively become almost the default diagnosis for all schizophrenia patients. Catatonic (dominated by disorders of movement, either excitement or stupor) is increasingly rare in the developed world, as is hebephrenic (early onset in adolescence dominated by thought disorder and a strange disconnected mood state). Simple schizophrenia was originally used to describe patients with severe negative symptoms (apathy, self-neglect, etc.) without any clear history of acute episodes, but was always suspect and has fallen from use.

Acute schizophrenia indicates the florid periods of relapse with prominent and positive symptoms (hallucinations, delusions, and disordered thinking). Chronic schizophrenia usually refers to the periods between such episodes where the patient demonstrates mainly negative symptoms (apathy, self-neglect, withdrawal) or less severe positive symptoms. While these are still useful terms, such divisions are far from straightforward. An attempt was made to classify schizophrenia on the basis of positive and negative symptoms (Crow 1980). It soon became clear that simplistic ideas of negative symptoms always coming after positive ones (the old idea of a 'schizophrenic defect state') did not hold up. Positive symptoms can persist for decades, negative symptoms can precede positive ones, and so on.

The current diagnostic system adopted by the World Health Organisation (Table 15.1), ICD-10 (World Health Organisation 1992), includes the clinical types alluded to here plus a fifth digit to clarify the course (e.g. episodic, continuous). Paranoid schizophrenia is now the overwhelmingly commonest type.

Table 15.1 ICD-10 classification of schizophrenia

Type	Course
F20.0 Paranoid	.0 Continuous
F20.1 Hebephrenic	.1 Episodic with progressive deficit
F20.2 Catatonic	.2 Episodic with stable deficit
F20.3 Undifferentiated	.3 Episodic remittent
F20.4 Post-schizophrenic depression	.4 Incomplete remission
F20.5 Residual	.5 Complete remission
F20.6 Simple	
F20.8* Other	.8 Other
F20.9* Unspecified	.9 Observation <1 year

* '8' is always used in ICD-10 for 'other', and '9' for 'unspecified'. Hence, missing numbers.

Data from *International Classification of Diseases* (ICD), version 10. Copyright (1992) World Health Organization.

Bordering disorders

Many patients present with a picture closely resembling schizophrenia but are not classified as such. These include the following:

+ *Persistent delusional disorders* are those in which the patient is usually disabled by a single delusional preoccupation, such as they have a misshapen body or they are the object of a specific plot. This may fluctuate over time but usually remains for years. What is striking is that the other features of schizophrenia do not develop.

+ *Schizotypal disorder* is rarely used and overlaps in an unclear manner with schizoid personality disorder. It refers to an odd, eccentric, and often aloof individual with strange thinking patterns. It reminds us of schizophrenia, but never develops any of that disorder's definite features.

+ *Acute and transient psychotic disorders* are, as their name suggests, brief, often with a rapidly fluctuating clinical presentation.

+ *Schizoaffective disorders* is a tricky diagnosis whose meaning has changed over time and whose use varies widely. It most often implies both evidence of major mood disturbance and clear schizophrenia symptoms concurrently in the same episode. The mood can be either manic or depressive, and it is still controversial how this disorder overlaps with bipolar affective disorder.

+ *Schizophreniform disorder* was once a very commonly used term which, although no longer officially part of the classification, is still used by clinicians who are uncertain and want to defer judgement.

Family factors in schizophrenia

The role of nature versus nurture, always a hot topic in psychiatry, has been most fiercely disputed in schizophrenia. Initially, the disorder was considered entirely genetic, although Bleuler took a more psychodynamic approach to understanding it. Genetic explanations dominated until after the Second World War. Then a period of confusion about diagnosis, predominantly in North America, driven by the ascendancy of psychoanalysis, emphasized experiential factors—particularly early childcare. The families of severely ill patients were often noted to be dysfunctional. This is not surprising, it is no easy task being the parent of someone who is very ill. A number of theories developed, many attributing the development of schizophrenia to family behaviour. These theories have now been fairly conclusively disproved.

Evidence from twin and adoption studies have incontrovertibly demonstrated the importance of inheritance in developing schizophrenia. The Danish adoption study (Rosenthal et al. 1971) was probably the key factor in changing opinion. Children of mothers with schizophrenia adopted at birth to healthy parents were followed up as adults and their incidence of schizophrenia was found to be 10 per cent. This is the same rate that would have been expected had they stayed with their mothers. Even more interesting, the researchers found that some of the adoptive parents with schizophrenic children demonstrated the 'over-protectiveness' thought to be one of the causal factors. It could be that such over-protectiveness is an understandable reaction of a parent to a struggling child. Similarly, twins separated at birth show the same risk for concordance for the disorder as those not separated.

Genetic risk is just that—'a risk', not a life sentence. Although having a schizophrenic parent raises the risk of developing schizophrenia tenfold, from 1 per cent to 10 per cent, that still leaves nine out of ten children who do not have a parent with the disease. Similarly, nine out of ten children of schizophrenic parents do not develop the disorder. There is little doubt that upbringing and experience can help protect against the development of schizophrenia. Even in identical twins, the risk of both developing the disease is just over 50 per cent, so experience counts for as much as heredity in each individual. When geneticists speak of a *hereditability* of 70–80 per cent, they refer to populations, not individuals. The genetics and hereditability of bipolar disorder are basically similar to those of schizophrenia, but the high-profile family theories were argued over schizophrenia.

Although these family theories have been effectively discredited within the professions, it is still important to know about them. They live on as part of our folk culture, and few parents of an individual with schizophrenia do not hear of them and blame themselves. Many continue to blame themselves, despite our reassurance, because of such theories. For staff working with families, it is best to acknowledge the theories and explain why they are not correct. Simply saying, 'The old family theories of schizophrenia are out of date' will not reassure effectively. Much better to discuss them explicitly and counter them.

Double bind

Probably the most well-known theory is that of the 'double bind' (Bateson et al. 1956). This states that contradictory communications between parent and child lead to confusion, which generates disorganized thinking about identity and relationships. The double bind is classically quoted as giving one message verbally and another contradictory message non-verbally: 'That's all right, I forgive you, it was nothing important' expressed with a face like thunder.

There is, of course, nothing unusual about such contradictions in human communication. Bateson argued that contradictory statements at different *levels* of communication were logically impossible and hence confusing. Bateson also proposed that these families were characterized by an unwritten rule of not challenging the contradictions. Although it was a fine piece of thinking, there has never been any confirmatory evidence that double binds are more frequent in families with a schizophrenic member than in any other families.

The schizophrenogenic mother/schism and skew

The *schizophrenogenic* mother is a particularly damaging concept because mothers are much more prone to blaming themselves and feeling guilty than any other family member. Coined by Frieda Fromm-Reichmann (1948), it meant an over-controlling but emotionally cold ('refrigerator') mother. Fromm-Reichmann was a psychoanalyst working with patients diagnosed with schizophrenia in 1950s USA. At that time, schizophrenia was diagnosed very liberally

Lidz met his patients' parents and concluded that there was a characteristic imbalance in their relationship (Lidz and Lidz 1949). He identified a skewed power relationship or a degree of separation (schism). Remarkably, this did receive some empirical verification, with Lidz able to identify affected families from listening 'blind' to tapes. However, it has not been repeated, and of course, association does not prove causation!

R.D. Laing

Laing was a brilliant writer whose books caught the mood of the 1960s and '70s, in particular, *The Divided Self* (Laing 1960). His views changed radically over time, but he is most remembered for explaining schizophrenia as our failure to understand the rich and often symbolic communications in which the patient expressed their view of the world. Laing believed that society was too unimaginative, responding with incomprehension and hostility to creative but tormented individuals who expressed different views.

The image of anxious, rigid parents (and parent figures such as doctors and nurses) denying the patient's authentic experience became a powerful stick to beat the professions with. Laing advocated treatment as a 'voyage of exploration'. It is the image of a struggle against an uncomprehending world, and the plea to just let the patient be, for which he is remembered.

Expressed emotion

Expressed emotion (EE) differs from the theories outlined previously in that it makes no claim for causation. The work by Leff and his colleagues is based on an earlier observation that intense family situations increase the likelihood of relapse and readmission in established schizophrenia (Brown et al. 1972). The result is a family treatment approach with several rigorous studies which confirm that combined with maintenance medication, it further reduces the relapse rate (Mari and Streiner 1994b).

Although EE work is considered non-controversial in the UK, it has been criticized in the US and Australia as apportioning blame to the family. It is described in more detail in Chapter 25 on psychosocial interventions, but if it is being considered, it is important to explore the families' understanding of it first. Despite education about schizophrenia (and hopefully dispelling old myths), we have found that parents still feel very guilty. While they may not blame themselves for causing the disease, they may understand EE as implying that they have failed to respond effectively.

Treatments in the community

We have dealt with schizophrenia at length because it is such an important and controversial disorder and because individuals suffering from it are likely to form a major part of outreach work. Because it is such a pervasive disorder and can affect all aspects of an individual's life, it is especially important to take a holistic approach. Although different treatments are classified and organized both in this and other chapters, they are not independent of each other. Currently, the most effective treatment in schizophrenia in terms of shortening relapses and reducing their frequency is undoubtedly the prescription of antipsychotics. However, this should not imply a simple reliance on drugs. Without attention to the personal and social needs of our patients, the drugs are not enough—even assuming they took them!

It is overly simplistic to decide that because the drugs are more effective than most psychosocial interventions, then most of our time should be devoted to optimizing pharmacotherapy. Successful engagement using effective psychosocial interventions takes time and energy, but it makes consistent cooperation with effective medication that much more likely.

Antipsychotic medication

The role of antipsychotic medication is addressed in detail in Chapter 7 and compliance in Chapter 11. Schizophrenia is the disorder par excellence where persistence with maintenance medication pays greatest dividends. There is no doubt that remaining on medication, whether oral or depot, for prolonged periods significantly reduces the rate of relapse. For most patients, it also improves functioning between relapses. They feel less vulnerable and less easily stressed, reducing friction with family and friends. Concentration is often better, although tiredness and a sense of mental sluggishness are common side effects.

Supporting individuals to continue with medication over periods often spanning years requires an honest approach. It is no good ducking the issues of how long the patient needs to continue. Although it can sometimes be necessary to be vague in the beginning, while developing a rapport, the fact that you will want an open-ended approach to continuation will have to be faced at some time. It is important to avoid being too gloomy but not to be dishonest:

'You will have to stay on them for a long time. I don't know exactly, but it's months, not weeks.' 'Things have stabilized now, but I wouldn't want to even consider a reduction for at least another year or so.' 'Yes, lots of people do stay on these drugs for life. Not all need to, but it's very difficult to predict. We'll just have to take it one step at a time.'

As pointed out in Chapter 11, we believe it best to take a 'normalizing' approach to problems with long-term medication. It is not easy for anyone to continue medication for years, and we should see our role as helping achieve it, rather than uncovering 'the reason' for non-compliance. It is important to explain, as thoroughly as possible, the role of the medicines. Comparisons with physical disorders can help destigmatize the whole process—but it is essential to choose the right comparison. We have often heard staff compare the process with the need for diabetics to take daily insulin, which is a poor analogy. If the diabetic patient misses a dose, they rapidly feel unwell and there can be dramatic consequences. In schizophrenia, if the patient misses a dose, then they often feel somewhat *better* immediately (the side effects disappear) and it will be some time, perhaps months, before the relapse. Much better is to compare to something like hypertension, where the side effects have to be endured to prevent long-term problems such as strokes and kidney failure (Chapter 11). As with all health promotion, this approach is generally more acceptable to older rather than younger patients. It is also very difficult to get a patient whose current life situation is pretty dire to think about the distant future.

With an empathic, normalizing approach to persisting with medicines, monitoring (as we remarked earlier) need not seem like snooping. Much depends on the outreach worker's own mind set. If you really believe that you are checking how many tablets are left in order to support your patient in taking them, then it will not come across like spying. If you are doing it to catch them out, then it will.

Collaboration has been shown to be the key to all forms of treatment compliance, not just medication. Patients who have genuinely been involved in the decision (nowadays referred to as 'shared decision-making') are much more likely to take responsibility for making the treatment happen. Even if the range of options is only which of two very similar drugs to take, any choice is better than no choice. This possibility of choice was vastly advanced with the advent of the atypical antipsychotics such as resperidone, Seroquel, and olanzapine. Whilst the therapeutic effects may be very similar to each other and to the older antipsychotics, there is a genuine difference in side-effect profile, and that is clearly a decision that belongs most with the patient.

The most obvious choice in relation to medication is usually that between oral and depot preparations. Depots were not abandoned with the arrival of the atypicals. For many patients, it was simply not possible to maintain regular oral medication and depots are the only way of ensuring cover. Now there are also several depot ('LAI', long-acting injectables) atypicals. A few patients prefer depots because it means they do not have to think about tablets and illness. However, many do find them quite demeaning and, even when well established on them, working towards oral self-medication can bring a greater sense of empowerment and dignity. For patients who have endured years of severe schizophrenia, anything that improves self-esteem is worth trying.

Clozapine

Clozapine is the only antipsychotic with a clear advantage over all the others in terms of clinical recovery. It is particularly indicated in resistant schizophrenia (Kane et al. 1988). Both patients and their families report improvements beyond simple symptom control, including a calming effect and improved clarity of thinking (Angermeyer et al. 2001). Despite this, only a fraction of patients who warrant a trial on clozapine get one. It is undeniably a more difficult regime to establish with its regular obligatory blood tests and the heavy early sedation. But once established, the results are often wonderfully rewarding.

Well-functioning community outreach can establish and maintain patients on clozapine in the community. Our Wandsworth team relied heavily on supervised medication, often with daily visits in the beginning. We even initiated clozapine for patients without hospital admission (which was not permitted at that time) and there were no serious complications (O'Brien and Firn 2002). Despite very successful results (and we observed several remarkable improvements), patients need ongoing support and encouragement to persist with the medicine.

Relapse signatures and early intervention

Clinical experience suggests that early intervention may abort incipient relapses, certainly shorten the duration of relapses, and also reduce their severity. Consequently, much attention has been paid to identifying early indications of relapse. For most patients there is a period of mounting anxiety and preoccupation as normal coping mechanisms become overpowered. This is referred to as 'affect dysregulation' by Hogarty (Hogarty et al. 1995). For some patients, this can be very specific—the resurfacing of old delusional ideas or bizarre hypochondriacal preoccupations. Helping patients and families recognize these warning signs may help and is prioritized in early intervention teams. There is probably stronger evidence for its value in bipolar disorder, but it has an intuitive appeal in all relapsing psychotic disorders. It has the added advantage of providing a joint exercise which patients and families value and which strengthens the therapeutic relationship.

With the emergence of these warning signs, the patient can increase the maintenance medication or take other previously agreed steps, such as to avoid known triggers (lack of sleep, illicit drugs), seek known supports (safe friends and families), or step up prearranged CBT practices. Such planning has the added benefit of reducing the overwhelming sense of helplessness which can be so damaging in this illness.

Psychosocial interventions

Stabilizing the living situation of individuals with schizophrenia by a range of psychosocial interventions is a core function of community outreach services. As the main feature of the disorder is a vulnerability to psychotic breakdown when overwhelmed by stress and anxiety, then interventions to reduce routine anxieties should help protect the patient. Most of these interventions are directed at reducing interpersonal stressors, such as avoiding friction with family members, neighbours, and acquaintances. While they are of value with the whole range of severe mental illnesses, they are particularly important in schizophrenia, in which interpersonal oversensitivity can be so crippling.

Few of the proven psychosocial interventions, however, can be applied in the middle of a crisis. They should be pursued when the patient is in remission, so it is essential that team mechanisms exist to ensure that they are routinely offered. It is rare, even these days, for the family of an individual with schizophrenia to ask directly for family work. They may ask for explanations and support, but rarely for help in finding new problem-solving techniques to reduce high expressed emotion. It is essential to routinely review the provision of complex psychosocial interventions such as family work, CBT, or relapse prevention routinely at regular multidisciplinary care reviews. Without this, the provision of such difficult procedures is usually very low indeed. The range of psychosocial interventions in psychosis is covered in Chapter 25.

Case study

Jonathon was referred to the assertive community outreach team following repeated hospital admissions with a diagnosis of schizophrenia. The referring CMHT had experienced great difficulty treating him. He was a highly intelligent man from an upper-class background whose relatives sometimes colluded with his paranoid beliefs about psychiatry and society. Jonathon did not believe he was ill and his family did not believe he was receiving the type of treatment that he deserved—namely, CBT or intensive psychotherapy.

He was extremely adept at intellectualizing and rationalizing his behaviour and beliefs (sometimes angry and threatening). Has previously had an incident of deliberate self-harm driven by the Capgras syndrome from which he suffers (a fixed notion that people were being switched by impostors).

On assessment by the team, we agreed that CBT may be offered to him as he was intelligent, cognitively intact, and able to discuss his experiences openly and understand psychological concepts. We were prepared to review his medication, but that given his history, he should not to stop antipsychotics despite his strongly expressed wishes. Intellectually, Jonathan was intimidating. When floridly psychotic, he was also quite threatening. He was allocated to the outreach worker with the most experience and training in CBT.

Following a further admission following non-compliance, we discharged him early, on daily supervised medication. He responded moderately well to prolonged treatment and his suspicions reduced to the point that he related well to his community outreach worker and other members of the team. He valued the CBT sessions, particularly as he was able to flex his intellectual muscles in debate about the nature and veracity of his beliefs.

Some of his beliefs became 'memories' of events that he insisted had really happened but were no longer occurring. In turn, his beliefs about the value of medication began to change and we could reduce the level of supervision. A relapse plan was negotiated which specified thresholds for intervention, including increased medication and joint visits (Table 15.2). A risk assessment was also completed (Table 15.3) that could be shared with the emergency department and general practitioner.

He is currently on surprisingly good terms with the assertive outreach team and holds down a part-time job. We have not been successful, however, in increasing contact with his family to help them better understand his illness and need for treatment.

Table 15.2 Summary care plan

Patient's name: Jonathon P.	CMHT: Wandsworth
Address: 15 Sudbury Walk, Battersea Estate, Battersea.	Phone: 020 8877 xxxx
	New patient: NO
Phone: none	If NO, date of review: ...... 17/04/15 .....
Date of birth: 12/10/85	Diagnosis:
GP: Givens	1 Schizophrenia F20.0
Phone:	2............................ F — —.—

Assessed needs or problem	Intervention	Resp. of
Psychotic experiences, mainly paranoid	◆ Maintain on risperidone 2 mg nocte. ◆ Monitor compliance openly and collaboratively. ◆ Monitor mental state at each visit. Observe for relapse signature: suspicion, unusual beliefs, and hostility. Repeat BPRS at 3-monthly intervals. ◆ Initiate relapse plan if Jonathon believes his brother or other member of his family has been substituted again, then increase risperidone to 4 mg nocte. ◆ Ongoing weekly CBT sessions aimed at modifying beliefs of Capgras syndrome.	AC
Risk of aggression when acutely paranoid	◆ Low threshold for joint visits. See risk assessment and contingency plan.	AC

Table 15.3 Risk management plan

Name: Jonathon P.

Categories of risk identified:

Aggression and violence	YES	Severe self-neglect	NO
Exploitation (self or others)	NO	Risk to children and young adults	NO
Suicide and self-harm	NO	Other (please specify)............	

Current factors which suggest there is significant apparent risk:

(For example: alcohol or substance misuse; specific threats; suicidal ideation; violent fantasies; anger; suspiciousness; persecutory beliefs; paranoid feelings or ideas about particular people)

No significant risk presently. Currently relatively well and accepting treatment of CBT plus medication. Paranoid beliefs mild, does not act on them.

Clear statement of anticipated risk(s):

(Who is at risk; how immediate is that risk; how severe; how ongoing)

No current risk.

Action plan:

(Including names of people responsible for each action and steps to be taken if plan breaks down)

Risk history of hostile and aggressive behaviour when acutely paranoid. Believes members of his family and health care team have been substituted by impostors. Has admitted to violent fantasies in past usually directed at his consultant psychiatrist. Has made one threat to kill consultant psychiatrist and has thrown chair at father (see risk history). If acutely paranoid or becoming suspicious of health care staff and family do not visit alone. Joint visits. Relapse plan to increase medication to 4 mg immediately following return of beliefs that people have been substituted with impostors. Supervision of medication may be required. Responds well to medication within period of 2–3 weeks. If increasingly hostile and resistant to intervention institute Mental Health Act assessment with view to compulsory admission.

Date completed: 17/04/15   **Review date: 17/10/15**

Conclusions

We have dealt with schizophrenia at length because it is such a complex and demanding disorder. It lies at the heart of much mental health practice. Because the experiences and symptoms of schizophrenia patients are so fascinating, they can become an intense focus of discussion, sometimes obscuring awareness of the whole person. Much of the earlier academic literature on this illness explored the minutiae of psychopathology at remarkable length. When structured assessments of schizophrenia patients' mental state, such as the present state examination, were used (Wing et al. 1974), they showed that more prosaic symptoms such as anxiety, panic, and depression are as severe as the delusions and hallucinations during breakdown. We simply overlook them.

We have found the stress-vulnerability hypothesis (Zubin and Spring 1977) and Hogarty's concept of affect dysregulation (Hogarty et al. 1995) enormously valuable guiding principles in community outreach. Rather than focus too much on individual hallucinations and delusions, we try to spot the stresses as they start to build up, and intervene to reduce them when possible. In this way, we hope to help our patients stay in control their lives and not be overwhelmed by their illness.

Chapter 16

Bipolar affective disorder

Introduction

Bipolar affective disorder is the term currently used for what used to be called manic-depression or 'manic-depressive psychosis'. Manic-depressive psychosis was one of the major mental illnesses that Kraepelin distinguished in his original studies (Kraepelin 1919) and, as defined then, it affects just under 0.7 per cent of the adult population (Weissman et al. 1996). He distinguished it from schizophrenia (then called 'dementia praecox') not so much by its symptoms as by its course. Dementia praecox was characterized by a gradual decline in functioning punctuated by episodes of severe disturbance. Manic-depression often showed full recovery between episodes, although the disturbed periods could be equally severe. French psychiatrists called it 'folie circulaire' (Falret 1854).

The linking of what appears to be such opposite mood states—the elation of mania and the despair of depression—arose from the clinical observation that they so often occurred in the same patient over time. Virtually all patients who had episodes of mania also had periods of severe depression, sometimes in close proximity. Indeed, even during the episodes of elation, patients displayed flashes of extreme sadness. These fluctuations in mood were (and still are) quite remarkable with a rapid descent from joy and overconfidence into bitter self-reproach and sometimes suicidal despair.

The term 'mania' and, with it, 'maniac', have acquired pejorative overtones. Hence the pressure to rename the disorder as bipolar affective disorder. Not all patients with severe mood (affective) disorders experience mania or hypomania. The two terms, mania and hypomania, are, in practice, used interchangeably, although hypomania should imply a much milder, non-psychotic form of the disturbance. This need only last a few days, during which the patient may retain both psychological and social control. While virtually all patients who experience mania also experience severe depressive episodes, many patients experience only the depressive episodes.

A series of family studies of depressed patients in northern Sweden (Perris 1969) showed that families 'bred true' as either 'unipolar' depressives (they had only depressed but not elated episodes) or as 'bipolar' depressives (they had both depressed and elated episodes). There were a very few families that had only elated episodes. Any patient who suffers an episode of mania is, therefore, diagnosed as suffering from a bipolar disorder, even if they have yet to experience a depression. Unipolar affective disorder is discussed along with the wider concept of depression in Chapter 18.

Causes of bipolar affective disorder

There is undoubtedly a significant constitutional element in bipolar disorder. It runs in families, with the children of affected individuals having about a 10 per cent risk of developing the disorder. This more than doubles if both parents are affected. As with schizophrenia, the risk increases to over 50 per cent in identical twins. Although controversial in the past, the importance of genetics in the development of bipolar disorder is now undisputed.

Elated and disorganized states are common with stimulant drugs such as amphetamines and cocaine. Similarly, depression can be caused by drugs such as reserpine or methyldopa which deplete the brain of neurotransmitters such as dopamine and serotonin. Combined with the observation that antidepressant treatment can precipitate manic episodes, this has given rise to various theories linking mood disorders to disorders of neural transmitters. Often these theories rather simplistically associate mania with raised and depression with lowered levels of the same transmitter. It is rare for such theories to survive unchanged for long, and there are regular amendments—which transmitter is involved, adjustments for receptor sensitivities, etc. It is likely, however, that such dramatic changes in levels of energy, affect, and cognition are associated with changes in brain chemistry.

As with all mental illnesses that run in families, the issue of nature versus nurture has been vigorously debated (see the discussion in Chapter 15, on schizophrenia). Psychoanalysts have suggested that mania acts as a defence against depression. Melanie Klein elaborated this most extensively (Segal 1983). Analysts' patients reported that they often dealt with potentially overwhelming depressive feelings by denying them and convincing themselves that they were happy. Most of us will have observed this mechanism, such as in recently bereaved individuals who hold their emotion at bay and remain active for a time before being overwhelmed. This is called a 'manic defence' against depression. This psychoanalytic explanation is endorsed by the regular clinical observation of flashes of misery that are so common within the manic state, and by the fact that most mania is both preceded and followed by depression. Mania also responds dramatically to ECT, the most powerful treatment for depression. The analysts' treatment strategy is to identify and interpret the depression that is being defended against. Few would now advance this as a causal explanation or as an effective treatment approach, but it may be a helpful way of thinking when working with a manic patient.

Clinical picture

The clinical presentation of hypomania is well described in standard textbooks. The patient is usually overactive, with boundless energy and reduced sleep. Thoughts are racing, often with rich and surprising associations. Many creative artists such as Handel, Schumann, and Spike Milligan have their inspiration during manic episodes and work on them further when more stable.

While the classical picture is of an elated, overjoyful individual, the more common experience is of someone who is irritable and impatient and who can become frankly hostile or paranoid if their wishes are frustrated. Delusions and hallucinations are not uncommon in mania, although, in contrast to schizophrenia, they tend to be overshadowed by the mood disturbance and to be 'mood-congruent'. This means that the strange ideas can be seen to flow from the feelings of grandiosity or despair. Severe mood swings may be associated with life stresses, but the relationship is not immediate, and the risk of relapse is usually some months later. The relationship to stressful life events becomes less obvious with repeated relapses. For many patients, there are specific times of the year when breakdowns are more likely, but often they appear to come out of the blue.

If mania was simply a matter of overactivity and poor sleep, there would be little reason for mental health services to get involved. Unfortunately, the most difficult aspect of mania to describe is its most damaging. There is almost invariably a deterioration in personal judgement. The patient may continue to deal with routine obligations, making business deals, seeing friends, and so on, but they lose the judgement needed in such activities. The result is often considerable damage to themselves and their families, damage which they bitterly regret when they recover. Foolish financial deals can lead to ruin, reckless sexual behaviour can devastate families and health, and disinhibition (particularly if the patient is also drinking excessively, which is not unusual in a manic episode) can lead to exploitation, abuse, and even criminal prosecution.

Case study

Janine worked for a national newspaper as a researcher in the fashion section. She was keen to become a journalist, and was usually described as 'bubbly' and enthusiastic. She was in her early 20s and still single, always very well presented and sought after by lots of men.

Over a period of some weeks her employers noticed that she was not so reliable about turning up on time, and there had been a couple of evenings when she had been 'outrageously' drunk with work mates. It was assumed that there were some boyfriend problems and this was, after all, an environment that prided itself on being rather bohemian.

She was seen by her GP who thought she was going high. Her mother phoned from Wales because she had experienced similar episodes with her late husband. Unfortunately, Janine laughed off the concern, did not attend her psychiatric appointment, and failed to show for work. The police picked her up in Manchester two weeks later, sleeping rough in a bus station at night. She was cheerful but dishevelled, and it became clear that she had run up over £2000 in debts in those two weeks, and had been exploited sexually by several men.

On admission to hospital in London, she rapidly settled with treatment but became profoundly depressed and humiliated, thinking back on what had happened. She refused to return to work (although they were happy to have her back) because of her embarrassment about the things she had done in the weeks leading up to her departure.

Treatment in the community

Perhaps one of the most important principles of treating bipolar patients in the community is to remember that early admission should not be considered a failure. Far from it, it may be in everyone's interest, especially if the situation is deteriorating fast. There are few psychiatric disorders in which insight is lost so quickly and the window of opportunity for collaborative work so brief.

Bipolar patients, unlike the majority of patients with severe psychotic illnesses, often have jobs and dependents and reputations. All of these can be irrevocably lost by a few weeks' disinhibited behaviour. This is particularly so as the early symptoms of a relapse are rarely perceived as 'illness'. The failing judgement may be very obvious to the key worker and family, but put down to enthusiasm, confidence, or even foolishness or heavy drinking by colleagues.

We will return to the issue of how to set thresholds in community outreach work with such patients.

Forming a therapeutic alliance

One of the paradoxes of working with these patients is that there often seems to be little justification for regular input between relapses. Unlike individuals with schizophrenia, for example, there is usually no established disability or persisting problems that need your attention. However, if you do not maintain contact between relapses, you end up with little opportunity to really get to know bipolar patients. We have found one of the most powerful advantages of outreach work is that it gives us a real opportunity to understand bipolar patients better and to form an effective therapeutic alliance.

Endorsement of the social care component of the team approach ensures that contacts can still be meaningful with patients in symptomatic remission. There is the opportunity to use them for supporting leisure activities and engaging in joint activities (cleaning out the flat, sorting out muddled finances) that the patient would find daunting, even if actually capable. Repeated hospital admissions can disrupt a patient's ability to plan ahead and to organize their housing, finances, and careers. Given that social and relationship stressors can precipitate relapses, bipolar patients will be more vulnerable if their lives are disorganized. The key worker can mediate and advise in stressful negotiations, helping to stabilize housing, finances, and work. It is often through these shared activities that greater understanding and enduring trust can develop. How feasible this will be, of course, depends on resources and caseloads. However, it can be a life-changing intervention.

Relapse signatures and early intervention

Relapse in bipolar disorder is fast—sometimes only a few days between normal functioning and the loss of insight and extreme elation. Increased contact with patients and increased familiarity with them means that community outreach workers can often spot the earliest symptoms of deterioration.

Case study

One of our patients always starts to wear hats when she is becoming unwell—this happens long before there are any other signs of her hypomania. Asked why she is wearing a hat, she will give an utterly sensible explanation, and certainly there is nothing in itself odd about the hats she wears. Long experience, however, has taught us and her family that within a few days of wearing a hat, she will start to sleep poorly and become aroused and erratic.

More often the indicator of an incipient relapse is some characteristic preoccupation that has featured in previous episodes that becomes prominent again. Not all patients, of course, have specific and reliable 'relapse signatures', but when they do, and when they can be agreed on between you and the patient as a signal for treatment, there is a real chance of being able to intervene very early. Sometimes this can prevent a relapse entirely.

Poor sleep is probably the commonest indicator of incipient relapse in bipolar disorder, soon followed by over-talkativeness and increased energy. Even then, it is not too late to intervene with an agreed 'relapse plan'. There is convincing evidence that spending time exploring the early indicators of relapse with patients when they are well can yield both an understanding of the predictors and a plan of intervention that either aborts relapses or substantially modifies them (Beynon et al. 2008). We talk many of our patients through the process of previous breakdowns to identify early signs. When we have agreement on these, we write them down (see Tables 16.2 and 16.3) and discuss with the patient what they want us to do when they occur. For most patients, the agreement is about taking added antipsychotic medication for a set period: for example, 'After two nights of disturbed sleep, add 2 mg of risperidone nightly for the next five nights.' It seems more acceptable and helpful if the intervention is linked simply to the experience, not to its implications (i.e. 'after two nights', not 'when disturbed sleep indicates a relapse'). Then there is less likelihood of argument about its 'meaning' and importance.

Discussing the meaning of these early signs needs to be done when the patient is in remission. The early stages of a mood swing is not the time if it can be avoided. It is also important to agree on how long the intervention should last. We advise to err on the side of caution. Taking the risperidone for two nights may be enough sometimes, but it is better to play safe. Inevitably, there may be times when the medicine is taken unnecessarily. There may be many other reasons for poor sleep, such as family worries or even indigestion, but the consequences of missing the 'window of opportunity' are considerably greater than a few days' medicine.

The balance of risks and benefits must be negotiated carefully with the patient. It has to make sense and seem proportionate, otherwise it will not be complied with. Although medication is the commonest early intervention— and was invariably one component of our Wandsworth assertive outreach team contingency plans—it is not the only one. For some patients, an agreement to stay with a family member for a period may work, or surrendering their car keys, or handing over credit cards to a member of the family for safekeeping.

On the whole, medication and increased monitoring and contact are the staples of such early interventions. Where there is an involved carer, then assessments and monitoring should include them if the patient allows it. That way, family members learn how we assess the level of overactivity, and they gain confidence in their own ability to judge improvement and deterioration.

Managing hypomania

Early intervention does not always succeed in preventing a hypomanic episode. It may still be possible to manage the patient without admission to hospital, and our patients tell us that, on the whole, they much prefer this. Even families prefer it—as long as admission can be swiftly arranged if needed.

There is no substitute, however, for frequent contact. If a hypomanic patient lives alone, then daily contact is probably optimal initially, and the support of the crisis resolution home treatment team can be negotiated in cases where hospital admission is a real likelihood. These contacts do not have to be long. Indeed, it is often best that they are not too long, as patients can become more aroused and irritable if they feel 'trapped' in the interview. Sharing visits across the team can be particularly helpful, as long as the patient knows those who visit them. Novelty is attractive to patients when they are high and can be used to gain cooperation when repeat visits from the same person may otherwise be viewed as 'dull' or 'boring'.

When sharing the burden for daily visits, it is important to introduce new members. One of the commonest patient criticisms of crisis resolution home treatment teams is having to answer the same questions over and over again with new staff. Hypomanic patients can find this particularly infuriating.

The ability to manage bipolar disorder was one of the real benefits of the Wandsworth assertive outreach team establishing a seven-day service. Missing medicines for even one day can rapidly undermine collaboration, and the situation can spiral out of control.

Negotiating and agreeing the direct care we provide for the patient is the core of such early intervention, but need not be restricted to it. We have found it very useful to agree with the patient who else we can involve should they start to relapse. Knowing what they did in previous episodes can help. One patient always goes to social services and creates a fuss when unwell, another explores his spiritual conflicts with the local priest. It can be enormously helpful to get the patient's agreement to give these people advice on what to do. It may simply be to inform you that the patient is there to save you time searching for them.

There is, rightly, much concern about respecting confidentiality in such issues. We advise obtaining the patient's written permission. However, sensitively approached, most patients see the point and are happy with it. This serves two functions: it makes us feel safer about doing it, and it helps the patient focus on the reality of their disorder. This is something that many bipolar patients are adept at avoiding, either by ignoring the disturbed periods altogether or by playing down their severity—'I suppose I was a bit cheerful'. If bipolar patients are not helped to confront the degree of disturbance associated with their elated periods, it is no surprise if they have 'little insight'. This can be a painful process and needs to be handled carefully. Memory during these hypomanic episodes may be genuinely hazy, so the business of discussing them can take time and may need repeating.

Getting a good night's sleep is essential to managing hypomania. It is both an indicator of recovery and also a prerequisite for avoiding admission. Even when taking antipsychotics, patients often need hypnotics to get off to sleep. Family members understandably worry about what the patient is doing if they are up and about in the middle of the night. Everything always seems worse in the night, and getting help is much more difficult. The family's emotional resources will be at a low ebb, and without sleep the situation rapidly becomes impossible. If disturbed behaviour continues through the night for more than one or two nights, and we cannot get on top of it, then a brief admission may be negotiated.

As mentioned in Chapter 7, we have experienced no problems (such as dependency) when using benzodiazepines with psychotic patients. Similarly, concerns about 'disinhibition' seem misplaced. After all, the patient is usually quite disinhibited when such sedation is being considered. We use them liberally with bipolar patients both in the community and in the ward, and have found this pragmatic approach to be common in successful community outreach services in much of Europe.

Mood stabilizers

Ensuring the use of mood stabilizers in bipolar disorder (Chapter 7) is an essential part of community outreach. The evidence is clear that such drugs reduce the likelihood of a relapse, although it can be difficult to demonstrate the impact for an individual patient. There is only limited evidence for the superiority of any one mood stabilizer above the others and, if anything, lithium has re-established its broad superiority with careful monitoring (Geddes and Miklowitz 2013). Choice is often dictated by patient response and sensitivity to side effects. Many patients are prescribed more than one mood stabilizer at a time, but there is little evidence that this really improves things.

The case manager's task is twofold. They must work with the patient to sustain compliance with the medicines over long periods. This involves early preparatory work, explaining the purpose, functioning, and side effects of the drugs involved. It may include structured support such as motivational interviewing (Chapter 11). All patients will need support, prompting, and encouragement. As many patients have complete remission between episodes, stressing the value of maintenance prophylactic medication needs to be convincing and can be an uphill task. The current range of mood stabilizers also requires careful monitoring. Lithium and carbamazepine necessitate regular blood tests to measure therapeutic levels and, for lithium, to monitor thyroid and renal damage. Local agreements and practice will vary about how blood tests are organized. Good general practices are able to monitor lithium in compliant patients, but even the best practices have difficulty recognizing and following up non-compliance. For patients needing regular outreach, it is usual for the case manager to help coordinate these routine blood tests whether through the GP, the team, or by prompting and even taking the patient to the clinic. It is optimal if the patient takes responsibility for this monitoring if they are capable of it, but you need to make sure it happens. This is no place for too much ideology.

The range of drugs licensed for treatment and maintenance in bipolar disorders has widened to include atypical antipsychotics such as olanzapine and Seroquel (Geddes and Miklowitz 2013).

In more unstable, disorganized, and non-compliant bipolar patients, low-dose depot antipsychotics can be a real lifesaver. With both antipsychotics and mood stabilizers, however, the patient should be regularly assessed for side effects. Bipolar patients seem more sensitive to drug side effects than schizophrenia patients; training all team members in routine side-effect screening is not that difficult (Chaplin et al. 1999).

Depression

Managing manic episodes in the community is a highly stressful activity. Not only must one anticipate and respond quickly, but there is the ever-present worry of them crashing down into depression. Depressive thinking and mood combined with manic energy and impulsiveness can be a lethal combination. Sometimes the risk is just too great and admission is indicated. Fleeting (but intense) depressive phenomena are frequent and characteristic of hypomania. Similarly, depression after the hypomanic episode is to be expected as the patient returns to sober reality, often to the memory of foolish and embarrassing exploits. Elated mood and overactivity are also, quite simply, exhausting for both patient and family. There is often a flat, joyless period to follow. Any decision to use antidepressants should be thought through carefully in such circumstances, both because of the natural course of the illness, and also because there is evidence that bipolar individuals' antidepressant treatment increases the risk of a further manic episode.

Psychological and psychosocial interventions

Bipolar patients often want extensive explanations of their illness and treatment. This is an illness where understanding and self-management can significantly improve the quality of life. Without such understanding, otherwise able individuals may stubbornly refuse to make minor adaptations to their lifestyle for which they pay an enormous price in repeated, devastating relapses. Sometimes it seems that some patients simply have to find out for themselves. However, remarkable changes can occur when 'the penny drops', especially following severe episodes when successful engagement has been maintained.

Case study

Jamie was the younger son in a family with an extensive history of bipolar illness. His father still managed to work, despite several breakdowns in his early life. He needed to take time off now and then, but remained on his lithium and out of hospital. His elder brother was living a 'hippy' life in a commune, was frequently depressed, refused medication, and had infrequent admissions for mania. Jamie's illness was much more severe and, by the age of 25, he had been compulsorily admitted six times and had twice nearly died (once from a drug overdose and once after falling from scaffolding when high). He was a talented musician, played in an amateur rock band, and would neither take the drugs we prescribed nor refrain from those offered by his friends.

During one of his admissions he became friendly with another, equally talented, bipolar patient with whom he shared the same key worker. For some reason, all three 'clicked', and by the end of that admission Jamie had acknowledged that he did suffer from a bipolar illness and agreed to continue on lithium and restrict (though not stop) his illicit drug use. He was surprisingly able to balance his anarchic artistic life with his treatment and has now stayed well for several years.

Jamie's summary care plan, risk management plan, and risk history are shown in Tables 16.1–16.3, respectively.

In all previous discussions, Jamie had equated treatment with the loss of his talent and personality. He had seen it as 'either/or'. Our protestations that the changes needed to protect him were fairly minor were to no avail—until that last admission. Education and information may simply need to be repeated over and over again.

The importance of relapse signal training and of compliance enhancement skills in the care of these patients has been mentioned earlier. Psychological treatments to enhance coping skills are also of great benefit. Relapses are often clearly stress related, so any treatment or training aimed at improving coping skills will help reduce vulnerability. Which coping skills are to be the target of such training are highly specific to the individual. For many patients, learning how to manage anger and frustration whilst still being assertive can be particularly beneficial. Social skills' training, though no longer fashionable, can sometimes make a major improvement in an individual's life. How to conduct a conversation and establish and maintain non-intimate, low-key friendships can make all the difference between a rewarding day and brooding loneliness. Community outreach workers have the advantage that they can deliver social skills' training *in vivo*—practising where, and with whom, the patient wants to use them.

CBT to explore and reduce depressive thinking and vulnerability is increasingly provided for bipolar individuals. Whatever the exact relationship between elation and depression in this disorder, there is no doubt that managing mood and how you feel is central to it. CBT has an established place in reducing depressive thinking. Many bipolar patients report that they find the depressions worse than the elations (although their families may not agree). Help in reducing the self-criticism and pessimism central to their depressive psychopathology is

Table 16.1 Summary care plan

Patient's name: Jamie S. Address: 52 Willerton House, Roehampton Phone: none Date of birth: 12/3/85 GP: Asquith Phone:	**CMHT: ACT TEAM** **Phone: 0208 877 xxxx** **New patient: NO** **If No, date of review: 25/5/16** **Diagnosis:** **1. Bipolar affective disorder .... F31.0** **2. .... F — —.—**

Assessed needs or problem	Intervention	Resp. of
Frequent relapse; manic relapse can appear over period of few days	◆ Frequent home visits, two visits per week to assess mental state and intervene early. ◆ Relapse signature and plan agreed—if no sleep for two nights and starts to believe he has special powers to take additional risperidone 2 mg twice daily. Depressive episodes largely managed in the community unless risk (see below). ◆ Provide regular psycho-education and advice about harmful use of drugs and effect on mental state and risk of relapse. ◆ Liaise with family and friends regularly during high-risk periods. Ensure they know how to access help easily from team and services day or night. Involve family in relapse plan.	BP
Poor compliance with medication	◆ Actively engage Jamie in care. Jamie interested in music. ◆ Reinforce messages of need for maintenance medication. ◆ Medication currently lithium 1200 mg nocte. ◆ Routinely assess for side effects, information on side effects of lithium. ◆ Ensure lithium levels monitored by GP 3 monthly.	BP

Completed

Table 16.2 Risk management plan

Name: Jamie S.			
Categories of risk identified:			
Aggression and violence	NO	Severe self-neglect	NO
Exploitation (self or others)	YES	Risk to children and young adults	NO
Suicide and self-harm	YES	Other (please specify)	

Current factors which suggest there is significant apparent risk:

(For example: alcohol or substance misuse; specific threats; suicidal ideation; violent fantasies; anger; suspiciousness; persecutory beliefs; paranoid feelings or ideas about particular people)

Currently moderately depressed. No current suicidal ideation.

Clear statement of anticipated risk(s):

Who is at risk; how immediate is that risk; how severe; how ongoing.

Attempted suicide by overdose when severely depressed.

Risk of accidental self-harm when high due to reckless behaviour.

Action plan:

(Including names of people responsible for each action and steps to be taken if plan breaks down)

Relapse signature and plan agreed with Jamie that if does not sleep for two nights and starts to believe he has special powers will take additional risperidone 2 mg twice daily. Provide increased visits and early intervention.

For mild episodes of elation increase contact, consider direct supervision of medication, and liaise with family if they can provide additional support and supervision at Jamie's house.

Depressive episodes largely managed at home unless risk. Assess mental state regularly using both BPRS and Beck Depression Inventory. If significant suicidal risk such as evidence of planning, hoarding of medication, etc. offer informal admission or assess for formal admission after discussion with team. For mild episodes of depression increase contact and liaise with family if they can provide additional support and supervision at Jamie's house.

Date completed: 25/05/16   **Review date: 25/11/16**

greatly appreciated. It helps protect from full-blown depressions (and perhaps from manic responses) and also cements the working alliance.

Stress reduction lies at the heart of many of the psychosocial interventions common to community outreach work with bipolar patients. Such interventions include work to protect the social framework around the patient, to enhance community tenure by ensuring that housing is secure, and to prevent

Table 16.3 Risk history

Client's name: Jamie S.

Give details of any risk behaviour shown by the patient (actual or threatened). Each entry must be signed and dated.

(E.g. previous violence; weapons used; impulsivity; self-harm; non-compliance; disengagement from services; convictions; potentially seriously harmful acts)

2005: Attempted suicide by overdose when severely depressed. Took 20 tablets of temazepam with bottle of spirits.

2006: Got into a fight when elated and abusive to people in pub. Suffered broken nose.
2006: Accidental self-harm by falling off scaffolding two storeys up when elated and abusing stimulant drugs.

the building up of enormous debts. Working with the informal network of social supports in the neighbourhood can be very rewarding, as most bipolar patients need company and do not thrive in isolation. The response of individuals within this network can be the difference between a successful early intervention and a compulsory hospitalization.

Working with the positives when the patient is well is the secret of community outreach with bipolar patients. It gives us insights into their personality and the strengths on which we can build a therapeutic relationship. It can also improve their quality of life directly and so increase their commitment to staying well. Only if there is something to get well for, and to stay well for, can we expect patients to put up with the treatments we offer them. Time and effort devoted to strengthening this is time well spent.

Conclusions

Work with individuals with bipolar affective disorder can be one of the most rewarding and successful aspects of community outreach. Initially, it may not seem like that, and we were rather despairing of our ability to help this group at the beginning of our Wandsworth assertive outreach team. We found that the benefits took a few years to become manifest and they were built on the team's experience of repeated relapses. It is in the period after a relapse that the therapeutic relationship can be developed and strengthened, using the range of approaches—social, psychological, and also pharmacological. From occupying the 'problem' slots in team reviews we found, some years on, that this group of patients became surprisingly silent.

Often these patients will have much to work with—families, interests, even jobs—so that the benefits of even moderate stabilization in mental state are visible and rewarding. The temptation to immediately reduce contact frequency once symptoms recede needs to be resisted. Persistence is all. Two years without a significant mood swing (not two years without an admission) was needed before negotiating a transfer of care back to the CMHT.

Chapter 17

Personality problems and disorders

Introduction

Personality is that which makes each of us different and unique. When we speak of someone's personality, we focus on those aspects which make them most memorable. We have an enormous range of terms to describe an individual's personality—strong, fiery, passionate, phlegmatic, intellectual, cold, ruthless, conscientious, etc. If we are to work successfully in long-term relationships with patients, we need to pay due attention to personality. Our patients' personalities profoundly affect how they deal with their illnesses and undoubtedly have a major impact on their overall outcome.

Not only do our patients have personalities, but we do as well. This means that, despite our professional training, there will be aspects of our work that we are better at than others and some patients we work better with than others. Even before we address the thorny issue of whether personality disorders are more than a set of pejorative labels, outreach work requires taking personality seriously.

There are several theories about personality formation. The very number of theories is a sure sign that we do not really know that much about why different people grow up to behave so differently. Nature versus nurture battles have generally given way to a recognition that both are important. Nowadays individuals divide more about which they think contributes most. Family resemblances in personality are balanced out by the wide variation we see within families. Most parents are struck by how different their children may seem right from birth— one placid and easy-going, another alert, inquisitive, and refusing to go to sleep.

It is probably safe to say that an adult's personality is the result of the interplay between their constitution and their experiences growing up. This is not the same as saying their 'upbringing'—there is more to growing up than what parents do. Peer-group norms and pressures, the rate of physical development and periods of illness have all been shown to influence personality. Constructing a 'personal narrative' may help to make sense of an individual personality, but it can be misleading. For instance, working with an elderly person who is anxious and unable to trust or form relationships and who had been in a concentration camp in their childhood, we would assume it was this horrific experience that marked their life. We have to remember, however, that the vast majority of victims of such atrocities appear to develop normally. Even when we find narratives helpful, we must remember that no explanatory model is conclusive or predictive. That said, we all need our models. Each of us must have some way of 'understanding' personality if we are to function in relationships. When the facts and the theory do not fit, however, we should trust the facts.

The diagnosis of 'personality disorder'

Even if we accept personality as a meaningful construct, do we accept personality disorder as a diagnosis? This has long been highly controversial in mental health—never more so than now. In an era of evidence-based practice, the reliability of personality disorder diagnoses is strongly questioned. The durability of the clinical descriptions of personality disorders is, however, quite striking. Schneider, who considered abnormal personalities to be 'constitutional variants that are highly influenced by personal experience', described ten specific types (Schneider 1923). Eight of these are still clearly distinguishable in DSM-V and ICD-10.

There is a marked hierarchy of reliability in psychiatric diagnoses. There is excellent agreement on organic and functional psychoses, fair agreement on neurotic disorders, but only very modest agreement on individual personality disorders.

In many ways this is not surprising, as the features of most personality disorders are essentially exaggerations (caricatures even) of the components of most of our personalities. The extreme forms of personality disorders, however, are usually recognized easily. While psychiatrists may have difficulty in agreeing on whether a patient suffers from one or another specific personality disorder, they do achieve good agreement on whether patients have 'a personality disorder'. One proposal for the upcoming ICD-11 is to abandon individual personality disorder diagnoses, and instead register the presence or absence of personality disorder, and then rate its severity from mild to severe (Tyrer et al. 2015). Whether clinicians will find this useful is unclear; we doubt it.

In the UK 1959 Mental Health Act (Department of Health 1959), personality disorder was recognized as having a different status from other mental disorders. Detention was only permitted if there was evidence of either danger or 'treatability'. This requirement for treatability reflected the doubts that existed within psychiatry then that it was a real mental disorder. While this distinction was retained in the 1983 Mental Health Act, it was abandoned in the 2007 amendment, when the catch-all term 'mental disorder' was introduced. All the previous subcategories of mental disorder—mental illness, mental handicap, personality disorder—were abandoned. The reason for this was to do away with the treatability clause and encourage psychiatrists to compulsorily treat individuals with severe personality disorders who were thought to be 'slipping through the net'.

Despite the introduction of provisions for the treatment of 'dangerous severe personality disorders' (DSPD), most UK psychiatrists have remained sceptical about the treatability of personality disorders. Certainly they have little faith in the effect of treatment imposed without the patient's consent and commitment. As a result, practice has not changed in response to the law, and psychiatrists are reluctant to use compulsion with this group. They still decline to offer treatment despite strong representations from GPs and families (and sometimes patients). The DSPD initiative, despite enormous initial investment, has shrunk to two small units in prisons. The tensions existing around compulsory treatment, and the doubts about the effectiveness of treatments, have resulted in the diagnosis of personality disorder being seen as stigmatizing, perhaps implying that they are a lifestyle choice not warranting treatment. This debate will continue outside the scope of this book. However, outreach workers need to be familiar with disorders of personality and be able to communicate effectively about them.

Current definitions

ICD-10

Current definitions of personality disorder emphasize description and avoid theories of development. The ICD-10 (World Health Organisation 1992) stresses the long-standing nature of the disorders and that they are usually discernible by adolescence but should not be diagnosed before adulthood. The broad ICD-10 diagnostic guidelines for a personality disorder are described in Box 17.1.

There are eight major personality disorders recognized in ICD-10. Of these, only two are particularly relevant to work in outreach workers—dissocial PD (F60.2) and borderline PD (F60.31) (see Table 17.1).

DSM classification

In DSM-IV (American Psychiatric Association 1994), personality disorders were placed in a second, parallel system called 'axis II' diagnoses (mental illnesses were often referred to as 'axis I'). However, they are broadly very similar to the ICD-10, with some differences in terminology (ICD-10: dissocial, anankastic, anxious; DSM: antisocial, obsessive-compulsive, avoidant); borderline was given its own category in DSM. DSM-V has abandoned the separation of

Box 17.1 F60—specific personality disorders

- Markedly disharmonious attitudes and behaviour involving usually several areas of functioning (e.g. affectivity, arousal, impulse control, perception and thought, relating to others).
- The abnormal behaviour pattern is enduring, long-standing, and not limited to episodes of illness; it is pervasive and clearly maladaptive to a broad range of personal and social situations.
- The foregoing manifestations always appear during childhood or adolescence and continue into adulthood.
- The disorder leads to considerable personal distress, but this may only become apparent late in its course.
- The disorder is usually, but not invariably, associated with significant problems in occupational and social performance.

Reprinted from *International Classification of Diseases (ICD)*, version 10. Copyright (1992) World Health Organization.

diagnosis into two axes, but still advises that personality should always be independently assessed. It recommends that if no disorder is identified, this should be recorded.

DSM, but not ICD, groups personality disorders into three clusters which reflect their broad characteristics (American Psychiatric Association 2013):

Cluster A: 'odd' or 'eccentric'

- paranoid
- schizoid
- schizotypal

Table 17.1 F60 Specific Personality Disorders

F60.0 Paranoid PD	**F60.1** Schizoid PD
F60.2 Dissocial PD	**F60.3** Emotionally unstable PD (**F60.31** Borderline type)
F60.4 Histrionic PD	**F60.5** Anankastic PD
F60.6 Anxious (avoidant) PD	**F60.7** Dependent PD
F60.8 Other Specific PD	**F60.9** PD unspecified

Data from *International Classification of Diseases (ICD)*, version 10. Copyright (1992) World Health Organization.

Cluster B: 'dramatic' or 'erratic'

+ histrionic
+ narcissistic
+ antisocial
+ borderline

Cluster C: 'anxious'

+ avoidant
+ dependent
+ obsessive-compulsive
+ passive-aggressive

Data from *Diagnostic and statistical manual of mental disorders,* 5th ed., 2013, American Psychiatric Association.

Proposed alterations

Close examination of the two systems shows that there are several minor differences—different names used for the same disorder (dissocial or antisocial), some disorders in one scheme but not the other (narcissistic in DSM, emotionally unstable in ICD). However, overall they are very similar, and the basic traditional ten personality disorders are enduring and have intuitive appeal.

Despite enduring popularity, there continue to be proposals to radically alter the approach, in particular emphasizing dimensions rather than categories. Tyrer et al. (2015) has proposed for the upcoming ICD-11 that 'absent' or 'present' is recorded and, if present, the severity noted. DSM-V suggested reducing ten PDs to six and classifying by disabilities and traits. It seems highly unlikely that either proposal will catch on. Personality disorder as a diagnosis, whilst intellectually suspect, is just too useful.

Treatability of personality disorders

Treatment is a difficult area. Opinions vary markedly about the treatability of personality disorder (particularly dissocial and borderline types), and there is little hard evidence (Bateman et al. 2015). There are imaginative, but still essentially experimental, treatments mainly for Cluster B—borderline and antisocial—disorders. Democratic therapeutic communities (Jones 1952) were developed for dissocial individuals (Lees et al. 1999). They continue to influence practice in prisons and drug units, but have faded from the NHS. Some forms of dynamic psychotherapy (Kernberg 1984; Ryle 1997; Mulder and Chanen 2013) and, more recently, adaptations of CBT in the form of dialectical behaviour therapy (Linehan et al. 1991), are proposed for borderline patients.

Much attention is currently directed to the treatment of patients with personality disorder in the UK. The government policy document 'No Longer a Diagnosis of Exclusion' (Department of Health 2003) directed both clinical activity and research energies to the area, and NICE guidance has been published for both borderline and antisocial PDs (NICE 2009; Gabbard 2007). Most of the development is centred on mentalization day hospitals which encourage borderline patients to pause and recognize their emotions rather than immediately act on them (Bateman and Fonagy 1999; Bateman et al. 2015).

The status of these treatments and the precise characteristics of who will respond to them are still uncertain. Clinicians may be reluctant to offer such treatments either because they remain unconvinced that they work or, even if convinced, they do not have the skills or resources. The result is that the diagnosis is still often seen by many as an 'excuse' to refuse to take on difficult patients.

We share the scepticism about the treatability of personality disorders as such. That does not mean that we refuse to take on the outreach care of these patients. There is a difference. Just as individuals with psychoses can also suffer from neurotic disorders and personality disorders, so personality-disordered individuals frequently have problems which both warrant treatments and which respond to treatment. Not only that, but people with personality disorder benefit from a thorough and honest assessment of their problems. An analysis of their behaviours, the likely triggers and risk areas, along with an exploration of difficult relationships, can often lead to very useful advice. Even being told that the issues are to do with personality, and not depression or some other mental illness, can be enormously helpful. It allows the individual to form more realistic expectations and engage in some sensible planning. Occupational or interpersonal stresses may be the result of failure to recognize the importance of personality. We remember one impulsive risk-taker who had been encouraged to get a clerical job to 'settle him down', but instead began to control his temper much better when he got a job much more to his liking in a fairground. Sometimes, fairly simple advice from a skilled and objective professional can make an enormous difference.

Personality disorder and community outreach

We have dealt with personality disorder at such length for two reasons. First, assertive outreach teams came under considerable pressure to take on patients with dissocial or borderline personality disorders. This is because they are often very high-profile patients, are frequently admitted, cause staff discord, and generate real concerns about safety. Their general reluctance to be consistently involved with care also qualified them on the grounds of 'hard to engage'. Similar pressures are brought to bear on CMHTs that offer outreach.

Our Wandsworth team resisted the pressure to accept referrals with a diagnosis exclusively of personality disorder. Our rationale was there was no evidence that outreach has anything specific to offer. Indeed, one of the few US studies of ACT that failed to find an advantage was with individuals with significant offending behaviour (Solomon and Draine 1995b). As assertive outreach was such an expensive treatment, we felt it should be restricted to those known to benefit from it.

The second reason we have focused on personality disorders is that the sorts of issues they present are so common in severe mental illnesses. The onset of psychotic disorders in early adult life (and there is increasing evidence that the prodromal phase stretches well back into adolescence) dramatically interferes with normal personal development. Interpersonal skills, vocational skills, and self-confidence are all disrupted. Not surprisingly, many psychosis patients struggle with personality deficits and disorders as a consequence of these early problems.

Dissocial personality disorder

Many young men with severe mental illnesses display clumsiness in their interpersonal relationships, relying on bluster and threat to make up for poor self-esteem and deficient social skills. Being socially marginalized, they may feel there is little to lose by delinquency, and for many this may be the norm of their peer group. Such delinquency and restricted social conscience should not surprise us given the multiple deprivations experienced by many of our patients. However, this is not the same as a dissocial personality disorder. Such men (not always men, but usually) require us to steer a path of support plus appropriate confrontation and, most importantly, encouragement and training to acquire the missing skills. Dissocial personality disorder (called antisocial in DSM) is a more pervasive problem and is characterized in ICD-10 by the characteristics listed in Box 17.2.

There will undoubtedly be a few patients on the caseload of any team who suffer both from severe mental illness and from dissocial personality disorder. These patients pose massive problems, both therapeutic and ethical. Most of these issues are touched on elsewhere (e.g. Chapters 8, 10, and 19). Needless to say, issues of safety must be uppermost. Regular team reviews are essential to protect individual workers from placing too much faith on the strength of

Box 17.2 F60.2—dissocial personality disorder

- Callous unconcern for the feelings of others.
- Gross and persistent attitude of irresponsibility and disregard for social norms, rules, and obligations.
- Incapacity to maintain enduring relationships, though having no difficulty in establishing them.
- Very low tolerance of frustration and a low threshold for discharge of aggression, including violence.
- Incapacity to experience guilt and to profit from experience, particularly punishment.
- Marked proneness to blame others or to offer plausible rationalizations for the behaviour that has brought the patient into conflict with society.

Reprinted from *International Classification of Diseases (ICD)*, version 10. Copyright (1992) World Health Organization.

their engagement with such patients. Realistic goals need to be set, and assumptions about the relative contributions of illness and personality to troublesome behaviours should be reviewed regularly.

Deciding when to protect the patient from the legal consequences of their actions and when to ensure that they face them is always difficult. Individuals with dissocial personality disorder do not learn well from punishment. It was this observation that gave rise to therapeutic communities. On the other hand, failure to allow the law to take its course may mean that the extent of the risk that an individual patient poses is not confronted. There is also the safety of others (both within the team and the public) to consider. On balance, we very rarely attempt to prevent prosecutions when there has been physical aggression, unless it is clearly associated with an acute psychotic relapse. The problem is more often the opposite—the police will not prosecute even if we ask them to because they do not consider it in the public interest.

Confidentiality and risk

Issues of confidentiality can be very difficult when the patient has a dissocial personality disorder. If there are risks to a third party because of illness, then the Mental Health Act can be invoked and a compulsory admission initiated. When callous disregard for others is not part of the illness, it becomes more problematic. For instance, what to do when a patient makes clear, non-delusional threats against a neighbour, and you have little doubt that they mean it? Similarly, we had a patient who worked as a minicab driver despite having no licence (and hence no insurance) and without admitting he was on heavy medication. Knowing what is going on, can one ignore it? In neither of these cases did we ignore it. We broke confidentiality and informed the neighbour and the minicab firm. We told both patients what we were going to do, explained our reasons, and had to live with the resultant fury. In the case of the minicab driver, our relationship remained strained for over a year and has probably never really returned to how it was before.

Issues of confidentiality are addressed in Chapter 12. Undoubtedly, this will remain a problematic area in mental health practice for the foreseeable future. Current professional guidelines are altogether too simplistic and simply out of touch with modern care.

Borderline personality disorder

Dissocial personality disorder is overwhelmingly diagnosed in men and borderline personality disorder in women. It is tempting to conclude that they comprise the same difficulties with relationships and impulse control filtered through the two differing gender roles. Although the introduction of borderline personality disorder led to extensive research, this has mainly been into treatment, not into whether it is a valid diagnosis. Its fluctuation and pattern of recovery in middle age continue to prompt speculation that it is not so much a 'proper' personality disorder but more an expression of a mood disorder. It presents more with self-harm and stormy relationships than does dissocial personality disorder (see Boxes 17.3–17.4).

A therapeutic approach

Clearly, helping such individuals is a daunting task, especially if they also suffer from a bipolar disorder or schizophrenia (though the latter seems rare with borderline but not dissocial personality disorder). Maintaining a non-judgemental approach is essential, but, while this is easy to say, it can be difficult in practice. Such patients have had more than their share of criticism and punishment, and may have little ability to make good use of either. Sometimes punishment may be inevitable but, when it is not, an honest but positive and supportive approach is really the only way. Confrontation may make us feel temporarily better, but rarely helps the patient (nor, in the long run, our ability to help them). Trying to distinguish what is personality and what is 'illness' (although this is a highly artificial distinction) can help develop different strategies.

Box 17.3 F60.3—emotionally unstable personality disorder

'A ... marked tendency to act impulsively without consideration of the consequences, together with affective instability. The ability to plan ahead may be minimal, and outbursts of intense anger may often lead to violence or "behavioural explosions".... Two variants ... are specified, and both share this general theme of impulsiveness and lack of self-control.'

Reprinted from *International Classification of Diseases (ICD)*, version 10. Copyright (1992) World Health Organization.

Team approach and reviews

In community outreach, patients with personality disorder have particularly benefited from a shared approach to care. The team can take the steam out of the relationship and the treatment, 'depersonalize' them, to good effect. Patients benefit from being visited by different members of the team with visits that are task-oriented rather than 'psychotherapeutic'. Such an approach requires meticulous care, planning, and clear boundaries. Good communication is essential to avoid the obvious 'splitting' that could arise. Such a team approach protects the individual team members faced with an emotionally unstable and demanding patient who phones them several times a day and demands crisis visits.

These patients need to be reviewed regularly in the team meeting. Reminding ourselves of the multiple disadvantages which most of them endured can help

Box 17.4 F60.31—borderline type

'Several characteristics of emotional instability are present; in addition, the patient's own self-image, aims, and internal preferences (including sexual) are often unclear or disturbed. There are usually chronic feelings of emptiness. A liability to become involved in intense and unstable relationships may cause repeated emotional crises with ... a series of suicidal threats or acts of self-harm.'

Reprinted from *International Classification of Diseases (ICD)*, version 10. Copyright (1992) World Health Organization.1

neutralize the moral disapproval that otherwise can so easily develop. It is also essential to acknowledge that, even with the best training, none of us is such a saint that we are immune to judgemental and even, occasionally, spiteful responses when pushed hard by patients. And pushed we will be—whether by accurately barbed comments about our personality or appearance, racist remarks, or physical intimidation. It is then that the team can support and protect us, and also rehabilitate the patient's reputation.

No staff member can help a patient if they have really decided against them. If there is a real personality clash between key worker and patient, this should be acknowledged and talked through. Sometimes it will be necessary to change key worker. This should only happen rarely however. It is generally better to work through such differences and learn from them.

Much of our work with personality-disordered patients is aimed at reducing overall stress (in exactly the same way we try to stabilize the environment to avoid psychotic relapses). For dissocial and borderline individuals, more of the focus needs to be on identifying potential flash points and finding ways of avoiding them. The use of alcohol or drugs is particularly risky in impulse-ridden patients. Where avoidance is not possible, then agreeing on some distracting manoeuvres can sometimes save the day.

Case study

A very handsome patient, with schizophrenia and an impulsive personality, is prone to violence. He is frequently approached by women but cannot cope with them. We have helped him to find activities that take place in a predominantly male environment (e.g. a gym, a music group that practises but does not perform). When he cannot avoid confrontation, we have taught him to simply excuse himself and leave without further explanation. When he begins to get stressed, he will work off his tension with a particularly punishing set in the gym.

Time spent on such problem-solving is well worth it. Even brief crises can wreak havoc and may take ages to repair. It is also experienced by many individuals as an acceptably collaborative approach—one that does not evoke a knee-jerk opposition to authority.

Conclusions

Personality problems and disorders are the daily bread of mental health professionals. We need to have a model of understanding personality that makes sense to us even if we do not necessarily believe that it explains it. One of us (TB) finds psychodynamic models helpful, while the other (MF) relies more on developmental and cognitive models. Whatever model it is, it needs to be robust enough to protect against moralizing. It also needs to survive when the facts do not fit, and to allow for an eclectic, pragmatic treatment strategy.

Arguments about the role of mental health services in the care of individuals with personality disorders (for which read 'dissocial personality disorder'!) are set to continue. There is a clear international agenda to explore how we can ensure some form of risk reduction and social policing.

Community outreach services are likely to best serve by focusing on what we know that they can do well, what there is evidence for, and avoiding too many forays into speculation and theory. We work with a group of patients who routinely face challenges and problems that the average person in the street would only expect to confront once or twice in a lifetime. Inevitably, this will mean that we learn how to help individuals with troubled and troublesome personalities. While we should not withhold our skills, we should be wary of overstating what we can do or of misdirecting our resources.

Chapter 18

Depression, anxiety, and situational disorders

Introduction

It is easy to forget that people with severe mental illnesses such as psychoses also suffer anxiety, depression, and grief just as we all do. Although the most prominent features of their illnesses may be their psychotic symptoms, careful examination of the mental state of individuals with schizophrenia often betrays very high levels of so-called neurotic symptoms. The management of situational and common mental disorders is not the primary focus of this book, as it is unlikely to be a major responsibility in community outreach. However, a familiarity with them, and a working competence with them, is necessary if we are not to fail our patients. Shy, anxious individuals with severe disorders are not easily referred to other services for specialist help.

Depression

Being alert to depression is essential in working with individuals with schizophrenia. Depression is common in such a devastating disorder with its loss of future ambitions, the exhausting stress of persecutory delusions and hallucinations, isolation, and damaged self-esteem. To complicate matters, depression can be very difficult to diagnose in schizophrenia. It has to be distinguished from the apathy and emptiness of negative symptoms and also from the inertia and sluggishness that can result from over-medication. Post-psychotic depression is, however, common, and there is increasing evidence that appropriate treatment with antidepressants can significantly improve recovery.

Rating scales

When antidepressants and antipsychotics are used concurrently in individuals with long-term disorders, we have found the use of structured rating scales particularly valuable in keeping track of progress (Chapter 7). The Beck Depression Inventory (Beck et al. 1961) is popular, but we find it long and quite demanding for our patients. The Hamilton Depression Scale (Bech et al. 1981) and the

Hospital Anxiety Depression Scale (Zigmond and Snaith 1983) are shorter and generally easier to use.

Making sure you use a structured assessment is more important than which scale you use. Distinguishing fluctuations in overall mental state, mood, and more general, personal life changes is a challenge for even the most skilled worker. Forcing some objectivity into the rating of mood helps you identify a response to treatment. Given the risks of long-term polypharmacy in our patients, we must be hard-nosed about the justification for antidepressants.

Cognitive behavioural therapy (CBT)

CBT has been shown to be successful in alleviating depression in non-psychotic individuals and is increasingly being used in the direct treatment of psychotic symptoms (Freeman 2015). This is not the book to dwell at length on the practice of CBT. There is no strong evidence of its value for depression in individuals with psychotic illnesses (Birchwood and Iqbal 1998), but we find our patients are receptive to CBT for depressive thinking and low self-esteem. Indeed, simply attempting such a collaborative approach (for CBT is nothing if not collaborative) can do wonders for a depressed and demoralized patient who for years has 'been done to' rather than 'negotiated with'.

A particular bonus with CBT in such patients is that the technique is broadly the same for the treatment of depression and for the treatment of residual psychotic symptoms. Once the approach has been established, it can be used across several areas as clinically indicated.

Case study

Diana suffered from bipolar affective disorder but had long periods of remission and normal functioning. This functioning, however, was compromised by chronic low self-esteem. As part of the CBT approach to this, Diana was asked to draw up a list of all her negative self-beliefs (e.g. 'nobody loves me', 'I am a bad person', 'I am unattractive'). In subsequent sessions, the task was to find objective evidence that contradicted or supported these beliefs (e.g. a letter or phone call from a friend or relative would contradict the belief that 'nobody loves me'). Each piece of evidence was written in a column for supporting the belief or contradicting it.

The therapist's task was to guide Diana and help her discover that the majority of objective evidence contradicted her beliefs. What supported her beliefs was her thinking.

Support and specific treatments

It is easy, with the current emphasis on evidence-based practice, to overlook the importance for depressed individuals of simple support and counselling. It makes a real difference when you are struggling with low mood (even if it may resolve without specific treatments) to have it recognized and talked about. Confirming that you can appreciate what the patient is going through—that this, for example, is a particularly difficult patch—can make a real difference. Not only does it reduce the isolation and fear that are such a feature of feeling depressed, it can legitimize a more measured approach to dealing with things. If your patient realizes that they are depressed, they may not drive themselves so hard and so give themselves space to recover. Sometimes this healthy use of the 'sick role' may be all that is needed.

Sometimes, patients with severe mental illness may need specific counselling, such as bereavement counselling or treatment for post-traumatic stress disorder. The indications for their use and their practice are essentially the same as for individuals without severe mental illness. However, greater sensitivity and judgement may be required to detect that need, and generally a slower, more supportive approach is necessary.

Bipolar disorder

In patients with bipolar disorder, there can be a risk with using antidepressants, as these may precipitate hypomania (Chapter 16). There is no easy solution to this. Patients may need the antidepressant, so the only approach is to be cautious and highly vigilant in monitoring. This is where proactive community outreach really comes into its own, as few patients complain of an elevation in mood—and families often interpret it early on as a welcome recovery from the depression. After hypomania, a period of depression is almost inevitable. Indeed, there are those who consider it an integral phase of the disorder. It is not normally necessary to prescribe antidepressants immediately.

Weeks, or sometimes even months, of hypomanic overactivity are understandably exhausting. We warn our patients to expect a collapse and to be optimistic that it will resolve fairly quickly. Side effects of drugs used to control the hypomania can also result in the patient feeling flat, exhausted, and apathetic. It is very difficult to get the balance absolutely right as sensitivity to both the therapeutic impact and the side effects of the tranquillizers changes rapidly as the hypomania resolves. The dose that may have been barely enough when the patient was high can suddenly cause overwhelming side effects.

The psychological aspects of recovering from hypomania also need to be worked through. Often, when high, the patient will have done things that later they deeply regret and about which they are embarrassed. These feelings will fade eventually but, in our experience, they are best acknowledged rather than skirted around. There is no formula for how to do this; judge each case individually. Broach the issue too early and it will be too painful to discuss and be hotly denied. Leave it too long and it may be stale and already resolved, and you may be accused of exaggeration. It is probably best to mention it fairly early and see how the patient responds. Tact is needed to air the issue without rubbing it in.

Avoiding talking about things can set up an unhealthy dynamic, introducing tension into the relationship. We have found that gentle, but penetrating, exploration of incidents that occurred during a period of florid illness can lead to a remarkable strengthening of the therapeutic relationship, especially if you and the patient were involved in them.

Anxiety disorders

Diagnosed agoraphobia and panic disorders seem relatively unusual in the severely mentally ill. Nevertheless, persisting high levels of arousal and tension are far from rare. Isolation resulting in becoming housebound is common, but it can be very difficult to be sure if such withdrawal is due more to apathy and negative symptoms or fear of confronting the world outside. The published literature on treating phobic disorders is generally unhelpful, as individuals with severe mental illness and psychotic disorders are almost invariably excluded from studies. Our experience is that the same principles of management apply, although they need to be used with discretion and sensitivity.

Most treatment of anxiety disorders is informed by behaviour therapy principles. Fears are understood as normal phenomena, albeit exaggerated in some patients. Time and energy are not expended in an exhaustive attempt to understand exactly how they arose but in helping overcome them. Support and encouragement are often enough: helping the individual face the worry by going with them to a new day centre, or accompanying them to a shop where they made a fuss when they were last ill.

Graded exposure

When this is not enough, then 'graded exposure' (often called 'desensitization' or 'reciprocal inhibition') can be very successful. This common-sense, simple approach consists of breaking the task down into small, manageable steps. The individual steps do not raise the patients' anxiety levels more than they can cope with. Having done it, you repeat the achievement together until it generates no significant anxiety before attempting the next step. There are several self-help books explaining the principles and practice of simple behavioural techniques.

The important lesson is to think through the steps with the patient, having explained and discussed exactly why you believe the approach to be a good idea and what it involves. The trick is to be very explicit, give clear recognition and praise when each goal has been achieved, and not to rush. Asking patients to rate their anxiety level on a scale during each attempt is now usual. We have found this overcomplicated and generally not that helpful with more severely ill patients who may find being asked to do the rating stressful in itself. Better, on the whole, simply to make sure that the arousal is tolerable. You should expect the odd bad days. Make sure that the patient is warned to expect them so that they are not misinterpreted as a failure of the treatment.

Most programmes of graded exposure involve a mixture of accompanied exercises and 'homework' in which the patient practises on their own what you have achieved together. Your presence reduces anxiety, so doing the same thing alone is still a challenge. Often with severely ill patients in outreach care, we downplay the homework and accompany the patient throughout each of the steps until the goal has been achieved. Only then do we encourage consolidation alone.

Medication

There is no conflict between taking a psychological approach to helping patients manage their anxiety and using medication; there is no 'either-or' about medicine or psychological interventions. Indeed, some early behavioural studies of graded exposure showed they were more successful if augmented by medications (either benzodiazepines or tricyclic antidepressants).

For individuals with psychotic disorders, the mild sedative effects of their antipsychotic medications can be utilized in managing anxiety. It is quite common for patients to ask us to increase their dose of antipsychotic temporarily when they are going through a stressful period. We do this often when there are family or external stressors, or even if there is nothing obvious but the patient reports increasing anxiety or poor sleep. The effect is probably both pharmacological and psychological—many patients see their medicine as a shield against stress, and simply knowing they are getting more helps.

Benzodiazepines have been severely criticized in the management of anxiety states because of the risks of dependence in long-term use. We regularly used them with the patients in our assertive outreach team and did not experience problems with dependence or abuse. The abuse problems we struggled with came more with anticholinergics, but this issue essentially evaporated with the advent of the newer antipsychotics. We used high doses of benzodiazepines in managing acute psychotic episodes in the community (Chapters 7 and 15) and often used them both as sleeping tablets and for short-term management of anxiety and situational stress without patients insisting on their continuation when the crisis was over. Perhaps severely ill patients are less hedonistic, or perhaps the sedative side effects of their antipsychotics are enough to contend with. Whatever the reason, we experienced very few problems either with dependence or disinhibition in the use of benzodiazepines.

Situational disorders

Post-traumatic stress disorder (PTSD)

Individuals with major mental illnesses are prey to stresses and crises as much, if not more, as other people. They can suffer bereavement or PTSD, and we need to be alert to these risks. Indeed, given the traumatic events experienced by many of our patients, it is surprising that there are not more cases of severe PTSD in individuals with long-standing mental illnesses.

One study showed that most of the symptoms of PTSD are present in patients with acute schizophrenia—but as part of general arousal, not as a discrete syndrome. Memories of traumatic experiences around admission to hospital and also on the ward can be powerful factors in determining patients' behaviour, although they may not amount to full-fledged PTSD. For some, it can lead to avoiding services, while for others, the vivid memory of the consequences of relapse can lead to improved treatment adherence.

Acknowledgement of the trauma is healing for the individual but also strengthens the therapeutic relationship. We, as staff, may have been part of the trauma, and we need to recognize it and take it seriously. As noted in Chapter 8 on the use of compulsion, we have found that our patients well able to relate positively to us while acknowledging that at times we may do things they do not want.

The development of an instrument to measure patients' perception of coercion—the MacArthur Admission Experience Survey (AES)—has stimulated research in the area of patients' experiences of compulsion (Gardner et al. 1993). One of the important findings of this research, which confirms our clinical experience, is that talking about these difficult events does help. 'Procedural justice'—one of the subscales of the AES, which measures whether the patient felt their opinion and concerns were sought (whether they had 'a voice')—made compulsion and admission less traumatic, even if they still disagreed with the decision (O'Donoghue et al. 2011).

Case study

Caroline became acutely paranoid following a protracted period of intermittent adherence to medication complicated by moderate use of cannabis. Within the space of a few days, she became convinced that someone was having an affair with her boyfriend. On one occasion she followed him to work after hearing people in the next-door flat discussing the details of the affair. When her outreach worker came to assess her with a doctor, she assaulted the outreach worker, believing that she was the one having the affair. Caroline was admitted to hospital with the help of the police. In hospital, she attempted to hang herself from a window bracket with her tights, seemingly in response to command hallucinations.

Within a few weeks, Caroline improved, gained partial insight into what had happened, and with good recall. She was shocked and frightened by what she had done. Her boyfriend had nearly left her as a result of her paranoia, she had nearly taken her own life, and she had assaulted her outreach worker. Helping her through this difficult time focused on rebuilding relationships and working on preventing such a dramatic relapse in the future.

Looking back, Caroline saw this admission as a watershed that forced her to acknowledge the diagnosis, the treatment, and the risks she took smoking cannabis. Her adherence and substance abuse improved to the extent that she has stayed out of hospital since.

Bereavement

An understanding of the process of bereavement—with its stages of shock and protest (including denial and disbelief), preoccupation, disorganization, and, finally, resolution (Bowlby 1961; Kübler-Ross 1969)—is essential for outreach. Even if your patient does not experience the loss of a family member, the illness itself constitutes a form of bereavement. Having to accept that their aspirations (university course, successful job, close family, etc.) have been profoundly, and often abruptly, lost with the onset of severe illness is very similar to a bereavement. Many patients (and families) never get beyond the phases of anger and denial in their grieving process. The result is an inability to adapt to the reality of the illness with the adjustments in their plans and routines that it requires.

Coming to terms with the reality and significance of the illness can be a long and painful process. Probably all of us have dealt at some time with angry young men with bipolar disorder who steadfastly refuse to discuss it, or cooperate with treatment until they have learnt 'the hard way'—that is, by experiencing several relapses. Usually, it is emotional resistance to the enormity of the change rather than any rational difficulties in understanding the facts or mastering the treatment regime. Recognizing the sense of loss that underlies the anger and denial is the first step to doing anything about it. Premature attempts at compliance enhancement strategies are unlikely to succeed until there has been some working through of these emotions. Patients will usually set the pace and determine when and how this can be done. We have to make clear to them that we are aware of what they have lost and that we are willing to engage with that loss.

Serious illnesses in the families of our patients can cause great distress. Anticipatory anxiety about impending loss can be as serious for patients as their families. Families (particularly parents, but sometimes siblings) describe a persisting worry about what is going to happen when they die. This is sometimes referred to as the 'WIAG' ('when I am gone') syndrome. Clinical experience often contrasts with this fear, and patients often survive the loss surprisingly well. Nevertheless, an impending loss can have a major impact on a patient.

We also need to be alert to the effects of a parent's grief, after the loss of a spouse, on the patient. We have had a small number of middle-aged schizophrenia patients who live with very aged parents who have devoted their lives to caring for the patient. Usually it is the mother. The patient's care can be substantially reduced or interrupted when the mother has to cope with her own grief over an illness or the death of her husband. It is important to ensure that she has the support and space to allow herself her own grief. Her concerns about now being the only one left to support her son or daughter will inevitably be heightened by her own loss.

There are a number of simple strategies to help. One is for us to spend more time with the patient, reassuring the mother that she can attend to her own emotional needs. Another is to spend time with the mother, encouraging her to talk through her grief and helping her with it. Alternatively, one might ensure that she gets prompt attention from a local bereavement service. Most of us will do a bit of all three!

Case study

John had lived at home with his parents for over 20 years, since his first breakdown. He led an ordered, if somewhat unexciting life. Without constant support from the team, he invariably stopped his medication and relapsed—neither he nor we could understand why, as he was generally satisfied with things when well.

His father suffered from severe asthma and hypertension and was housebound. He was taciturn and rather critical of his son, but otherwise had nothing to do with him. His mother was an energetic and outwardly happy individual who did everything for John. She said that she had long since come to terms with his illness, thought he was a 'lovely lad', and took pride in how she and her two daughters looked after him.

His father died suddenly (though not unexpectedly) and John seemed unperturbed by it. In the months following the funeral, he began to deteriorate and we had difficulty understanding this—he denied any worry or grief. Only slowly did it dawn on us that, although his mother was still as committed to him, she was struggling to deal with her own grief and loneliness. Whilst John was still getting his meals cooked and his washing done, he was not getting the same input and support he was used to.

Helping John's mother to take her own needs seriously was not at all easy. Only by engaging his sisters were we able to make any progress at all. Even then, things remained rocky for over a year, and John had his first admission for several years.

'Neurotic disorders'

We have emphasized in this chapter that individuals with severe and psychotic disorders are prey to most things that can befall those who do not suffer from them. Not surprisingly, they may be less concerned about symptoms that would worry us—they have much more serious problems to contend with. They can, however, display a range of 'neurotic' symptoms, either the so-called non-specific neurotic symptoms embodied in depression and anxiety, or more specific problems such as obsessive-compulsive symptoms, somatization, or eating disorders. Again, the research literature is rarely helpful, as most specialist units exclude patients with severe mental illness.

Obsessions and compulsions

A significant proportion of psychotic patients display repetitive thoughts or actions. For most, these cause no distress and are often considered 'mannerisms' or, occasionally, 'stereotypies'. For a smaller number, the repetitions and intrusions are distressing and have the quality of obsessions or compulsions, although they may not be resisted as strongly as in usual cases. There is a small group of schizophrenia patients whose hallucinatory experiences demonstrate obsessional features (i.e. they are 'obliged' to hear the voices repeatedly).

We take a pragmatic approach to trying to help with such complications. For a couple of patients, we found some improvement with SSRIs, but it has not been spectacular. The behavioural approaches we have used have been aimed more at reducing the impact of the thoughts and actions on the patient's life and minimizing their impact on those around them. CBT is increasingly being employed for persisting, distressing symptoms in psychosis. We are not aware of any formalized reports of its use with this problem, but it would seem worth a try. If the patient is not distressed and there is no social impact from the symptoms, we generally think it is best to leave well alone.

Eating disorders and diet

Patients can develop all sorts of strange eating habits—but then, so can any of us. We have a number of patients with very specific diets, some of which are quite healthy and some of which are not. Some of these have delusional origins—we had one patient in our Wandsworth assertive outreach team who has delusions about China and will only eat what he considered to be 'Chinese' food, although most of us would not recognize it as such.

Concern about weight and diet is increasingly common in all our patients, particularly women, because of weight gain from atypical antipsychotics. A number develop a form of bulimia nervosa as a consequence of repeatedly trying and failing to diet. Dietary and exercise advice is clearly necessary in these instances, although we have had little success, and sadly the literature seems to confirm that we are not alone (Phelan et al. 2001; Osborn et al. 2007). We have had some modest success with younger male patients who can use exercise and training both as a control for their weight and as a source of self-esteem. Overall, however, the aim must be to try to prevent weight gain.

Case study

Marie suffers from severe bipolar affective disorder, manic type, and requires intensive interventions to manage her at home during periods of elation. She sees her main problem, however, as her attempts to control her weight and the consequent binge eating. It took two years of working with Marie, around her 'core' psychiatric symptoms, before she first discussed her eating disorder. She describes binge eating, vomiting, guilt, and use of stimulants (coffee, smoking, and procyclidine) to excess—all to reduce her appetite.

Conclusions

Working in community outreach with the severely mentally ill requires us to achieve a fine balance. We must develop and maintain the specialist skills appropriate to this patient group, but must also not lose sight of the fact that they are, in important ways, more like the general population than they are different. Our main task is to help them manage their psychosis so that they can lead as normal a life as possible. For this reason, we must focus on the complexities of these long-term disorders. We must use techniques such as structured assessments to ensure that we do not become so embroiled in their day-to-day existence that we fail to see the wood for the trees. On the other hand, we need to have a sensitivity to their own unique problems, including the time-limited disorders (such as depression and anxiety) that affect the severely mentally ill as they do all of us.

We would argue that being alert to these 'less technical' aspects of management serves another purpose beyond making sure our patients get the treatment they need. It constantly reminds us that we are dealing with *people* not *disorders* or *illnesses*. It reminds us also that the people we are dealing with are more like us than they are different. The history of psychiatry teaches us that even the best-intentioned staff can lose sight of this when constantly working with very dependent and disabled individuals.

Substance misuse/dual diagnosis

Introduction

Psychotic illnesses are increasingly complicated by alcohol and drug misuse, as patients no longer spend long periods restricted in hospital or residential institutions. When patients are treated in the community, the benefits of social inclusion can be offset by greater exposure to drugs and alcohol. The term 'dual diagnosis patients' will be used throughout this chapter to refer to people with a psychotic illness plus harmful or hazardous substance misuse, which includes alcohol, any legal or illegal drugs, or both. 'Dual disorders' is commonly used in the US, as is the term 'co-morbidity'. Diagnostic classification systems differentiate between people with a primary psychotic illness moderated (usually negatively) by substance misuse, and people who have shorter psychotic episodes (beyond the expected effects of intoxication) induced and attributed to recent substance misuse. In community outreach teams, our work is usually with people with a primary severe and enduring mental illness complicated by drug or alcohol misuse.

Dual diagnosis carries additional problems for both patients and services. Integrating substance abuse strategies and more traditional mental health interventions in the same community team is an essential response for these individuals.

Service responses

One very real problem for these patients has been the reluctance of either community mental health services or addiction services to work wholeheartedly with them. The response of services was often one of 'passing the buck'. Interviewing key professionals and reviewing local strategies in the UK, Rorstad and Checinski (1996) concluded:

> Where major disabling mental health problems co-existed with an addiction problem, intervention strategies appeared to be based on the assumption that until the mental health problem had been addressed there was little or nothing that could be done by a substance misuse service to help the patient. The problem with dealing with psychoses or other major and disabling mental health problems was seen

as beyond the training and resource competence of a substance misuse service even where that service was staffed by qualified mental health nurses and medical personnel.[1]

Patients with dual diagnosis straddle the divide between general and addiction services. Treatment in parallel systems appears to be ineffective and inefficient as clinicians fail to modify their models of working (Drake et al. 1995).

The conflicting assumptions of the models of care that traditionally operate in addiction and mental health services are outlined in Table 19.1. These differences hinder the establishment of partnerships, and patients have great difficulty finding their place within the system even when motivated. The most fundamental conflict arises between outreach care (taking the service to ambivalent individuals) and clinic-based treatment programmes (designed to test that patients are motivated). For addiction services, attendance at appointments is expected, and discharge from the service will usually follow repeated non-attendance.

In the wider social care context, dual diagnosis patients are often excluded from housing and residential facilities, especially when illicit drug use is involved. Possession or use of cannabis in a mental health hostel is unlikely to lead to the involvement of the police but is likely to jeopardize that placement,

Table 19.1 Differences in approach between addiction services and community outreach

Substance misuse services	Community outreach services
◆ Confrontational approach	◆ Emphasis on engagement and collaboration
◆ Clinic-based	◆ Outreach is standard
◆ Motivation important element of entry criteria	◆ Optimistic about developing motivation
◆ Psychotropic medication is discouraged	◆ Antipsychotics actively prescribed
◆ Treatment episodes are focused and time limited	◆ Comprehensive and not time limited
◆ Defaulters not normally followed up	◆ Assertively follow up patients who do not engage
◆ Compulsory treatment not used	◆ Compulsory treatment a common feature
◆ Group therapy widely used	◆ Groups poorly tolerated by severely ill psychotic patients

[1] Reproduced from Rorstad, P. and Checinski, K. (1996) *Dual diagnosis: facing the challenge*, Wynne House Publishing, Guildford.

because the hostel needs to protect its legal status. Conversely, drug rehabilitation programmes rarely tolerate residents with severe mental health problems. Homelessness or prison are frequent consequences (Lehman and Dixon 1995). Guidance has helped to clarify the desired service response: mainstream mental health services take the responsibility for meeting the needs of people with a dual diagnosis, but they seek support and expert input from addiction services where required (Department of Health 2002). Integrated care from a single team is more effective than parallel care from both services and sequential approaches to treatment (NICE 2011). Such a model is also more affordable and sustainable.

Incidence

In the US, 40–60 per cent of patients with severe mental illness are estimated as also having a problem with alcohol and drug abuse (Mueser et al. 1995). The large CATIE medication trial of 1493 patients with chronic schizophrenia found that 37 per cent of participants met diagnostic criteria for substance use disorder (Swartz et al. 2006). A South London community team study identified substance abuse in 36.3 per cent of 171 psychotic patients in contact with the service (Menezes et al. 1996). Alcohol abuse was most common at 20.5 per cent; 4.7 per cent had a problem with drugs only; and 11.1 per cent with both. Cannabis was the most common of the drugs abused. Men were twice as likely as women to suffer substance abuse. Among men, there was a trend for drug use, but not alcohol use, to decrease with age. Both decreased with age for women. The authors acknowledge that these findings cannot be widely generalized, but they give a benchmark to compare local experience. The market choices and availability of drugs changes over time in the general population and is mirrored in the habits of the people we work with. For example, we saw a rise in the use 'crack' cocaine by our patients some years ago, and now the so-called designer drugs or 'legal highs' are new players in the old drama (Zawilska 2011). Cannabis and alcohol use, however, constitute the bulk of our work in dual diagnosis.

Associated findings for dual diagnosis patients

Many of the outcomes, service use, and demographic associations shown in Table 19.2 interact with each other. For example, the greater use of inpatient services will also be related to the association between dual diagnosis and poorer compliance with medication. But even those patients who regularly take their medication but abuse substances are readmitted to hospital sooner

Table 19.2 Associated findings for dual diagnosis patients

Characteristic	Study findings
◆ Greater use of inpatient services	30 per cent more likely to stay in hospital more than 60 days and three times more likely to stay more than 120 days (Menezes et al. 1996)
◆ Worse clinical outcomes	Greater symptom severity (Lehman et al. 1993)
◆ Worse social outcomes	Poorer housing and occupation stability (Lehman et al. 1993)
◆ Greater incidence of violence and aggression	Strong association between violence and polysubstance misuse in psychosis patients (Witt et al. 2013; Steadman et al. 1998; Fazel et al. 2009)
◆ Greater incidence of suicide	Among people with schizophrenia, a three times increased risk in patients with coexisting drug misuse (Hawton et al. 2005)
◆ Demographically younger and male	Male patients are twice as likely as female to have dual diagnosis. Drug abuse diminishes with age in men, but not alcohol abuse (Menezes et al. 1996)
◆ Poorer compliance with prescribed medication	Medication non-compliance significantly higher (Owen et al. 1996)
◆ More contact with the criminal justice system	Offending generally of low severity—theft, alcohol offences, driving offences (Scott et al. 1998)
◆ More use of A&E services	Greater utilization by current abusers (Bartels et al. 1993)
◆ Increased costs for services	'Core' psychiatric costs increased by £1046 per annum (McCrone et al. 2000)

compared to medication-adherent patients who do not use substances (Hunt et al. 2002).

Assessment

Structured assessments for the presence and degree of substance misuse, of harmful use, and of dependence will help target interventions appropriately and guide treatment. Inadequate assessment can lead to both a neglect of substance abuse interventions (e.g. education, detoxification, and counselling) and over-treatment of the psychotic illness through misdiagnosis (Drake and Mercer-McFadden 1995).

A brief drug and drink history carried out in a non-judgemental, 'matter-of-fact', and confidential manner will maximize disclosure. Acutely ill patients, or those with cognitive deficits, may significantly under-report use. We find that well-engaged patients will acknowledge alcohol and cannabis use but rarely admit to the use of crack cocaine, opiates, and amphetamines. Although we know our patients well, we are still surprised by revelations of covert drug and alcohol misuse. Urine drug screens for patients admitted to hospital can often provide unexpected information. Similarly, liver enzymes can indicate recent heavy alcohol use. Simply smelling alcohol on a patient's breath is a cheap guide to alcohol use, as is the observation of pupillary changes, behaviour changes, or drugs paraphernalia and empty beer cans in the home. Family and friends are often keen to provide information on drug and alcohol use and to express their concerns.

A realistic approach to sensible drinking and harmful use of illicit drugs is necessary. Many of our patients regularly use alcohol and cannabis and describe broadly positive effects of reduced arousal and improved social interaction and mood. Others patients show clearly detrimental effects from their alcohol abuse, such as aggression and disruption of relationships, gastric problems, impulsive behaviour, depression, and forgetfulness. Cannabis is associated with a worsening of psychotic symptoms, especially paranoia, for many vulnerable patients.

For alcohol, one unit is equivalent to half a pint of ordinary-strength beer or lager, one small glass of wine, or a single measure of spirits. Safe drinking guidance was lowered in 2016 for men from 21 units per week, so that now men and women are advised not to regularly drink more than 14 units a week and to spread this drinking over three days or more.

Co-morbid substance abuse disorder is diagnosed not only on the quantity of intake but on the basis of the adverse social, psychological, vocational, or medical consequences (Drake and Mercer-McFadden 1995). With dual diagnosis patients, the substance misuse history may need to be brief and tailored to what the patient can reasonably tolerate.

There are a number of alcohol and drug misuse assessment resources and questionnaires available online from public health agencies and charities that can be performed with people in their homes. Typically they help calculate risk from self-reported intake, patterns of use (such as bingeing or persistent use), and consequences and behaviours of use (such as being unable to remember what happened the night before) (see Box 19.1). For a detailed account of components required for a full assessment, see NICE (2011).

Community outreach for dual diagnosis

Outreach is a good foundation for delivering specialized interventions aimed at combating the harmful and hazardous effects of substance misuse. Over and above the ambivalence about their habits, patients with alcohol and drug abuse are poor at attending outpatient clinics (Burns et al. 1993b). This is not

Box 19.1 Elements of a full substance misuse history

Past and current alcohol and drug use

◆ age when started misuse (including nicotine)
◆ types and quantities of alcohol and drugs taken
◆ frequency of misuse
◆ awareness of effects on mental state—positive and negative
◆ routes of administration, use of clean equipment and sharing habits if injecting, HIV/hepatitis B or C status, knowledge of modes of transmission, use of condoms, supply of needles and syringes
◆ experience of overdose
◆ periods of abstinence and triggers for relapse
◆ symptoms when unable to obtain alcohol or drugs
◆ cost of use

Medical history

◆ complications of misuse—abscesses, gastric and liver problems, hepatitis B or C/HIV
◆ accidents or head injuries
◆ cognitive effects of alcohol—Wernicke's encephalopathy, Korsakoff's syndrome, peripheral neuropathy
◆ diet
◆ previous addiction treatment or rehabilitation

Social history

◆ high-risk peer group
◆ drug or alcohol misuse in partner or family
◆ effect of use on relationships, family, work, housing

Forensic history

◆ currently offending
◆ past contact with criminal justice system

surprising given periods of intoxication when good intentions are easily forgotten. Further barriers arise if the patient has a chaotic lifestyle and disorganized thinking from a psychotic illness. At its very least, outreach can help the patient deal with the practical problems that prevent them getting treatment. In addition, stable living conditions, symptom management, daytime activity or distraction, and development of a non-abusing peer group are part of a comprehensive approach to harm minimization and treatment.

The New Hampshire model (McHugo et al. 1999) incorporates these elements of assertive engagement, attention to basic needs such as housing and finance, and harm reduction delivered through case management. Non-confrontational approaches to the management of substance abuse are preferred and supported by experience and research. Treatment goals are often limited to harm reduction and compromising on drug or alcohol use rather than abstinence. Principles of collaboration fit the needs of dual diagnosis patients well. This integrated model consists of a self-sufficient assertive outreach team set up to work exclusively with dual diagnosis patients. Expertise in addiction is incorporated into a team that has a clear remit to focus equally on substance abuse and psychosis. The approach rests on the assumption that dual diagnosis patients should be treated within the mental health system and not the addictions system.

The New Hampshire model uses a four-stage approach to individual and group treatment of substance abuse:

1. engagement stage
2. persuasion stage
3. active treatment
4. relapse prevention (Osher and Kofoed 1989)—similar to the motivational interviewing approach (Miller and Rollinick 1991)

Motivational interviewing

Motivational interviewing is particularly useful for dual diagnosis patients in that it guides interventions with those who lack 'insight' and motivation to change their behaviour. (The traditional model refers to this as the 'pre-contemplative phase'—the patient is not yet considering reducing or stopping harmful use.) The goal of the therapist is to guide the patient from pre-contemplation towards a readiness to change and beyond to reduction and possibly eventual abstinence.

The emphasis is on helping the patient review their beliefs and behaviours and to expose cognitive dissonance between their goals and their current substance abuse in order to generate motivation. The 'pre-contemplative' patient is

---

Box 19.2 Stages in motivational interviewing

1. Pre-contemplative—the patient is not ready or interested in behaviour changes.
2. Contemplative—the patient is uncertain or ambivalent about change.
3. Preparation—the patient is ready for change.
4. Action—change is occurring; interventions assist change.
5. Maintenance—interventions aimed at maintaining healthy behaviour.

---

given information and education to help them contemplate change and move to the 'preparation stage'. One method is to ask the patient to draw up a list of positive and negative aspects of their drug or alcohol abuse. When the ratio of perceived costs and benefits tips towards costs (e.g. crisis or hospitalization resulting from drug abuse), the patient may be motivated to change, and is then guided to the 'action stage' of how to proceed with changing their behaviour. Finally, the 'maintenance stage' is about securing abstinence and positive behaviours (see Box 19.2).

Such sophisticated approaches are hindered by the cognitive impairments that affect some patients with severe mental illness. Impairments of memory, attention, and information processing put the onus on case managers to make the intervention process clear and unambiguous, with frequent repetition of educational information and checking for understanding. We all suffer from denial of the consequences of our current behaviour—paying tomorrow for what we can have today. Making these links between the present and future may be difficult for our patients. Living marginalized and impoverished lives, they may feel they have less to lose. Potential losses can act as motivating forces for others (Carey 1995).

Further substance abuse interventions

Alcoholics Anonymous

The classic intervention for addiction is the 12-step approach of Alcoholics Anonymous (AA) and Narcotics Anonymous. AA groups are underused by persons with dual diagnosis, and mental health professionals are cautious about referring patients to AA because of fears that the AA group will discourage them from taking prescribed medication (Meissen et al. 1999). In addition, AA is founded upon a self-help, moral, and spiritual model, which can seem out of step with mainstream psychiatric practice. It is a much more pervasive approach in the USA than in Europe. Advantages of the model, however, include a powerful support network available to members. New members can obtain a 'sponsor' from the group and experienced members act as guides.

Pharmacological treatment

The use of medication in the management of dual diagnosis can be for the clinical management of detoxification; to prevent relapse; to control side effects; or to treat any causes of substance misuse, such as depression.

Detoxification using substitute medication is necessary for patients with physical dependence. Substitute medication (usually tapering doses of benzodiazepines and anticonvulsants) reduces the risks of delirium tremens and grand mal convulsions associated with alcohol withdrawal. Outreach provides the supports for a home-based detoxification with frequent or daily calls, supervision of substitute drug administration, and longer detoxification time scales. This may not be a safe option for all patients. Poorly motivated patients may need to get away from the home environment for it to succeed. Availability of carers at home may be a critical factor. Psychological support of the patient during and after detoxification is vital to prevent relapse into addiction and for their concurrent mental illness. Inpatient detoxification may be safer for those with severe physical problems, but pressure on the availability of hospital beds makes this a difficult choice.

The pharmacological treatment of cocaine and amphetamine dependence and craving has not been established (Vocci and Montoya 2009). Benzodiazepines for alcohol detoxification, and methadone (a synthetic opiate agonist) for opiate dependence, are safe and effective. The current guidelines are beyond the scope of this book and will vary between clinicians.

Antabuse (disulfiram) has been widely used in the treatment of uncomplicated alcohol abuse. It causes uncomfortable headache and flushing if the patient drinks alcohol. It has little place in the care of dual diagnosis patients, as it can exacerbate psychosis and be dangerous. Patients can drink safely only several days after stopping treatment with antabuse. It is therefore most effective in highly motivated patients or where daily supervision of the medication is available from a family member (Schwartz and Lehman 1995).

Relapse prevention

Relapse is a hallmark of addictive disorders, and is the rule rather than the exception after a successful course of treatment.
(Carey 1995)

'Keep away from people, places, and things related to addiction' is a slogan used in AA as a relapse prevention technique. Identify the relapse scenarios and triggers, and rehearse coping strategies. In our work we can turn talking into behaviour by enacting situations and asking the patient to say how they would refuse an offer of drugs or alcohol or an invite to the pub. For dual diagnosis patients, this involves contingency planning for how to cope should their mental health deteriorate and inhibitions or judgement become affected. Unstable bipolar patients have marked problems when going high. Family education and support will be an integral part of both treatment and relapse prevention.

Harm minimization

Harm minimization concentrates on reducing the damage that substance abuse brings to the patient and their networks. The concept originated from helping opiate abusers with strategies such as needle exchanges, where the abuse is tolerated but assistance given to reduce very serious associated risks. For the 'pre-contemplative' patient, this may be the only approach possible. Intervention on behalf of a patient to protect their tenancy, diffuse a conflict, or prevent offending behaviour likely to lead to prosecution helps to minimize complications and preserve supportive networks still available to the patient. Even helping a patient change from spirits or high-strength lager to normal-strength beer, or providing meals on wheels and vitamins, are potent harm minimization strategies.

Case study

David drinks 20 cans of Guinness a day, suffers from schizophrenia, has a poor diet, diabetes, liver damage, severe tremor, memory loss, and is vulnerable to exploitation. The team had never known David when he was not drinking this amount.

David's main concern was the amount of money he spent on alcohol, and this functioned as the key motivating factor. Individual counselling and motivational approaches proved unsuccessful because of his poor ability to retain and understand information. After lengthy negotiation, David agreed to inpatient detoxification, as he believed he would save money. We felt that a routine detoxification and return to his flat, even with daily contact, would not make a lasting impact, as he lived alone and had no other activities besides drinking. However, he was someone who would follow 'no drinking' rules in day centres, hospital, hostels, etc.

We delayed admission and detoxification in order to explore the option of residential accommodation on a permanent or rehabilitative basis with David. We started taking him to a mental health resource centre daily, where he could get a meal and a bath and spend periods of time, up to five hours, abstinent.

Given his level of psychiatric illness, a rehabilitative 'dry' house was difficult to find. David was ambivalent about leaving his flat, even for a few months, fearing he might lose it.

Eventually, we were able to identify and finance a three-month residential placement in a dry house. David was detoxified in hospital and went directly to the dry house. We were able to assess his mental state, physical health, and tremor more accurately once he had dried out. The outreach team continued to be intensively involved throughout. Whilst David was in the hostel, we applied for appointeeship of his benefit money. This acted as a further safeguard against relapse, as money to buy alcohol was controlled and limited.

The team continues to see David frequently now he is back at home. We help supervise his psychiatric and physical medication, check his blood sugars, help him maintain his flat and finances, and support him in staying off alcohol. David still has periods of binge drinking but has not returned to regular use or physical dependence. His physical health has been stabilized and his mental health, ability to retain information, and interaction with others has improved somewhat.

David's care plan and risk management plans are shown in Tables 19.3 and 19.4, respectively.

Table 19.3 Summary care plan

Patient's name: David G. Address: 21 Harvest House, Savona Estate, Battersea Phone: 0207 622 xxxx Date of birth: 30/7/61 GP: Alexander Phone: 0207 535 xxxx	CMHT: ACT TEAM Phone: 0208 877 xxxx New patient: NO If NO, date of review: ...... 22/5/16 .... Diagnosis: 1 Schizophrenia .... F 20.0 2 Alcohol dependence syndrome F 10.2	
Assessed needs or problem	**Intervention**	**Resp. of**
Poor adherence with medication and treatment due to cognitive deficits	◆ Periods of supervised medication, ◆ Psychiatric and physical medication dispensed in dosette box. Supervise on each visit. ◆ Assist with monitoring blood sugar by BM stick on each visit.	AC
Risk of relapse of severe alcohol abuse	◆ Accompany to resource centre two times weekly to develop non-drinking environment and activities. ◆ Liaise with appointee to manage David's money, limiting amount available to buy alcohol. ◆ Reinforce David's goal to save money and other psycho-educational and motivational messages about risk to health of alcohol binges or return to regular use. ◆ Give practical assistance with maintaining accommodation, dealing with correspondence, personal care, and household tasks.	AC
Difficulty managing personal and household affairs	◆ Home help once per week.	AC

Table 19.4 Risk management plan

Name: David G.			
Categories of risk identified:			
Aggression and violence	NO	Severe self-neglect	NO
Exploitation (self or others)	YES	Risk to children & young adults	NO
Suicide and self-harm	NO	Other (please specify)	

Current factors which suggest there is significant apparent risk:

(For example: alcohol or substance misuse; specific threats; suicidal ideation; violent fantasies; anger; suspiciousness; persecutory beliefs; paranoid feelings or ideas about particular people)

David has been exploited by local drinkers who have threatened him, used his flat, and taken money from him.

Clear statement of anticipated risk(s):

(Who is at risk; how immediate is that risk; how severe; how ongoing)

David is at risk of assault from other residents of his estate who abuse alcohol and have intimidated and extorted money from him. Low risk to staff of assault by these people during home visit to his flat.

Action plan:

(Including names of people responsible for each action and steps to be taken if plan breaks down)

David encouraged not to allow access to these people. Police to be informed when further incidents of extortion occur. Allocated team member not to visit alone when it is known others are in his flat, phone to check this before visiting each day.

Date completed: 22/5/16	Review date: 22/11/16

Conclusions

Compared to the general population, people with severe mental illness have an increased risk of developing substance abuse and dependence disorders (Regier et al. 1990). This is particularly evident for young male patients. Reasons for this are complex and include social isolation and high rates of unemployment. Some develop substance abuse because of the distress from their psychiatric symptoms or due to cognitive impairments. Involvement with substance abuse peer groups may also appear less stigmatizing to them than involvement with psychiatric patients.

Psychotic patients also appear to be more sensitive to drug and alcohol use—smaller amounts destabilize them. They may suffer greater consequences of substance misuse such as more frequent hospitalization and difficulties finding a place within separate treatment systems for dealing with the two disorders.

Accepting responsibility for this group of patients within one integrated treatment team is recommended. Most substance abuse treatments can be incorporated into community outreach practice with appropriate training and commitment. These include harm minimization strategies, relapse prevention strategies, housing protection, motivational interviewing, individual counselling, practical assistance, pharmacological treatment of withdrawal, and family work. We should, however, be cautious about assuming that substance abuse interventions are unambiguous, evidence-based strategies with a high success rate. Real life is more complex. Many of our patients have freely chosen patterns of drug or alcohol use for which they do not want our help, however much hardship and conflict arises from their use. In addition, many mental health staff find this 'volitional' aspect of substance abuse sits uncomfortably with our approach to mental illnesses where tolerance often relies on the recognition that the patient has no direct control over their illness. We have, however, a responsibility to manage these two somewhat conflicting models and to offer help and seek out practical and effective interventions.

Chapter 20

Finance and appointeeship

Introduction

Many patients with severe and persistent mental illness will identify money as their main problem in surviving in the community. If the key worker and team can help with this problem, then they have a head start. It is an invaluable engagement tool, as well as ensuring the patient can survive outside hospital.

In community outreach, one soon recognizes that financial crises are a frequent cause in themselves for patients to self-present at hospital, or that the stress they impose increases the risk of relapse. We neglect finances at our peril. Do not assume that because the patient has not informed you of any problems, that they are receiving their full benefit entitlement or that the rent or electricity is being paid. Look out for unopened brown envelopes by the door and make sensitive enquiries—especially with patients with a history of neglecting to pay bills or to reapply for benefits.

Much of a case manager's time will be spent assisting and advocating for patients' personal finance. High rates of unemployment due to the disruptive effects of frequent illness and hospitalization limit independent means of support. Complex, frequently revised, and often bewildering rules for eligibility and applications for welfare benefits require intervention or advocacy for even the most able of our patients.

This chapter will describe the broad sweep of benefits, other sources of help, and practical interventions such as appointeeship (also known as representative payeeship) to help people manage their money and keep their community tenure. Because of national specificities and frequent amendments to the names and rules applied to state benefits, we will not attempt to describe the fine detail.

State welfare benefits

The state offers financial protection for people because of either low income (means-tested) or against specific criteria such as disability, maternity, age, and previous contributions through taxation (non-means-tested).

Means-tested benefits

Means-tested benefits are designed to ensure an individual's or family's income does not fall below the poverty line. Income support and housing benefit are both means-tested. Savings and any other income must be declared. Depending on this assessment, payment can be either a 'top-up' or meet the entire cost of living or rent. The following examples taken from a mental health charity fact sheet (Rethink Mental Illness 2015) indicate the complexity in the UK context for people able to work (Universal Credit) and those unable to work through illness or disability (Income-Related Employment Support Allowance) (see Box 20.1).

Non-means-tested benefits

If a patient is unable to work through illness or disability according to the rules outlined in Box 20.1, and has paid enough contributions through taxation in the relevant years, they can qualify for contribution-based Employment Support Allowance (ESA), regardless of other income. Many patients with severe mental illness, though, will be eligible for Personal Independence Payment (PIP), because their health condition or disability is long-term and they need help with personal care, daily living, or getting around. PIP applies to people with physical or mental disabilities. They do not need to have paid contributions through tax to qualify, and earnings and savings are not assessed. PIP can be claimed whether they are in work or not. Most of the time, the full amount of PIP is paid on top of other benefits or tax credits. PIP has two components: care and mobility, paid at two different levels, standard or enhanced. Enhanced-level payments provide for higher need. Depending on need, payment for both components is not uncommon.

A patient can claim PIP if they:

♦ are between the age of 16 and under pension age

♦ have a long-term condition or disability (existed for three months and expected to last for at least nine months)

♦ live in Great Britain and are not subject to immigration control

Needs are decided through the following:

♦ answers put on the application

♦ evidence and information from health and social care professionals

♦ possible face-to-face assessment with an independent health care professional commissioned by the benefits agency, who will provide the Department of Work and Pensions with a report

Box 20.1 Universal Credit

Universal Credit (UC) is being introduced to replace some existing benefits in some parts of the UK. In time, UC will replace all of the following benefits:

◆ Housing Benefit

◆ Income Support

◆ income-based Job Seeker's Allowance

◆ income-related Employment and Support Allowance

◆ Child Tax Credit

◆ Working Tax Credit

◆ Budgeting Loans

UC can be claimed if:

◆ you are aged between 18 and under the pension age; if you are aged 16 or 17, you may be able to get UC

◆ you live in Great Britain and not subject to immigration control

◆ you are not in education

◆ your household income is low and you don't have much in savings or capital

At the moment UC can only be claimed if you are:

◆ single

◆ childless

◆ able to work

◆ making a new claim for benefits

A work allowance enables some money to be earned without it affecting the amount of UC received. Money can be reduced depending on your living arrangements and whether you have children. For every £1 you earn above a certain limit, you will get 65p less UC.

Income-Related Employment and Support Allowance (ESA-IR)

Income-related ESA can be claimed if you have an illness or disability and have not paid enough contributions through taxation to qualify for contribution-based ESA. In this circumstance, the means test looks at income and savings or capital (over £6,000). Eligibility requires that you are:

(continued)

Box 20.1 Continued

- aged between 16 and under the pension age
- live in Great Britain
- not getting Statutory Sick Pay (SSP) (you can get a top-up of ESA-IR if in receipt of SSP)
- not getting Statutory Maternity Pay (SSP) (top-up as above)
- not getting Job Seeker's Allowance
- not getting Universal Credit

To get ESA, the Department for Work and Pensions has to understand that you cannot work because of your disability. They use the following information to decide:

- Work Capability Assessment/self-assessment
- supporting evidence or information from health and social care professionals
- face-to-face assessment with an independent health care professional from the approved centre, who will provide the Department for Work and Pensions with a report

To encourage people to gain skills, be socially included, and test their ability to work, there are conditions where you can claim ESA and perform 'permitted work'. Permitted work means that you need to follow certain rules on hours and amounts of earnings. Permitted work might, for example, include working on a voluntary basis, caring for a relative, or working as part of a treatment programme under medical supervision—as long as you don't earn more than £107.50 a week.

- Etc., etc.!

Initial claims to PIP are 'triaged' by telephone. If the basic entitlement conditions are met, a claimant questionnaire is issued, unless it is felt that mental or cognitive impairment makes this impractical.

Assessment covers the following activities:

- preparing food
- taking nutrition
- managing therapy or monitoring a health condition
- washing and bathing
- managing toilet needs or incontinence

- dressing and undressing
- communicating verbally
- reading and understanding signs, symbols, and words
- engaging with other people face-to-face
- making decisions about money
- planning and following journeys
- moving around

The assessment may feel more relevant to physical disability to many patients who may be put off by questions relating to ability to stand and distances able to walk, aided or unaided, in the mobility component. It is important to reassure patients that problems with planning and following journeys may be because they need prompting to do things due to poor motivation; need support because of anxiety and poor social and daily living skills; or because they might get distracted by voices, feel paranoid, or get lost. The assessor will be trying to determine if the claimant needs prompting to be able to undertake a journey to avoid overwhelming psychological distress.

Claimants can be supported by family members, carers, and community outreach workers. The benefits agency recognizes some patients will have additional support needs through the bureaucratic process of assessment, for example, by not being automatically disqualified if the forms do not come back on time.

The purpose of PIP is that extra money is paid to make a contribution to the extra costs incurred in living with a long-term condition or disability. The benefit allows patients to pay for assistance in the form of nursing care, meals on wheels, takeaway food, or any item to help them lead full, active, and more independent lives.

In reality, most psychiatric patients do not use their money directly for these purposes—though we did have one patient who placed an advert for someone to watch over her and keep her company through sleepless nights. Help with psychiatric problems for PIP purposes may include the following:

- prompting and reminding
- accompanying a patient to an activity or place
- supervision to ensure the patient remains safe or takes prescribed treatment
- emotional support
- practical help with shopping, eating, paying bills, reading mail, and the like

Benefits for carers

Caring for a friend or family member with severe mental illness clearly has financial costs, not least in reduced hours in paid employment. The state recognizes this with benefits aimed at carers. Carers also provide a valuable service, which would otherwise cost the state many times what they may claim in benefits.

In England, Scotland, and Wales, carers who look after an individual for at least 35 hours a week may be entitled to Carer's Allowance if the person they care for is entitled to benefits due to a long-term condition or disability. The carer must not be earning more than a set amount, and not in full-time education or studying more than 21 hours a week. There is also a scheme for carers to get a credit towards their state pension whilst not making any contributions because of their caring role, and to have a carer's premium to certain other benefits such as Universal Credit.

It is usually advantageous to make a claim for Carer's Allowance even though claiming can impact on other 'overlapping' benefits such as housing benefit. It is worth getting good benefits advice and a full benefit check, as you may be entitled to extra premiums within other benefits, and to ensure that the best combination of allowances is claimed for your circumstances.

Local sources of income and help

Despite the plethora of state benefits, they are inflexible and often paid infrequently. PIP is paid every four weeks, and budgeting across a long period can prove difficult for many patients. Teams need ready access to a small fund of money to help patients out in difficult situations, as well as to provide for some activities of social inclusion that might enable patients to engage or even work towards fostering treatment goals. We have used team finances to pay for a patient's dog to be boarded in kennels whilst he was in hospital. We have arranged with a local day centre that certain patients from our team, who cannot pay for meals, will still get them, and the team will be invoiced periodically.

Our knowledge of other external sources of financial assistance will help patients both to survive and to have a better quality of life. Examples are disabled travel permits, holiday grants from charities, and voluntary organizations able to provide furniture at minimal or no cost. Many leisure centres and cinemas give concessionary rates at off-peak times to people on benefits. Knowledge of such local resources should be shared with the team. Constructing a resource file at the team base containing charities' digests and information on local organizations and funds is a valuable investment of time.

Helping patients manage their money

The key worker is often directly involved in giving advice and practical help in personal finances. Along with relatives and carers, they are in the best position to know patients' needs and circumstances. The key worker must, however, be aware of their limitations and encourage the patient and carer in seeking expert welfare rights advice.

The recovery approach to daily living skills mean that, when possible, we should encourage patients to take control of their benefits, and offer support and advice only when needed. Even if the patient fills in only their name, address, date of birth, and personal details, this is preferable to the patient just handing you every envelope that comes through the door, unopened, for you to deal with. Spend time going through letters with patients so that they come to understand, and be less scared of, the jargon used. Similarly, coaching people on how to communicate with the benefits agency over the telephone enhances survival skills and encourages growth and responsibility.

Budgeting

Help with budgeting is a common and helpful intervention. Few patients, however, will be receptive to written budgets involving excessive calculations. Making the complexity of financial management easy by reducing budgeting to a set amount to spend on a daily basis can be helpful. For example, if a patient's total disposable weekly income is £120, they can afford to spend £17 per day. A written daily or weekly shopping list may be of more value than a written budget, in monetary terms. Daily disposable income can be broken down further to represent one packet of cigarettes, one takeaway meal, purchase of bread and milk, and money towards weekly toiletries and clothing or luxuries.

Practical steps to making limited money go further may involve accompanying the patient to their local shops and learning how to solve the problem of buying necessities from a limited budget using staple food items and the use of budget stores. The patient should be encouraged to prioritize and delay gratification for some items. For example, although a patient may want a mobile phone, it may not be possible to get it from one week's money and still have money for food. Spreading the cost over several weeks and, for instance, suggesting they buy a 'pay as you go' phone will ensure that crises over bills and food are less likely to occur.

Helping the patient to set up standing orders for any rent or bills means they only need to manage disposable income. In recent years, payment of welfare benefits by giro or cheque has been replaced by payment into a named bank account. Problems arise for patients unwilling or unable to open an account. In these circumstances, a scheme exists to collect payments from nominated outlets. The individual is issued with a card that doesn't need a PIN but requires a memorable date and proof of ID in order to collect. It is possible to have money deducted and redirected at source from people's benefits. This is often done by housing departments for rent arrears. Gas and electricity can be paid for on a 'pay as you go' basis through key- and card-based meters. This system avoids arrears but can be expensive and may also leave patients without necessary utilities at times.

Debt

Debts for overdue utility bills are not uncommon and can generally be dealt with by asking the company to accept payment by instalments. Banks and companies operate confidentiality policies for personal finances. The company will generally ask for written requests for payment by instalments signed by the patient, and often a letter from the patient authorizing the company to discuss details with the key worker, before they will even consider the matter. Local agencies such as the Citizen's Advice Bureau are free and offer expert assistance on debt and other matters.

For example, multiple and complicated debts involving so-called pay day loans, as well as store card and credit card debts, can quickly compound and may require an intervention plan. Advice bureaux can help set up debt management plans, non–legally binding arrangements managed by a third-party provider to deal with creditors for certain debts. These plans allow the debtor to pay back one monthly amount which is agreed between the creditors, and divided between them.

There are also online debt remedy tools that ask a set of questions and can provide advice and action plans dependent on responses. For example, the algorithm asks if you have recently received court papers or a bailiff's letter, and takes you through personal circumstances such as income, priority and other spending, living costs, assets, and the nature and extent of the debts.

In cases of acute and serious mental illness at the time of the purchase or contract, it is important to query whether the patient was clearly mentally ill and the creditor aware of their incapacity to understand the transaction. In that case, there is no binding contract and the debt cannot be enforced (e.g. a manic patient displaying multiple bizarre behaviours and delusions who orders a wedding dress and a pram from a department store).

Fraud

Benefits agencies take a tough line on fraud, which can easily be committed unintentionally by our patients. Failing to tell them about a change in your circumstances or care needs, failing to declare other income for means-tested benefits, and, especially, working whilst claiming benefits all constitute fraud. In general, we will advise a patient on their obligations when it becomes apparent that they have not fully informed the benefits agency of their activities. We will also advise them of the legitimate methods of returning to work and ways of preserving their benefits. They must also be advised that they run the risk of losing their benefit altogether if they deliberately mislead officials.

It can be tempting to turn a blind eye to benefit fraud—after all, our patients are often poor and disadvantaged—and some case managers even describe it as a form of advocacy! It is risky for the patient and risky for the therapeutic relationship (which only flourishes in conditions of honesty and trust). Whilst we do not actively report on our patients' exploitation of the benefits system, we do make it clear that we will not collude. At times this has created tension but, usually, in the long term, we have been able to work through this.

Case study

Roger started working casually for a bicycle courier company. He did not declare his income or work to the benefits agency and continued claiming Income-Related Employment Support Allowance (ESA).

He informed his key worker of what he was doing and asked his advice. Roger was advised that the nature of his work may not satisfy permitted work criteria as it was not arranged as part of a support and treatment programme and therefore would be in conflict with his claim for ESA. If he wished to pursue this job, he would have to earn enough money to effectively replace the benefits. Furthermore, any subsequent claim, if he lost the job, would be jeopardized, because he had shown capability to work. Any new claim would have to be on the basis that his current condition has got a lot worse or he was claiming for a new condition.

Eventually, the benefits agency found out about his earnings and his benefits were stopped. Roger then asked his key worker to write supporting letters asking for the benefits to be reinstated, saying that the work had only been voluntary. We had to say to Roger that we could not write letters that were not factual.

Managing other people's money

Appointeeship (representative payeeship)

When a patient is mentally incapable of managing their own affairs, another person can become their appointee (referred to as a payee in the US) for the purposes of their state welfare benefits. The appointee can make claims, collect or receive payments, and spend the money on behalf of the patient. This person can be a relative, friend, hospital or local authority administrator, or nursing home manager. In our locality, the local authority administers the appointee arrangement and the patient's key worker liaises closely with the appointee to request money or make adjustments as circumstances change.

The appointee is responsible for paying rent and bills, collecting benefits, informing the benefits agency of changes, and allocating spending money to the patient. The appointee role is quite time consuming and involves setting up bank accounts and standing orders. It may be easier if the appointee and key worker are different people, as conflicts inevitably arise over the withholding of spending money.

The advantages of appointeeship are considerable, not least that it ensures financial and housing stability. The removal of these two potential sources of crisis and stress allow the key worker and patient to concentrate on making life more satisfying. Patients subject to appointeeship often build up savings which can be used periodically for holidays, televisions, and other luxuries. On a more prosaic note, appointeeship can be used to restrict access to income that would be spent on harmful drug or alcohol use.

Dixon et al. (1999) looked at case managers' and the patients' perspectives on a representative payee programme with 54 individuals in an assertive outreach service in the US. Both parties could perceive the advantages for housing, substance use, and budgeting. Nearly half the case managers said they had been verbally abused over management of the money. However, there was little evidence of the working alliance being damaged. Clients' satisfaction with the representative payeeship increased over time: the longer the arrangement lasted, the greater the satisfaction and the fewer the problems.

Lasting Power of Attorney

The patient must be capable of understanding the consequences of delegating this power over their financial affairs even if they may not be capable of performing the tasks themselves. A power of attorney cannot be made by a patient incapable of understanding what they are doing. The Lasting Power of Attorney extends beyond the management of state benefits and must be registered through the Office of the Public Guardian. This is a legal intervention—appointing another person (the attorney) to act in respect to property and financial affairs. It can be general or limited to certain aspects. This could be useful when an individual with bipolar disorder is concerned that when they become unwell they might go on a spending spree and spend more than they can afford. We have not taken on this function. It is a relatively expensive and fiddly process. It is usually delegated to relatives and most typically used for individuals with dementia.

Court of Protection

For individuals who do not have capacity to make financial decisions, a relative can apply to the Court of Protection to become their deputy. As an office of the

Supreme Court, this is a real court, capable of resolving legal disputes. The court must be satisfied, by medical evidence, of mental incapacity and that appointeeship or powers of attorney are not sufficient or possible. The court can authorize someone to look after property, financial affairs, and the day-to-day needs of the patient and their dependents. Applying to the Court of Protection is a very protracted and expensive process and seldom used in adult mental health. More often it is restricted to elderly persons with considerable assets.

Conclusions

Helping patients with their finances is a vital part of our job. Nothing is as important to most of our patients as their money. Most patients do not have savings to fall back on when claims are delayed. The most important piece of advice, when dealing with the benefits agency, is to always keep copies of correspondence and to always ask for the name of the person that you are speaking with. Files and claims go missing with alarming regularity, and promises of action often fail to materialize. Likewise, if you tell the patient that you will contact the benefits agency for them, or post a letter, do not forget!

Whatever a patient's source of income, teaching them more effective budgeting skills will be a worthwhile investment. Clearly, we all learn from our mistakes, and we must not be over-prescriptive in a person's personal financial choices. We do have a duty, however, to ensure that, as far as possible, major arrears and debts do not occur through simple neglect. Having access to some regular, disposable income is an essential component of anyone's quality of life. Our patients usually have precious little. So, the more we can increase it and help them to manage it, the more we improve their lot.

Chapter 21

Housing and homelessness

Introduction

Where you live has an impact on well-being, but not having a place to live has more serious implications for health. Social factors like housing together with socio-economic, employment, and educational inequities play a role in determining general and mental health. Housing is high on the patient's agenda, and homelessness causes major difficulties for services wishing to discharge a patient from hospital who is clinically ready to leave but has nowhere to go.

Prevalence of homelessness and serious mental illness

As we might expect, those people in the most unstable accommodation have higher rates of psychotic illness, substance misuse, co-morbidity, and severity of symptomatology. An extensive literature review by Rees (2009) observes that mental illness is both a cause and a consequence of homelessness, and therefore the prevalence of mental illness in this group is greater than for the population as a whole. People with major depression, schizophrenia, and bipolar disorder make up 25–30 per cent of adult street homeless and those in direct access hostels, with higher rates in the US than in Europe. In the European schizophrenia cohort (Bebbington 2005), 33 per cent of the British sample had experienced homelessness in their lifetime, with 13 per cent having experienced 'rooflessness' (sleeping rough on the streets). This compared to 8 per cent having experienced homelessness in Germany and 13 per cent in France.

It is a myth that the closure of psychiatric institutions has dumped long-stay psychiatric patients on the street. Although many people sleeping on the streets have mental health problems, they are not a consequence of the closure of long-stay psychiatric hospitals (Leff 1993). An Audit Commission report has suggested that the problem relates to a combination of the decline in acute psychiatric beds, agencies failing to work together, and community mental health services failing to provide adequate support (Audit Commission 1994).

There are degrees of homelessness. One classification has been used by Stergiopoulos et al. (2015) in measuring housing status and outcomes in a trial of intensive case management. 'Absolute homelessness' describes rough sleepers and those with little prospect of shelter in the coming months. Those in 'precarious housing' have had briefer episodes of homelessness but are currently in or moving between rooms and lodging houses. People classified as 'relatively homeless' are facing problems due to being reliant on informal arrangements on friends' sofas, living in transitional emergency shelters, or in plainly overcrowded and squalid circumstances.

Types of housing and residential provision

Community mental health teams generally work with patients living in independent accommodation. Indeed, the rationale for outreach is partly to provide home-based care to enable people to survive in their own homes. If a patient is referred to us who is living in staffed residential accommodation, we need to think carefully about what advantage specialist community mental health care brings over and above the work of the team of residential social workers or hostel nurses over the longer term. This is simply because the majority of their needs should be met through the hostel staff. In effect, they are already receiving an intensive service from the hostel, but they may legitimately ask for more skilled support for behavioural interventions and in managing crises.

There are, however, different levels of staffed residential provision and a range of providers. A 24-hour staffed hostel managed as part of a health and social care rehabilitation service will be capable of meeting patients' daily needs (a patient on methadone or with an active forensic history being typical exceptions). A hostel managed through the charitable sector, or a housing association with a non-specialist peripatetic ('floating') support worker who calls in every few days, will need a collaborative relationship with local health providers in primary and secondary care. Cost varies with the level of staffing, with the estimated average cost of providing floating outreach at around £150 per week per tenant in England, compared to £500 per week for residential care (Killaspy 2016).

The emphasis on independent accommodation is one of the characteristics that differentiate community outreach from rehabilitation services. Rehabilitation services provide long-term 'hospital hostel' accommodation and group homes for more chronically disabled patients. These are typically patients who have not recovered adequately to the extent that everyday functioning is severely impaired and problematic behaviours present challenges to social inclusion in community settings. Over half the NHS mental health trusts in England have a community rehabilitation team (Killaspy 2014). These teams provide clinical input to local supported housing and residential services.

In some more dispersed or rural settings, this function is combined within a standard community team or as a component of an assertive outreach service.

Independent accommodation and social housing

Mainstream housing is the goal for most patients. In the UK, decent, appropriate, and affordable housing is a scarce resource even for the working population. Increasingly, local government has become reluctant to be directly involved in housing, and in the UK, the 'right to buy' policy resulted in the sale of a large proportion of state-owned social housing to tenants in the 1980s. At the same time, successive governments have sought to promote housing associations as alternative major providers of social housing.

Low housing supply means that eligibility criteria for access are ever stricter. Homelessness is the primary criterion, but even this is no longer a guarantee of a social housing tenancy. Legal entitlement to housing in the UK means that people must be accepted by a local authority as 'statutorily homeless', according to the following criteria:

- They are 'eligible for public funds' (dependent on immigration status).
- They have a 'local connection' to the council concerned (subject to a fixed legal definition).
- They are 'unintentionally homeless' (specific criteria must be met).
- They are in 'priority need' due to various factors, one of which is 'vulnerable as a result of old age, mental illness or handicap or physical disability or other special reason'.

Since 2011, local authorities are able to fully discharge their statutory duty by offering a tenancy in the private rented sector for 12 months, without the consent of the prospective tenant. Previously the local authority had to offer a social home (i.e. owned by a council or registered social landlord), unless the tenant opted for the private sector. While waiting to be housed, homeless people are entitled to temporary accommodation. Both the temporary accommodation and the subsequent offer may be a long way outside the area in which the individual applied to be housed, making mental health follow-up a challenge.

Hostels

The level of care offered by hostels varies considerably, as does the range of providers. Few hostels are provided solely by health services, except in rehabilitation services. Social housing is a local authority obligation in the UK, and most hostels are commissioned by social service and housing departments. This means that hostels are not staffed by health professionals. The needs of the severely mentally are sometimes not well understood, and hostels have tended to 'cherry-pick' more stable and cooperative residents. Substance abuse, in particular, is not tolerated or addressed in many hostels.

Types of residential care arranged by intensity of care provision include the following:

+ high/medium-staffed hostels and nursing homes (24-hour nursed care units), provided in and outside the NHS; staffing 8–20 per unit, typically 6–12 residents or larger if a nursing home for older adults
+ low-staffed hostels (day cover or peripatetic only), mainly run with unqualified staff
+ supported lodgings/landlord-run care homes
+ core and cluster flats, often run by voluntary and independent sector providers
+ individual care packages developed around an individual's needs

A criticism of hospital hostels run by health care staff (usually nurses) is that they can become 'mini-institutions', with institutional practices transferred from the ward. An advantage of these hostels, however, is that patients can be detained under the Mental Health Act, which can act as a safeguard when stepping down patients from inpatient care.

Nursing homes

Most nursing homes are set up to meet the long-term needs of elderly and infirm patients with dementia. Few are registered to take patients under the age of 65. Occasionally, patients under 65 can suffer a stroke or have other physical health and nursing care needs (such as dressing, bathing, or feeding due to frailty) beyond those which can be met in a mental health hostel. In rare instances, individuals may meet the threshold for continuing health care and have funding agreed through the health commissioners. Typically, though, patients with more severe and complex care needs (in England, those covered by Section 117 of the Mental Health Act, which places a duty on statutory bodies to provide support) will get funding shared between health and social services. Otherwise, funding responsibility is based on the balance of health versus social care needs.

Patients waiting for decision can easily remain on an acute ward for extended periods. A full package of home care, meals service, district nurses, and daily visits can be attempted if the patient retains some mobility or has family support. One alternative for less frail elderly patients is sheltered accommodation. These are independent flats with warden supervision and alarms.

Emergency accommodation

Housing crises are common. Knowledge of immediate resources for the homeless patient, in the form of bed and breakfast accommodation or night shelters, is essential. The use of these resources is a last resort and proper risk assessment is a prerequisite. Short-term bed and breakfast can sometimes be arranged in a day through the hospital bed service for patients in hospital fit for discharge. If a patient is unintentionally homeless, the local authority homeless persons' unit may agree to place them, but they seldom do this for patients in hospital. They will certainly not place patients who they deem to have made themselves intentionally homeless through eviction for rent arrears. Neither will they place patients with more severe support needs under specialist care. They regard these patients as the responsibility of the mental health services and look to them for both funding and placement.

Patients can self-refer to a homeless persons' night shelter. These are usually run by charities and offer dormitory-style accommodation for those sleeping rough. They tend to be rather intimidating places and our experience is that patients can get exploited or assaulted. Most large cities run a homeless persons' telephone line which offers information, on a daily basis, on available night shelter places.

Service approaches

We have described how homelessness can be a consequence of serious mental illness. People find themselves homeless as a result of their symptoms and behaviour, eviction for rent arrears, substance misuse, self-neglect, or even exploitation.

Dual diagnosis patients are highly likely to become homeless, often because their substance abuse results in disruptive behaviour, loss of social support, and financial problems (Drake et al. 1997). Housing First (Tsemberis 2010) offers an alternative approach to the typical stepwise pathway of preparing someone who might be considered 'hard to house'. The programme is aimed at people with long-term homelessness and severe mental illness. Instead of transitioning through outreach treatment, attempts and failures at sobriety, shelters, accommodation conditional on treatment adherence, and so on, the person is offered rapid dignity and hope by being offered housing first. In return, they sign up to the programme by agreeing to the payment of rent and weekly visits by the Housing First case management team. A large randomized study of 1198 participants in four Canadian cities showed greater housing stability among Housing First persons than those receiving standard care at two-year follow-up, but was unable to show a statistically significant difference between the two groups in quality of life (Stergiopoulos et al. 2015).

The advantage of a community outreach approach is that the intensity of care delivered in the patient's own home can be stepped up at times of need, rather than the patient having to move through different locations and teams. More assertive outreach can not only be an alternative to hospital admission, it also reduces the need for other institutional residential services. The UK700 intensive case management study (UK700 Group: Burns et al. 1999b) demonstrated that utilization of costed services such as home care and meals service is less for intensive care than for usual care. Key workers give practical help to assist patients in shopping, cooking, and cleaning, as described in the chapter on daily living skills. We have patients receiving regular home care because of severe motivational, physical, or behavioural difficulties, but we try not to accept their long-term dependence on these services. Our experience is that continued engagement and symptom management help preserve tenancies in ordinary housing, as do substance misuse interventions.

The value of home-based interventions and assessment and frequent home visits means that housing difficulties, repairs, and faults come to light quickly. Broken windows and faulty or insecure door locks require prompt attention. Many difficulties are financial (for discussion, see Chapter 20). Our ACT team had a vacuum cleaner that we were able to loan to patients.

It is worth getting to know the housing officer in the housing association or council who deals with your particular area. Explanation of the patient's circumstances usually produces a more sympathetic and rapid response.

Furniture schemes are a good resource for cheap second-hand furniture. To aid resettlement, the local housing support project can provide cheap starter packs for single people. For a patient moving out of hospital or bed and breakfast accommodation into their own flat, a starter pack includes a second-hand bed, cooker, fridge, and chair. Furniture is donated, then collected and delivered by volunteers to the patient. Many such schemes exist across the country to put unwanted furniture to good use.

Case study

Tony had lived in a succession of hostels and temporary accommodation since the breakup of his marriage. His wife had no longer been able to put up with his increasingly unstable mental state and manic episodes, during which he would drink and sing Elvis songs all night. He was 50, and had had a traditional marriage where he was unaccustomed to cooking, paying bills, or looking after himself. Having lived in a family home for most of his life, he could not settle in a hostel, and became demotivated and depressed. As his mental health became more stable he started asking for independent accommodation.

An assessment of, amongst other things, daily living skills and finances, was made in readiness for the resettlement. Tony was motivated to move but knew little about the practicalities of running a home. He had done some preparatory work with the hostel staff—learning to iron, shop, and cook basic meals. Since the hostel did not allow drinking on the premises and most of his money went in contributions to the rent, he seldom drank, but was looking forward to having more money and being able to drink at home. Tony was advised to try to save some money in the intervening weeks for moving expenses and in anticipation that his benefits would be disrupted with changes in address and circumstances.

Once the offer was made, Tony and his key worker went to view the flat. Some minor repairs were needed and these were arranged before the move date. A community care grant was applied for and a starter pack from the housing project obtained so that he had a bed and a cooker from day one. On the day he moved in, he was assisted in contacting the benefits agency to notify them of his new address. An application for housing benefit was also made.

Over subsequent visits, Tony was introduced to local shops and facilities, whilst basic plans were agreed for weekly expenditure and shopping lists. His key worker helped him put up curtains and pictures. Both Tony and his key worker spent time trying to work out the complicated key-meter system for the electricity and where to charge up the key. He was registered with a local GP that the team knew had a good understanding of mental health problems.

Tony enjoyed having his own place and his self-esteem improved. He tended to eat out more than cook, and kept the flat in a reasonable condition. He did get drunk occasionally, but it did not lead to a more unstable mental state or any behavioural disturbance for the neighbours.

Conclusions

Most people consider moving house a stressful event. Homelessness is more stressful and furthermore robs people of their dignity and hope. Tsemberis (2010) quotes one client:

> 'I walked around for years without a single key: a key to a car, a key to a house, a key to anything…. I do not think people understand what a key typifies. It is something that belongs to you. It is something huge.'

Stable and secure housing really is a basic need. Morgan (1993) outlines how the stress-vulnerability and social-drift models apply to housing, with unstable housing increasing the stress on vulnerable patients. For psychotic patients, unstable housing is rarely the cause of their illness but can exacerbate arousal and precipitate relapse. Patients with severe mental health problems drift into deprivation and bad housing. Bad housing usually means socially isolating and dangerous estates, inter-tenant disputes, and damp or poor conditions—all with negative consequences for long-term outcomes.

Because assertive community outreach employs a direct and comprehensive approach to care, allowing frequent and daily contact, patients can be maintained in their own homes much longer than would otherwise be the case. The root causes and the consequences of bad housing can be tackled in a coordinated manner. Problems arise when patients are of 'no fixed abode' and must be placed in whatever hostel or temporary accommodation is available in the locality. This is the traditional brokerage problem of fitting a square peg into a round hole—if there is anywhere available at all! We always resisted the temptation to place people outside the team's geographical boundary, however temporarily, as flexibility of response and particularly the availability of support may be limited.

Housing is one area of practice which is entirely dependent on local knowledge. There are no structured assessment tools or theoretical models to guide novices. The team as a whole will contain considerable expertise through contacts with bed and breakfast owners, hostel staff, and other patients. Patients will tell you which hostels provide the better service. We stopped using one hostel in the borough, despite a chronic shortage of places, because successive patients reported poor standards. The impact of an appropriate housing placement on a patient's satisfaction, well-being, and community tenure can be immense. We only wish there was more housing to choose from.

Chapter 22

Physical health care

Introduction

People with severe mental illnesses suffer much worse physical health than the general population. They are significantly more likely to die early. Their standardized mortality is 1.6, which means that their risk of dying at any given age is 60 per cent above the average (Harris and Barraclough 1998). Put more simply, their overall life expectancy is estimated to be 15–20 years below average (Thornicroft 2011). This is currently a major focus for improving mental health services and achieving parity with physical health care with the slogan 'mind the gap'. While suicide contributes to increased mortality, the main causes are respiratory and cardiovascular. Over a quarter of 101 severely mentally ill patients, studied in 16 general practices, were significantly obese, and over half were regular smokers (Kendrick 1996). In addition, 11 were hypertensive, 21 had persistent cough or sputum, and 24 suffered shortness of breath! Changes in lifestyle or earlier and better treatment could prevent many of these problems. Working closely with this patient group means that we need to understand more about why their health is so poor and what we can do about it.

The problem is not that severely mentally ill patients do not register with a GP or visit them. Kendrick's findings were based on patients registered with good practices, and he found that the severely mentally ill attended their GP more than the average. They had about eight contacts a year compared with an average of three for an age-matched control group (Kendrick et al. 1994). Of course, most of these appointments are for repeat prescriptions rather than specific treatments and, sadly, the level of preventive health care (e.g. blood pressure checks, cervical smear, advice on smoking or weight) is very low for individuals with psychosis (Burns and Cohen 1998). These failings of medical care are particularly striking given such regular contact with both primary and secondary care. There are several factors contributing to such poor care.

Help-seeking behaviour

A regular clinical observation is that individuals with severe mental illness, particularly psychoses, simply do not complain about physical illnesses. They appear to tolerate in silence signs and symptoms that would alarm most of us.

Why this should be so is unclear, but it is very striking. It is probably one of the reasons the 'annual medical' was a requirement in long-stay wards in mental hospitals. Occasionally, patients may tolerate manifestations of diseases for delusional reasons. One of our female patients has refused to have a benign ovarian cyst operated upon because of her belief that she is pregnant. This is rare, however, and the inactivity seems more often to be simply to do with overall self-neglect and shyness, or just lack of motivation in seeking help.

It is easy for us in mental health to forget that, in most medical practice, if the patient does not ask for help, they are assumed to be well. Studies in primary care demonstrate repeatedly that consultations are patient-driven. It is the patient who sets the agenda, not the doctor. 'Open-ended' questioning has long been promoted as the desirable consulting style. Even in secondary medical care, where the approach is often more structured, the doctor will not actively pursue the patient if they do not attend for treatment. Except in the case of mental health and some infectious diseases such as tuberculosis and sexually transmitted diseases, the responsibility for seeking help is left entirely to the patient (Robson and Gray 2007; O'Callaghan et al. 2010).

Failure to register with a GP

The vast majority of severely mentally ill people in the UK are registered with a GP, who is responsible for ensuring their general medical care. Nonetheless, the rate of non-registration is higher than for the general population. The group of unregistered patients is a particular concern as they are most at risk.

There appear to be several reasons for not registering. The seriously mentally ill often have unstable accommodation and move from place to place, particularly within cities. This makes remaining registered very difficult. They may also quarrel and fall out with their GP and be removed from the list. Although there are mechanisms for allocating a new GP, this depends on the patient pursuing it. The most important reason for non-registration is these patients simply cannot be bothered, either because they do not see the point or because of the inertia and apathy that can be part of their illness. Our patients may also lack many of the social prompts which bind adults to their GPs, such as getting insurance medicals and taking children for vaccinations. Given poor physical health shown even in mentally ill patients with a good GP (Kendrick 1996), being without one is clearly a disaster.

Homeless patients

One group rarely registered with a GP is the homeless. 'Homeless' refers to individuals who lack stable permanent accommodation, so it includes those living in bed and breakfast establishments, shelters, and (in many countries) cheap hotels. 'Roofless' is the term reserved for those who are actually living on the streets. Most homeless outreach teams target the roofless, often with the initial aim of finding them temporary accommodation.

These patients have very significant physical health problems and there are often local initiatives to try to reach them (Hwang and Burns 2014). Many night shelters and drop-in facilities for the homeless and those sleeping rough have clinics providing assessment and treatment by visiting GPs. There are particular problems relating to infectious diseases such as tuberculosis and hepatitis with this very disadvantaged group. In assertive outreach teams that target the homeless, trying to get the patient to register with a GP can be one of the most important early interventions. When this proves impossible, the use of outreach clinics in shelters or attendance at an A&E department may be the only feasible alternative.

Causes of increased physical ill health

In outreach to individuals with severe mental illnesses, we therefore need to be highly vigilant to the risks of poor physical health and, particularly, untreated physical problems. Some form of structure helps in assessing the risks and spotting such problems. There are generally three main causes for concern—although it will be immediately obvious that there is considerable overlap between them.

Consequences of self-neglect

The most obvious of these are poor teeth, obesity, and respiratory problems. Some patients have very poor dental health simply because they do not brush their teeth. However, good dental hygiene is particularly important in our patient group who are at increased risk of caries because of the dry mouth which is a side effect with several drugs. This is not just a cosmetic issue—bad teeth can lead to abscesses and pain. They can also add to social marginalization if they look off-putting or cause bad breath. One of the more rewarding experiences with the Wandsworth assertive outreach team was a man who, after a couple of years persistent coaxing, started and responded very well to clozapine. As a consequence of his improved mental state, he allowed us to help him get his massive inguinal hernia repaired and have several months' dental work completed. This quite transformed his appearance and delighted his long-suffering mother.

Obesity is increasingly common in our patients and is probably now the number one problem. Much of it is, of course, because of the newer antipsychotic drugs which increase the appetite. It is also driven by poor eating habits, especially a reliance on fast food in younger patients. In such a deprived group, obesity also can lead to marginalization because clothes do not fit, people feel 'a mess', and self-respect falls even further.

Individuals with psychoses start to smoke at about the same rate as the general population. The difference is that now the majority of adults stop smoking after a few years, whereas our patients rarely do. Their smoking may be ignored because helping them stop is considered too difficult (the well-established public health initiatives depend on supporting motivation and consistency—hard to achieve with this group). Alternatively, there is a common assumption that smoking is 'trivial' compared to their mental illness. It was once even believed that schizophrenia patients had a lower risk for lung cancer! Cigarettes were also a common currency of social exchange in mental hospitals, sanctioned by staff in the past. Smoking also impacts pharmacokinetics with smokers needing higher drug doses (Tsuda et al. 2014) and often reporting that it reduces drug side effects.

Smoking cessation programmes are now top of the agenda of physical care for psychosis patients (Gelenberg et al. 2008) along with strategies to prevent weight gain (Álvarez-Jiménez et al. 2008) or, failing that, to lose weight by increasing activity and controlling diet (Faulkner et al. 2007). The limited success with cessation programmes in this group is in stark, and disappointing, contrast to their success with the general population.

Even when conditions have been diagnosed and treatment prescribed, patients may simply not comply. We experienced the tragic consequences of a relatively young woman suffering from both schizophrenia and very high blood pressure who was inconsistent in her compliance with antihypertensives. She suffered a series of strokes, leaving her permanently dependent on nursing care in her 30s. Disorders such as diabetes, which require strict monitoring of blood sugars, medication, and dietary control, present a challenge to most people without the multiple deprivations of mental illness. Unless we can find novel and effective interventions, the immediate prospect of 'closing the gap' looks gloomy.

Consequences of treatment

Most psychiatric drugs have side effects. A dry mouth, increased appetite, and variable degrees of sedation are common. All three contribute to obesity.

Some of the newer antipsychotics are associated with 'metabolic syndrome' with raised triglycerides, significant weight gain (notably abdominal fat) and consequently a very high risk for Type 2 diabetes. Regular checks of triglyceride levels and glucose metabolism, plus girth measurement, are now considered essential routine parts of treatment with the new antipsychotics. Patients often drink high-calorie soft drinks because of their dry mouth (which also increases their risk of dental caries), they eat more, and they are less active. It is not surprising that they put on weight, which is bad for their health and self-esteem.

Older drugs also have their own health risks. Thyroid and renal problems associated with lithium are perhaps the most serious, and require regular monitoring.

Co-morbid conditions

Co-morbid use of alcohol and drugs is a major cause of poor health in individuals with severe mental illness. It is associated with a range of problems, including infections from HIV and hepatitis through to local abscesses from unhygienic syringes. Intoxication is associated also with a raised risk of trauma, whether it is falling down stairs when drunk, getting into a fight in a pub, or being threatened and assaulted by drug dealers when debts have not been paid. Long-term consequences of chronic use—such as neuropathies, cognitive impairment, and deteriorating liver function—are easy to miss, as they develop so gradually. Life-threatening conditions such as delirium tremens or a chest infection presenting with confusion and irritability can be misdiagnosed as relapses of the psychotic disorder. The consequent delay in instituting appropriate treatment increases the risks.

Role of the outreach worker

Most mental health professionals take a holistic and inclusive view of their obligations to their patients. Whether we are social workers, nurses, doctors, psychologists, or occupational therapists, we recognize that if the patient is physically unwell, then something must be done about it. Outreach workers inevitably accept a commitment that stretches beyond their narrow professional training. In the Wandsworth assertive outreach team, physical health care was a sizeable component of the work. It was regularly addressed in team reviews and featured as an identified need on at least 15–20 per cent of care plans.

Physical health assessment and team responses

Given the weight of evidence on poorer health outcomes for the people we work with, it is incumbent on us to systematically assess for physical health in community patients and to work with the patient and primary care where modifiable risk factors are identified.

The National Audit of Schizophrenia (Royal College of Psychiatrists 2014) includes a standard for a minimum of annual monitoring and recording of five physical health indicators:

- smoking
- body mass index (BMI)

- blood glucose control
- blood lipids
- blood pressure

Suggested arrangements to coordinate assessment and monitoring with the GP are helpfully covered by NICE schizophrenia guidance (NICE 2014b). Mental health teams should assume lead responsibility for the first 12 months of care or until the service user's condition has stabilized. Unless there are established local agreements, primary care should subsequently take lead responsibility.

It is no use monitoring unless we have some idea of appropriate interventions. The most commonly used response framework is the Lester Positive Cardiometabolic Health Resource (Shiers et al. 2014). This simplifies responses using a red, amber, or green scoring system according to each assessed indicator. For example, a BMI measurement of over 25 (23 if South Asian or Chinese) or more than 5 kg weight gain over a three-month period would score red. This would trigger actions including a medication review and lifestyle advice on diet and exercise. Brief interventions for smokers include combined nicotine replacement therapy using patches or gum and/or varenicline. Some patients are now switching to electronic cigarettes; individual or group behavioural support will be necessary for people with high dependency.

Taking people to hospital

Many patients need support and supervision with treatment through forgetfulness or chaotic lives driven by more immediate survival needs (Chapter 11). If we consider a dosette box necessary for the psychiatric medicines, then it is probably equally necessary for the antihypertensives. Similarly, if we need to visit daily to supervise clozapine administration, then why would it be less urgent to supervise administration of glibenclamide?

The principles of encouragement and motivational enhancement transfer equally to other long-term medications. We had two patients with chronic renal failure under our care. For one, we had to supervise all the medicines and often took him, grumbling and resentful, to the hospital for dialysis. For the other, we encouraged her to tolerate what is a demanding regime, but only needed to accompany her to consultant appointments.

Using the team doctors

Sometimes patients simply will not go to their GP or to hospital for an assessment. It is important to remember that psychiatrists are qualified doctors. While consultants may have lost touch with many of their general medical skills, trainee psychiatrists should be able to diagnose and, if necessary, treat most common minor physical disorders. We try to avoid this when possible. Receiving comprehensive health care from a GP is one of the benefits of life in the community that we want patients to access. It helps in affirming their normality and reduces stigma and isolation. Emphasizing such common needs and rights reminds all involved (patient, doctor, and the other patients in the waiting room) that people with mental illness are more like the rest of us than they are different. However, a doctrinaire refusal to treat, for example, a chest infection or hypertension in a patient with no GP seems counterproductive.

When the patient has a GP but will not go, it is, of course, essential that the plan of action is agreed with the GP. We have rarely found GPs to be resistant to this approach. When we have had to treat physical health problems directly, patients have usually been very positive. It makes their lives easier and they know that it is not something they would routinely expect from us. They often experience it as us having made a special effort for them.

Problems with providing physical health care directly

Mental health workers often get considerable satisfaction from helping patients with their physical health care—and so they should in our opinion. There are immediate and obvious benefits for the patient's comfort and quality of life. Family members are often very appreciative and, in a quieter way, so are the patients. There are, however, some issues which need to be thought through. These relate mainly to how to manage the relationship with general health care services, but also touch on ethical and professional obligations.

Confidentiality

The role of the case manager as advocate and support can be a tricky one. Most clinicians are quite flexible about family members being present during consultations, and answer their questions directly. It is surprisingly uncommon for a physician to ask an adult patient if they mind their relative being present—they take the patient's acquiescence as permission. We are much more likely to ask about it in mental health where family relationships can be very complex.

When the person attending a clinic appointment with the patient is not a family member, there does not seem to be any accepted practice. We tend to ask our patients if they want us with them for support. For those who have real difficulties understanding or managing their physical illnesses and treatments, we definitely want to be present. We want to know what is involved because we will be responsible for prompting or delivering it. We negotiate this with the patient beforehand and explain it to the doctor or nurse they are consulting. Usually it is fine, but sometimes it causes uncertainty and discomfort. Some doctors respond with a dogmatic 'no' and exclude us. We never found it useful to challenge this. If we cannot be present, then we may have to wait for the letter to the GP to find out exactly what is the problem.

Withdrawal of support by primary care

One unwanted risk with intensive community support may be that the primary care team withdraws from engagement with the patient. They may see us as more competent—especially if the patient is very difficult or hostile. Knowing we have general medical skills, they may wish to pass over some of their responsibilities to us. In some cases this is fine, but in others it may be unfair to the patient and to us.

Case study

Ed was a 45-year-old man of Italian extraction who suffers from long-standing paranoid schizophrenia. He had responded well to one of the newer antipsychotics and no longer experienced active hallucinations or delusions. He was, however, very isolated and self-neglecting. He required frequent visits to ensure his treatment and also to keep his flat acceptable and to 'turf out' local drug addicts who exploited him. His major problem was that he drank to excess (his father died of alcoholism) and had developed moderate cognitive impairment and diabetes, which he totally neglected. Because we visited him two or three times a week, the local district nurses refused to visit him and administer his insulin in the way they did for several other cognitively impaired patients. They insisted that as he could get out to buy his vodka, he was not 'housebound' and therefore did not warrant home visits. Because we saw him regularly, we became obliged to manage his insulin, and the district nurses refused our request that they visit on the days we did not. The result is that we had to visit daily to manage the insulin.

While we had been flattered by the GP insisting that without our input this patient would be dead, we are unhappy that he was denied visits from a district nurse. The arguments they present are fairly strong, but we remain convinced that had this man received less support from us he would, in truth, be getting more appropriate support from primary care. The reality, of course, is that we may simply have to accept the responsibility. We could not visit him and manage his antipsychotics and insulin one day, knowing that he would not take his injection the next.

Ethical dilemmas over compulsion

The UK Mental Health Act allows us to compel someone to have treatment for their mental illness but gives no authority whatsoever to compel treatment for physical conditions. Knowing this does not necessarily make it easy to work with a patient who is neglecting their physical health. It can be one of the most difficult aspects of our work to suffer the frustration of watching someone we know well and care about deteriorate, and to be unable to intervene in the way we could if the deterioration was psychiatric. Team support and discussion are essential. Discussion provides the opportunity to ventilate some of these frustrations and reaffirm the realities of our position. We have usually found that families fully understand our position (they may for years also have experienced a stubborn refusal from their ill member to take simple advice). Other professionals are sometimes not so understanding. The primary care team involved with Ed were very critical of us, insisting that we should move him to a nursing home. Perhaps to spare their own consciences, they consistently refused to recognize that the Mental Health Act gave us no power to force him when he was so resolutely unwilling to go.

Maintaining skills

What would we do for a family member? That is the rough benchmark we used in the team when we discuss what was an appropriate level of support to offer our patients. There are few 'professional' guidelines established for these decisions. This rather simple benchmark works well when deciding how active to be in taking patients to and from appointments, but it does not help with deciding on which specific medical interventions we are competent to provide.

Even if a family member often takes responsibility for direct care, society expects—and if anything goes wrong, will insist upon—higher levels of accountability from us. If mental health staff do deliver physical health care, they need to be certain that they have received the appropriate skills and training. More important is to make sure that skills are adequately maintained. Most nurses will have been trained in diabetes care, but those working in mental health care will not be delivering such care very often. Our memories of the implications of the different blood levels will be rusty. What is the level to test for ketones? What is the level to omit the insulin injection?

Each professional member of the team is responsible for ensuring that they keep their skills and knowledge up to date. The team leader has a responsibility to make sure that each of the team is competent in what they are asked to do. If a team does not have a culture of openness and trust, it is possible that a member may not admit that they 'aren't up to' a procedure if many of their colleagues seem comfortable with it. Making sure that such concerns are acknowledged and addressed—and not seen as failings—is an essential task for a team leader.

Conclusions

Help with physical health care is a core component of community outreach with the severely mentally ill. They have greater than average needs and the barriers to accessing adequate care are daunting. Insisting on a very rigid demarcation of our 'mental health role' is neither in their interests nor, as we have found, in ours. Help with overall health care improves engagement and delivers an often immediately obvious improvement in quality of life that is mutually rewarding for outreach worker and patient. There are complex 'border' issues that come with this work, often raising important ethical and resource concerns. Honestly handled, we have found these challenges strengthen the team's understanding of its function and can also improve relationships with other health care providers. All of this can only be in the long-term interests of our patients.

Chapter 23

Employment

Introduction

Along with where we were born, where we went to school, and where we live now, work is an important social determinant of health (Marmot 2005). Vocational programmes are not new. Victorian asylums recognized the moral and constitutional benefits of work. Nowadays the case for employment for people with severe mental illness is driven by the recovery approach but also by an economic case (Sainsbury Centre for Mental Health 2009). Gone are the days of sheltered employment and industrial therapy units in favour of individual placement and support (IPS), a form of supported employment which helps patients into paid competitive work. Embracing competitive employment was driven by US practice in outreach and case management services, where real employment is very much higher on their list of priorities than in the UK. Employment law and welfare provision differ there. US teams have a longer history of employing vocational workers with the remit to develop opportunities and to support patients in jobs.

Compared to the US, most of Europe provides better safeguards for employees. The downside of such legislation is that employers may consider it risky to take on workers with long-standing health problems, since it is not easy to sack people on health grounds once hired. State benefits for the unemployed and those less able to work through sickness are relatively generous in Europe. This means that there is often little or nothing to be gained financially from seeking employment if you qualify for higher rates of disability allowances. The inflexibility of the benefit system creates a 'catch-22' situation where if you become employed you lose your benefit. Then if your employment is terminated, or you leave on health grounds, your case for having welfare benefits reinstated can be undermined by having worked! Transitional employment schemes exist, but do not seem to have a high take-up rate within our patient group.

This chapter presents the relevant evidence base for positive vocational interventions, strategies, and a case study. Helping our patients to structure their day through non-work activity is covered in Chapter 24, on daily living skills. Welfare benefits to support people in the transition to work, and those unable to work, are reviewed in Chapter 20, on finance and appointeeship.

Employment rates for people with severe mental illness stand at 8–9 per cent according to government statistics (Department of Health 2013), with men having a lower rate of employment than women. It has been estimated that 50–90 per cent of people with ongoing mental health problems wish to return to work (Grove 1999; Rinaldi and Hill 2000). Surveys of relatives report that structured daytime activity is viewed as the most pressing unmet need (Steinwachs et al. 1992).

Models and approaches

> In the past, extensive resources have been directed towards pre-vocational activities, with little demonstrable impact. (Bond 1992)

'Place then train' is the approach recommended by the evidence. Training people and then placing them, often via a stepwise exposure to work, is less effective in the short and long term. Table 23.1 arranges work-related interventions in an approximate hierarchy, based on the evidence base for effectiveness, ranging from one-to-one specialist assistance with mainstream employment, through volunteering, to work preparation groups at mental health resource centres.

Specialist programmes

Specialist one-to-one work programmes exist purely to help individuals find and keep appropriate work. They may exist in the voluntary or statutory sector, and availability varies markedly. The best programmes are integrated into mental health services. Schemes may offer a range of placements from voluntary to fully paid, mainstream work. The most successful programmes simply take patients 'as they are' and develop or find suitable jobs. This approach is preferable to trying to mould the patient to fit an existing job. Such schemes rely on direct contact with employers, rather than on advertised vacancies.

The individual placement and support (IPS) programme is the dominant evidence-based approach and recommended for use in both the NICE guidance on schizophrenia (NICE 2014b) and bipolar disorder (NICE 2014a). An early example in the US (Drake and Becker 1996) built extensive links with local employers. The programme uses techniques such as job shadowing, where the patient can follow a regular employee for a day or two, observing and learning the job. There is no obligation for the employer to hire at the end. The targeted jobs' tax credit acted as an incentive for employers in the IPS locality. If the patient is hired on a permanent basis and is disabled, the employer can 'write off' the first $2400 of wages. IPS employment specialists join case management teams and directly assist in searching for jobs. On securing employment, they

Table 23.1 Hierarchy of work-focused models and approaches

Intervention	Description	Example
Individual placement and support (IPS) programme	Intensive one-to-one assistance with finding, starting, and maintaining real work placements	IPS programme with integrated employment specialists in CMHTs (Rinaldi and Perkins 2007)
Vocationally focused outreach or rehabilitation	Intensive one-to-one assistance with finding, starting, and maintaining real work placements as part of a wider care plan delivered by an outreach or rehabilitation team	Training in community living (Test 1992)
Clubhouse model	Mental health day facilities focused on work and user/member involvement	Fountain House, New York (Beard et al. 1982)
Sheltered employment	Social firms or workshops run in partnership with health or social care agencies and with explicit remit to employ disadvantaged groups	Industrial therapy units; Remploy
Voluntary work	Voluntary placements often consisting of only a few hours per week	Volunteer bureaux; hospital volunteer programmes
Work training	Courses in basic skills aimed at the long-term unemployed or people with disabilities	Vary by locality with multiple third-sector providers.
Vocational counselling	Individualized job, interview, and career advice	Disability employment adviser at local job centre
Work groups at resource centre	Job clubs providing advice, support, and resources for job search and application; work activities, such as gardening, typing, word processing, secretarial skills training	

provide ongoing support to enable the service user to maintain the job. They may provide support with difficulties on the job, difficulties outside of work that impact on work, and help work out reasonable adjustments and negotiating them with employers. Employment specialists have a caseload of 20–25 (see Box 23.1).

The literature confirms little relationship between employment outcomes and the individual's diagnosis, severity of impairment, and social skills. This tells us that we should push against low expectations from staff, patients, and families about the likelihood of work. Motivation in the form of wanting to work and believing that you can are the best predictors of work outcomes in people with severe mental illness (Rinaldi et al. 2007).

Box 23.1 The key principles of individual placement and support (IPS)

- Competitive employment is the main goal.
- Everyone who wants it is eligible for employment support.
- Job search is consistent with individual choices and preferences.
- Job search is rapid.
- Employment specialists and clinical teams are integrated through location and working together.
- Support is not time limited and is individualized to both the employer and the employee.
- The person is supported through the transition from benefits to work.

Adapted from *Psychiatric Rehabilitation Journal*, 31, Bond G.R., Drake R.E and Becker D.R., 'An update on randomized controlled trials of evidence-based supported employment', pp. 280–289. Copyright (2008) American Psychological Association.

The employment specialist role does not require a mental health professional, and in the UK they are more likely to be individuals with experience in vocational rehabilitation or occupational psychology, or they may have personal experience of mental health problems (Rinaldi et al. 2007). They do, however, need the ability to relate positively to employers and to be able to identify an individual's interests, strengths, skills, abilities, and coping styles in order to match them with jobs. Applying technical knowledge regarding the welfare benefits system and employment law in relation to disability entitlements, such as reasonable adjustments in the workplace, are other competencies for the role.

Most of the research into IPS has come from the USA with its low level of welfare benefits and 'hire and fire' culture. A European RCT in six countries, EQOLISE (Burns et al. 2007), confirmed its effectiveness under European conditions. Over 300 patients with schizophrenia who had been unemployed for a minimum of one year were randomized either to IPS or high-quality, well-established stepwise vocational rehabilitation. The rate of return to work was double in IPS (55 per cent versus 28 per cent). It was noticed in this 18-month trial that of the patients who found jobs in either arm, few found them beyond nine months. A trial of limiting IPS support to nine months (IPS-LITE) compared to standard IPS was conducted in the UK. It found the rate of employment basically the same in both (41 per cent in IPS-LITE and 46 per cent in IPS) (Burns et al. 2015). However, IPS-LITE released much more capacity, increasing throughput such that its overall effectiveness (had that capacity been utilized) would be increased by 17 per cent in the 18 months of the trial and presumably much more as time went on. IPS-LITE has been proposed as a more effective and rational use of resources, ensuring that more patients are afforded the opportunity for the service with the same number of staff.

The User Employment Programme (Perkins et al. 2000) is a modified approach that places patients in existing clinical and non-clinical positions within our local mental health Trust in South West London. Mental health services are major employers, and if other employers are to be persuaded to offer work to people with severe mental health problems, we have to lead by example. The Trust includes personal experience of mental health problems as a desirable quality on all job specifications. Through this programme, the community support worker with one of the assertive outreach teams in the Trust was employed full-time and on a full salary. This integrates the concept of expertise by experience into working in mental health, and was very successful for us in terms of job performance, team culture, and skill mix.

Vocationally focused outreach

The 2015 Care Quality Commission community mental health survey found that when respondents were asked whether NHS mental health services gave them any help or advice with finding support for work, 47 per cent said 'No, but I would have liked help.'

In the absence of a dedicated employment specialist, encouraging a team member to take on responsibility for the vocational focus will enhance the priority given to employment.

Case study

Marion is a young woman with schizophrenia who was highly motivated to get back to work. She had gone on training courses and attended day centres for a number of years, but wanted mainstream employment. She presented as a likeable and cooperative patient with noticeable movement disorder as side effects from her medication. These had the effect of exaggerating the perception of her functional difficulties.

Marion was highlighted as being motivated for work at her review meeting (see Table 23.2). Her key worker and the team's vocational worker carried out a formal assessment. Issues highlighted on assessment were the following:

◆ Marion's over-enthusiastic expectations

◆ limited work history, which included loss of jobs, associated with relapse

◆ her sufficiently high functional capability to try mainstream work

The team's vocational worker approached a local supermarket and arranged an appointment with the personnel manager who was having trouble motivating and keeping staff in

Table 23.2 Summary care plan

Name: Marion W. Address: Flat 3, 49 Smith Square Phone: 0208 645 xxxx Date of birth: 22/6/90 GP: Morgan Phone: 0208 767 xxxx	CMHT: Wandsworth West Phone: 0208 877 xxxx New patient: NO If NO, date of review: 29/5/16 Diagnosis: 1 Schizophrenia F 20.0 2 .... F— —.—

Assessed needs or problem	Intervention	Resp. of
I would like to work and have more occupation. I want a part-time job.	◆ Assess mainstream employment preferences with team employment specialist. ◆ Active assistance with job hunting and application subject to assessment. ◆ Approach appropriate employers directly and explain advantages to them of employing Marion. ◆ Support Marion through process but give realistic appraisal of difficulties involved. ◆ Provide advice on impact of work on benefits.	MW and JF MW and employment specialist
Dystonic side effects of medication	◆ Review medication and side effects. ◆ Provide education on medication and side effects. Give written information.	TB/ JF

specific jobs (e.g. putting shopping into bags from Internet shopping orders prior to delivery). Marion liked the sound of this job—it was not that different from doing her own shopping. The vocational worker on the team spoke to the personnel officer about the maximum number of hours and pay that would enable Marion to still qualify for welfare benefits.

On the day of the interview, Marion was smartly presented and excited. She had worked on presentation and practised interview questions with her key worker. The vocational worker who was familiar with the personnel manager took her to the interview. Marion got the job and continues to work at the store 16 hours a week. She has recently started working on the checkout tills. The personnel officer is delighted to have at least one person who actually wants to be there!

The clubhouse model

Unlike 'recovery colleges', which focus on education for self-management, and are often run by provider organizations with peer trainers, 'clubhouses' have a particularly peer-run ethos together with a focus on employment as well as education and social activities. The early clubs, such as Fountain House in New York (Beard et al. 1982), were set up as self-help psychosocial centres in large cities in the US. One of their chief aims (aside from mutual support) is to provide employment opportunities for members through pre-vocational work groups operating from the clubhouse itself (e.g. gardening and catering) and also through external individual work placements. Clubhouses incorporate a belief in empowerment and the potential for productivity of the most disabled.

There are now more than 300 clubhouses that subscribe to the model across the world, according to the International Directory of Clubhouses. Staff at new centres are trained by those from existing sites according to an agreed set of standards. Although we must bear in mind the limited effectiveness of pre-vocational work preparation compared to IPS, clubhouses constitute a valuable resource for social inclusion.

Sheltered workshops and social enterprises

'Remploy' was set up by the UK government in response to the 1944 Disabled Persons (Employment) Act, mainly to serve people with physical disabilities sustained in the Second World War. Remploy runs traditional, manufacturing-based sheltered workshops. In 2015, its funding and relationship with the UK government was ended, in part because of concerns about supporting segregated work for disabled people rather than promoting mainstream work and social inclusion. Social enterprises provide work and training opportunities for people otherwise excluded from work because of mental health problems, homelessness, or other disadvantages, including addictions and a history of offending. These small businesses include cafes, restaurants, garages, and printers, and describe themselves as socially responsible traders which typically promote people moving on to genuinely mainstream employment. Social enterprises have a long history in Italy, where they are called 'B-Cooperatives' and have been very successful indeed. This stems from much more favourable tax incentives and regulations about the awarding of contracts. It means that not only the employer but also the other employees value the presence of their colleagues from socially excluded groups. Everybody benefits by the arrangement.

Voluntary work

Voluntary work can be a valuable strategy during an initial period of a work placement. The employer or social enterprise can assess the employee's competencies and motivation before starting paid work. More often, voluntary work consists of donating a few hours a week to a good cause such as a charity or public service. The idea of working for a few hours a week for altruistic reasons with only expenses paid is anathema to many of our patients. One advantage of voluntary work is that it does not affect volunteers' welfare benefits. Also, valuable skills and social contacts can develop in a non-threatening, non-contractual environment.

Volunteers are free to leave, arrive late, and work to their abilities without sanction. Most areas have a local volunteer bureau, often linked to the local council for voluntary services that helps coordinate local charitable organizations. The volunteer bureau acts as a job centre for voluntary work. The patient or key worker phones up the volunteer bureau, is invited for a simple interview to ascertain skills and interests, and discusses local opportunities. Many volunteer bureaux are skilled in developing places for people with mental health problems and providing some form of support for the duration of the placement. Activities vary from helping at children's adventure playgrounds and youth or elderly luncheon clubs, to filling envelopes for charity fundraising or lobbying.

Work training

So-called pre-vocational training schemes in catering, computer skills, and administration, for example, are available, and some are set up specifically to help people with mental health problems and other disabilities. We refer patients sparingly to such courses because of high dropout rates. Patients report that training often caters to the lowest common denominator and rarely leads to real work opportunities. Some work training is offered to those who have been long-term unemployed—conditional on continuing to receive welfare benefits—commissioned through voluntary organizations and social firms. If a patient is receiving disability benefits, they are unlikely to be called up by the benefits agency for retraining aimed at the long-term unemployed.

Vocational counselling

Most of us are familiar with the drawbacks of vocational counselling from our encounters with careers officers whilst at school. If we want to be a teacher, then chances are that the careers officer will look at our school reports and then suggest that plumbing might be more realistic. Local job centres employ disability employment advisers (DEAs) whose role it is to assess employment prospects, provide advice and coaching on job opportunities, develop placements, and provide advice on how work will affect welfare benefits. DEAs have access to certain training schemes and are up to date with changes in the benefits system.

Work groups at mental health day centres

Gardening and activity groups are often recreational in nature. Groups that have a more mainstream work focus, such as job clubs, provide telephones and stamps to assist in job searches, practice interviews, and foster self-help and advice among participants. The disadvantage is the remoteness from the labour market and the potential lack of an individualized or highly motivating environment.

Welfare benefits and work

Benefits often represent the biggest psychological and practical obstacle to switching to competitive employment. Uncertainty and change in the UK benefits system mean that outreach workers need to keep abreast of developments or have access to good welfare rights advice.

Currently if you are receiving employment or disability benefits in the UK and start paid work of 16 hours or more per week, you should seek advice and a 'better-off' calculation about the impact on benefit entitlement. This would include eligibility for in-work benefits and tax credits you could apply for.

Working to strengths

Factors relevant to work can be conceived in terms of a patient's strengths or by their impairments. The strengths model of case management (Rapp 1992; Ryan and Morgan 2004) is particularly helpful in working with a patient's aspirations and goals, since it emphasizes abilities over deficits and collaboration over brokerage. Furthermore, just as in the broader recovery approach, people with severe and enduring mental illness are seen as possessing the ability to learn, grow, and change. The local community is viewed not as an obstacle but as a resource containing many opportunities. Even if the aspirations of the patient to work seem remote, or the choice of work somewhat grandiose, there are worthwhile shorter-term steps on the way to these ultimate goals. 'It is likely that the client generally regarded to be unmotivated is more likely to respond to a positive focus than to a negative focus which highlights the problems' (Morgan 1993).

Case study

One patient with severe bipolar affective disorder has aspirations to be a supermodel. In many respects, Gloria is well suited. She is slim and has no appetite, she is offhand and belligerent with people, and she smokes and drinks heavily—perhaps the characteristics of an established rather than an aspiring supermodel.

Initial work with Gloria involved not dismissing this aspiration, but breaking it down into more achievable goals—healthy eating (as opposed to not eating), negotiation and presentation (as opposed to making demands of other people), and establishing a daytime pattern of activity mirroring that of a working day. Gloria did eventually participate in a charity fashion show organized by the local mental health resource centre.

The strengths approach does not ignore the assessed needs of the patient, but starts from the patient's agenda and list of 'wants'.

Conclusions

The evidence consistently favours direct and rapid exposure to mainstream competitive employment over stepwise pre-vocational activities (Drake et al. 1999b). Such supported employment is more effective than pre-vocational training in helping patients find and maintain competitive employment (Crowther et al. 2001). Studies that have looked at whether the potential stress of rapid exposure to competitive employment increases the risk of relapse have shown no association (Bond et al. 1997; McFarlane et al. 2000). Indeed, a surprise (and possibly random) finding in the EQOLISE study (Burns et al. 2007) was that readmissions were significantly reduced, not increased, in the IPS group despite their higher rates of employment.

The value of targeting and assessing patients for employment support is less clear, but would seem sensible when jobs are scarce. Studies of employability show that patient characteristics such as diagnosis, severity of impairment, and social skills have relatively little impact on employment outcomes (Grove 2000). Having a history of employment, being motivated, and believing that employment is achievable are the positive predictors of employment outcomes.

Community outreach teams, especially if enhanced by an employment specialist, can provide employment interventions as part of an overall care package. There are significant structural differences affecting the UK labour market that may appear to make our job harder compared to our US counterparts. Significant unemployment rates for people with severe mental illness challenge us. We should remember the contribution of work to our own self-esteem and well-being, and support the aspirations of patients and their families towards greater social inclusion.

Chapter 24

Daily living skills

Introduction

Social inclusion and survival in community settings require that people are able to engage in everyday domestic activities, and ideally in social activities, sports and hobbies, personal leisure interests, and learning. Most of us take the skills required to negotiate these for granted, but they are a struggle for people with severe mental illness. We are no longer dealing with institutionalized patients moving out of long-stay wards who may never have used a pedestrian crossing or supermarket. We are more likely to be working with people who find cooking or shopping difficult due to motivational, cognitive, and information-processing deficits. To help patients develop daily living skills, we must resist the temptation to simply do everything for them, as happened in long-stay institutions. This involves listening to the patient's agenda, goal setting, collaborating, and focusing on empowering steps to self-management.

The programme for assertive community treatment (PACT) was originally called training in community living (TCL). Stein and Test (1980) saw the core task of their outreach team as teaching patients the skills to survive with their illnesses outside hospital, and believed this task would be time limited. Medication management, shopping, cooking, and other household and interpersonal tasks were taught *in vivo*. Skills learnt in one context, such as a day centre, did not transfer readily to the context of the patient's own home. Also, unless comprehensive psychosocial help was provided directly in the patient's own environment, they often did not engage with services.

Stein and Test felt strongly that traditional aftercare services underestimated the range of skills and assistance that severely mentally ill people needed to survive. The term TCL did not survive because it became clear that the improved community tenure, employment, social relationships, symptomatology, and satisfaction with their lives during the 14-month experimental service were lost soon after the service was withdrawn. This is an important finding; Stein and Test recognized the need for ongoing community support and skills training for these patients:

> It must be concluded that even very intensive community treatment models do not provide a cure for severe mental illnesses, but rather provide a support system within

which persons with persistent vulnerabilities can live in the community and grow. It appears these supports must be ongoing rather than time limited. (Test 1992)

We must remember that Stein and Test were working with some of the most hospitalized, disabled, and severely mentally ill patients in their PACT programme. In the intervening years, opinion and evidence, influenced by the recovery approach and longitudinal outcome studies, mean that we no longer subscribe to the necessity of indefinite support, but recognize that social and clinical recovery from severe and enduring psychosis is reachable for a significant proportion of patients (Hegarty et al. 1994; Jääskeläinen et al. 2013; Menezes et al. 2006; Sainsbury Centre for Mental Health 2008).

The impact of cognitive deficits

The most important principle in support of *in vivo* daily living skills training is the recognition that many patients with severe psychotic illness have difficulty transferring skills learnt in a therapeutic setting to their natural environment of the home, family, and community. Neurocognitive deficits are associated with poorer longer-term functioning in the community (Fervaha et al. 2014; Green et al. 2004). Undoubtedly, these can have a profound outcome on the ability to acquire new skills and problem-solve, and on prospects for community living. As shown in Box 24.1, certain aspects of cognitive functioning have been shown by Green (1996) to impede functional and community outcomes.

Some of these deficits relate to specific outcomes. For example, verbal memory and vigilance are required for skill acquisition. The ability to remember instructions or stories both in the short and long term are necessary

---

Box 24.1 Neurocognitive factors associated with poor outcome

- poor verbal memory
- poor concentration, vigilance, or attention
- difficulty processing information
- poor transfer of learning
- poor concept formation
- poor cognitive flexibility
- negative symptoms

when learning a new skill or task. Negative symptoms may reduce the ability to form social networks, but they do not appear to hinder skills acquisition. Information-processing deficits are likely to hinder communication and social behaviour. Poor cognitive flexibility can mean that patients transferred to settings where they have more choice and challenge become more symptomatic.

NICE (2014) reviewed the evidence from well-conducted studies for techniques aimed at improving cognitive functioning, such as attention, working memory, and executive functioning. Of these, only cognitive remediation ('brain training') techniques have yielded limited evidence for improving social or vocational functioning in people with psychoses.

Assessment

Before we embark on individualized and *in vivo* interventions, we usually need to establish some baseline through structured or semi-structured assessment. We prefer a naturalistic assessment over time to establish a patient's strengths and weaknesses in daily and social living skills. Regular home- and community-based contacts soon make these apparent. There may, however, be value in exposing newer patients to routine functional assessments to gauge global abilities and deficits.

The purpose of assessment is to guide the process of change. Goals should be identified and documented in the care plan and they should be based on the patient's wishes for role functioning. For example, the patient expresses a desire on prompting to meet more people and expand his range of social activities. The key worker can then enquire about social and cultural preferences, and establish with the patient agreed and achievable goals. For example, a patient may express a desire for mainstream social activity rather than attendance at a drop-in centre for mental health patients. His cultural norms may be more based on going to the pub or a snooker club. A possible goal may be going for a Sunday pub lunch with a parent or friend. Single-issue goals such as the use of public transport or using the launderette will not require the use of a structured assessment tool, as progress can be readily evaluated.

There is no single definitive assessment tool or interview process appropriate for comprehensive functional assessment of daily living skills. One particularly thorough scale is the Social Functioning Scale (Birchwood et al. 1990). This scale was developed for assessment of social and daily living skills as a baseline for schizophrenia family work. Table 24.1 summarizes the areas covered in this scale. Newer evaluation scales include the Personal and Social

Table 24.1 Assessment of social and daily living skills from the Social
Functioning Scale

Functional area	Sample questions
Social withdrawal	On average, what time do you get up? How often will you start a conversation at home? How often will you leave the house for any reason?
Relationships	How many friends do you have at the moment? How easy or difficult do you find talking to people at present? Do you feel uneasy with groups of people?
Social activities	Over the past three months, how often have you participated in the following activities—going to the cinema; visiting places of interest; visiting friends; sport; going to a pub; eating out; visiting relatives; etc.?
Recreational activities	Over the past three months, how often have you done any of the following—reading; gardening; a hobby; shopping; listening to music or the radio; watching television; etc.?
Independence (competence)	How able are you at doing or using the following—public transport; handling money; budgeting; cooking; shopping; washing clothes; personal hygiene; etc.?
Independence (performance)	How often have you done the following in the past three months—buying an item from a shop alone; washing up; washing own clothes; looking for a job; doing the food shopping; cooking a meal; using buses or trains; etc.?
Employment	Do you think you are capable of some kind of job? How often do you make attempts to find a job? If not employed, how do you spend your day?

Data from *The British Journal of Psychiatry,* 157, Birchwood M., Smith J., Cochrane R. et al. 'The Social Functioning Scale: the development and validation of a new scale of social adjustment for use in family intervention programmes with schizophrenic patients', pp. 853–859, 1990.

Performance Scale (Morosini et al. 2000), which is clinician- or researcher-rated from interviews with the patient and care givers across four domains of functioning: personal and social relationships, socially useful activities, self-care, and disturbing and aggressive behaviours. It is sometimes worthwhile quantifying daytime activity for evaluation of interventions or as part of goal setting. The Time Budget Measure (Jolley et al. 2006) is designed particularly for people with psychosis, can be completed as a structured interview, and is sensitive to change over time.

Occupational therapists have extensive training in this area and can assist members of community outreach teams in conducting more formal functional assessments.

Specific interventions

Activity analysis

All activities that we wish to teach or rehearse with patients are best broken down into their constituent parts. This is to understand what is involved, to identify critical elements that may require reinforcing, and to not overwhelm the patient with too much information at once. Information on materials needed, time required, the suitable environment, and stages to completion are all relevant. For example, in order to use a washing machine at a launderette, consider the following questions:

- Which is the nearest launderette?
- When is it open?
- What do you need to take with you—powder, conditioner, laundry bag, newspaper to read while waiting, the correct coins for both washer and drier?
- Which clothes can be washed together—whites and coloured, cotton and synthetic? How can you tell from the label?
- Where do the coins go in the machine?
- How do you select the correct cycle?
- How long does it take?

This task demands physical ability, numeracy, organization and preparation, patience, and motivation. The patient needs verbal memory and information-processing skills. Stage one may be simply to identify the location, opening times, and coins needed by going with the patient. Stage two might be sorting out the clothes into appropriate categories for washing, and so on.

Daily living skills

Following Maslow's (1954) hierarchy of needs, the most important skills for community living are the ability to cook and feed oneself, keeping safe, maintaining stable accommodation, and financial security. In terms of the Personal and Social Performance Scale (Morosini et al. 2000), which is rated out of 100, an extremely low score of 1–5 would indicate survival risks, such as death due to malnutrition, dehydration, infections, and inability to recognize situations of marked danger. As scores increase towards moderate and mild it becomes harder to disentangle ranges of normality from something that might reasonably be of concern for social functioning. This is why shared goal setting is so important. We do not overly prioritize the physical tidiness of patients' accommodation because it is often a matter of personal choice and poses little or no risk. We are often reminded of this deviance from social norms of cleanliness or tidiness when taking visitors or students on home visits. They often comment that we are too tolerant!

Many people are poor at cooking for themselves, and a whole industry of convenience food has grown up as a result. Convenience and takeaway food can, however, be unhealthy if the sole source of nutrition. Helping patients investigate their choices and use their local convenience shops, supermarkets, takeaways, and food delivery services may be all the patient wants. The starting point for cooking may be using the principles of motivational interviewing to encourage patients to recognize that cooking may be both cost-effective and an enjoyable skill. Often patients may lack the materials necessary to cook for themselves. Obtaining grants to buy cooking implements and crockery may act as further encouragement. Cooking does require patience and concentration in order to be a safe activity. If the patient is not prepared to wait until an item is cooked, or forgets to turn off the hob, or leaves the pan unattended, then interventions aimed at improving attention and delaying gratification will be required before trying to cook.

For some patients, properly assessed and negotiated, it may be reasonable to organize a meals delivery service, especially for elderly and frail patients. Likewise, home care, from once to several times a week, can be organized to help patients with cleaning the house, shopping, collecting benefits, etc. These costed services, however, present new challenges. Some patients do not allow others into their home; some behave in such a way that home carers are reluctant to provide the service. Patients who are hard to engage with outreach services are unlikely to be able to cope with such external services.

We generally find that direct service provision from the team or utilization of the patient's family, plus daily living skills training where appropriate, works best. Doing everything for the patient does not motivate them to acquire new skills and may promote unhealthy dependency. A balance between direct support, prompting, and training is required. We refer to this as developing realistic interdependence. We are all dependent on others to some extent for affection, company, or money. The realistic goal of community outreach may not be complete independence in all functional areas.

Social skills training

NICE guidance (2104) is clear in its recommendation not to routinely offer social skills training as a specific intervention to people with psychosis or schizophrenia. By this they mean structured group or individual psychosocial interventions aimed at coping and functioning in social situations, with training and rehearsal of tasks such as identifying and acting on verbal and non-verbal social cues. The accumulated evidence is that such structured interventions are no better than generic social and group activities. It does not mean that in specific situations and with specific individuals some work should not be attempted, but do so judiciously with regard to other interventions with a stronger evidence base. For example, working with patients on basic assertiveness skills to avoid exploitation by others could be worthwhile. We have encountered a number of patients who are exploited by others for money or the use of their accommodation. Persuasive and socially skilled acquaintances (often met in hospital) talk their way into the home and then use it for drug-taking activities, at the expense of our patient. If the patient can rehearse assertion strategies and identify the reward in denying access, then these consequences may be avoided. At the same time, practical interventions enable and support the skills training. We can ensure that the patient's doors and windows are secure, they have not lost their key, and they have a spy hole and chain fitted. Role play in the patient's home is one method of rehearsing responses. The key worker can play the drug dealer at the door, and the patient is required to respond assertively to requests to come in.

Social skills training can, for some patients, include more basic skills such as establishing normal eye contact and other non-verbal behaviour, reducing the amount of 'psychotic talk', asking leading questions and responding to questions, or asking for additional information. Setting homework tasks is common in social and daily living skills training. The patient can then report back how the homework went and how they felt. For example: 'When you go to the post office tomorrow, as we did on our last visit, practise looking at the counter clerk and establishing normal eye contact. Also take your gas bill and ask if this can be paid out of your benefit money.'

Case study

Jerome had lived in a low-support hostel for many years and wanted his own flat. Because of his marked negative symptoms of schizophrenia, and the lack of any skills training in the hostel, it was not felt that this was a realistic proposition. Jerome spent most of his time in bed, would often appear confused, had difficulty managing his finances, and showed little motivation to change.

Functional assessment showed that Jerome often stayed in bed until early afternoon; he only went out to the hospital to play pool or to visit patients on the wards; he had a few superficial relationships with other patients, no hobbies; he did not use public transport, wash his clothes, cook, or manage his money well. Jerome did not want to work but did want to manage and keep his own flat and develop his daytime activities (see Table 24.2). He had poor concentration, motivation, and verbal memory.

The initial work centred around the priorities of keeping his finances in order and ensuring that he made his flat safe, locked the door, and knew how to use the heating. Jerome was introduced to local shops and places to buy food. He liked West African food, and he and his key worker were able to locate a shop that sold some African vegetables and products. This

Table 24.2 Summary care plan

Name: Jerome D.	CMHT: ACT team
Address: Flat 2, Eden House, Kampala Estate	Phone: 0208 877 Xxxx
	New Patient: NO
Phone: None	If No, Date of Review: 6/6/16
Date Of Birth: 17/08/85	Diagnosis:
GP: Reynolds	Schizophrenia F20.0
Phone: 0208 228 Xxxx	2..................... F ——.—

Assessed needs or problem	Intervention	Resp. of
I want to keep my accommodation safe and secure.	◆ Practise assertiveness and security skills. ◆ Frequent visits, twice weekly (plus phone calls) in initial resettlement period. ◆ Ensure finances are in order to pay rent through housing benefit and utility bills.	BJ /JD
Work on daily living skills.	◆ Visit local facilities, shops, leisure facilities, day centre, cafes, post office. ◆ *In vivo* training of managing money, budgeting, shopping, cooking, medication management, relapse planning. Work on concentration and memory. Training to be brief and repeated. Ask Jerome to practise tasks as homework and report back at next visit. ◆ Practical assistance where necessary to resolve difficulties.	BJ/JD

enabled work to begin on showing him how to prepare and cook basic rice and vegetable dishes and to clean up after himself. In order to cook he needed gas, and a lot of time was spent going through bills and showing him how and where to pay them, as well as how to budget and save money for future bills.

Unfortunately, while this skills training was going on, a group of acquaintances starting visiting Jerome, taking money from him and using his flat to abuse drugs. This necessitated a shift in priorities to teaching Jerome assertiveness strategies to refuse access to these people.

Conclusions

We have discussed daily living skills and social skills training as one topic because they are both part of the adjustment, adaptation, and rehabilitative process of helping people stay in their own homes. Community outreach eschews traditional group approaches to the training process in favour of direct provision of *in vivo*, individualized intervention. This form of psychosocial intervention is valuable as a component of comprehensive care in helping patients cope with the additional demands of community living. Research evidence for significant improvements in community functioning, however, is not robust.

We must also recognize the cognitive demands that such complex interventions and skills require of our patients. This leads us to provide intervention packages that are not time limited, have realistic goals, and include reinforcement and rehearsal. Interventions are aimed at improving the quality of life of community patients by opening doors to mainstream activities and opportunities.

Chapter 25

Psychosocial interventions with families, carers, and patients

Introduction

Psychosocial interventions emphasize the broader, non-drug approaches to mental health problems while, at the same time, distancing themselves from the older, ideologically overburdened and 'less scientific' psychotherapies. Psychosocial interventions are framed by an understanding that psychoses have a genetic component exacerbated by stressful life events and emotional environments. They comprise psychological and behavioural treatments focusing on the here-and-now and practical problem-solving strategies.

Psychosocial interventions also share a commitment to working together (staff, patients, families, and carers) to understand problems better and develop strategies to reduce their impact. These strategies can combine psychological strategies (e.g. challenging automatic thoughts in cognitive behaviour therapy), behavioural strategies (families avoiding expressing criticism in response to symptoms), or simple advanced planning and decision-making strategies (taking increased medication in response to an agreed relapse signature). NICE guidance (2014) is clear that psychological interventions are more effective for people with both first-episode and subsequent phases of psychotic illness when delivered in conjunction with antipsychotic medication. The procedures and interventions vary between the approaches and for individual patients within approaches. All, however, build on dialogue and collaboration.

Although a simple, satisfactory definition for psychosocial interventions may not be readily available, most of us recognize the areas and the individual techniques attracting interest and research. There are three broad areas of activity usually implied by 'psychosocial interventions':

1. psycho-education
2. behavioural family management
3. cognitive behaviour therapy (CBT)

The gulf between theory and practice

The vast discrepancy between what is preached and what is practised is striking. In no other area is the failure of research findings to translate into routine practice so obvious. The volume of high-quality research in CBT and behavioural family management in psychosis (NICE 2014b) is remarkable. Yet even in the centres of excellence (where much of this research has been conducted), the interventions are rarely part of routine local service. In a large national audit of schizophrenia care in England and Wales (Royal College of Psychiatrists 2014), services reported that 23 per cent of patients not in remission were offered family intervention and 45 per cent of patients not in remission were offered CBT. Some 12 per cent of patients said they had received a family intervention; 18 per cent reported that they had received CBT. Nurses with comprehensive training in these approaches—on specialized postgraduate schemes such as accredited Thorn courses (Gournay and Birley 1998)—rarely apply them routinely (Fadden 1997). This is frequently blamed on resource limitations. One problem is that many Thorn graduates are rapidly promoted out of the direct clinical arena. Positive outcomes from training are maximized by ongoing supervision of staff following such courses (Brooker et al. 1994). Undoubtedly there is a resource issue, but we doubt that it explains the extent of the gulf between theory and practice; we believe the reasons are more complex.

Efficacy and effectiveness

First, there is the difference between treatment *efficacy* and clinical *effectiveness*. Treatment efficacy is how successful a treatment is under optimal experimental conditions (e.g. all the staff are excellent, all the patients get all the treatment, the patients only have one problem, and there are no drop-outs). Clinical effectiveness, however, is how the treatment fares in the real world (where patients may not comply fully with treatments, staff may vary in skill, and other external factors complicate the process). Even with simple drug treatments, there is a significant difference between efficacy and effectiveness.

Resistance

Second, psychological and behavioural work requires motivation from both sides. Despite the trend towards briefer talking therapies, exemplified by the UK Improving Access to Psychological Therapies programme for mild to moderate mental health problems (Clark 2011), these are still relatively labour-intensive interventions. They require us to enter more formal programmes with patients structured over many sessions. In classical psychodynamic psychotherapy, the patient brought the commitment—the therapist's job was to understand and interpret what was brought (even if it was silence!). In most of the current psychosocial interventions, patients and their families may be convinced that it is the right approach, but they will rarely seek out the treatment and insist on it. It is we who are usually pushing the intervention, often driven by our awareness of our own failing to follow best practice guidance (NICE 2014b) and standards (HQIP and The Royal College of Psychiatrists 2014). Patient and family resistance can be considerable—and for quite understandable reasons. Families may, over time, have achieved an uneasy truce, a pragmatic working agreement, with the patient and do not want it disturbed. Both they and the patient may be exhausted and demoralized by years of struggle with the illness.

Modern psychosocial interventions, with their emphasis on behavioural change, homework, and targets are also very hard work. They give the therapists more control over the pace of change. It should not be forgotten that even the most diplomatically phrased exercise implies a tacit criticism of previous functioning, and can cause resentment. Think about it. How do you feel if someone suggests you change one of your habits? Traditional psychotherapists took understanding such resistance to change very seriously and had complex theories about it and strategies to deal with it. In modern teaching, it is often rather glossed over, implying that the obvious benefits from the treatment will overcome any doubts. Early dropout is high n CBT approaches in psychosis.

Supporting psychosocial interventions in community outreach

Despite the problems previously outlined, it is possible to work towards more routine provision of evidence-based psychosocial interventions for patients with severe mental illness. A first step is to make sure that they are taken seriously within the team. The most effective way of ensuring this is to provide high-quality teaching and supervision. When possible, staff should be encouraged to attend courses accredited through the Thorn initiative (Gournay and Birley 1998) or their more recent local equivalents. These courses cover best practice in psychosocial interventions for the care and treatment of severe mental illness. We established a day-release course locally when we ran the Wandsworth assertive outreach team, based closely on the official Thorn syllabus.

Such courses are equally applicable to case managers from non-nursing backgrounds, and we have had both social workers and occupational therapists on our course as well as mental health support workers and nurses.

Access to such a course may not be readily available for all staff (as it was not in the first few years of our service). One can still raise the profile and quality of such work by ensuring that one or two staff attend, and then using professional development slots within the team to share skills and supervise ongoing practice. Taking time to review the psychosocial management of individual patients during routine reviews continues to reaffirm their importance. For most mental health practitioners, these skills carry high professional status, and there is a real hunger to discuss them and improve them. Making sure they are discussed in detail in reviews is rarely a problem.

One way to ensure that our patients do benefit from these approaches, however, is to be honest about which ones work for us and which we can deliver. There is a tendency for the most complex and demanding treatments (those that require the highest level of skill) to have the highest status. We have decided, as a team, to emphasize the simpler, more feasible interventions that should be routinely available to all our patients and their families. Once they are being consistently applied, then there is scope for the more recherché treatments.

Being honest and realistic about what you can achieve is much more likely to produce results than exaggerated claims about 'cutting-edge practice'. What follows is an overview of what we routinely did in the Wandsworth assertive outreach team and support in community outreach services. It is not comprehensive, and other teams will go further. We consider some of the interventions, however, to be essential components of acceptable practice, without which we would be failing our patients.

Family and carer interventions

Evidence for family interventions for adults with schizophrenia is clear. NICE (2014b) recommends that specific interventions are offered to families of people with psychosis or schizophrenia who live with or are in close contact with the patient. NICE states that family interventions should be conducted according to the following guidelines:

◆ include the person with psychosis if practical with consideration for family relationships
◆ be at least ten sessions, lasting between three months and one year
◆ consider preferences for single-family or multi-family group intervention
◆ have specific supportive, educational, or treatment functions
◆ include negotiated problem-solving or crisis management work

These recommendations stem from the beneficial effect of family intervention on relapse rates which remain significant in NICE meta-analysis of well-conducted studies with at least 24 months' follow-up.

Before any successful psychosocial interventions with families or carers can be contemplated, they first have to be engaged with the services. A supportive family (and most carers in mental health are families rather than friends or neighbours) can be the most powerful determinant of outcome for individuals with severe mental illness. Contrary to previous theories, which have implicated families in the genesis and exacerbation of psychoses (Chapter 15), the overwhelming evidence—both scientific and clinical—is that patients living with families do better than those without them. Of course, this does not prove that families *cause* better outcomes. It is highly likely that less ill patients stay with families and more severely ill ones cannot tolerate the relationships—and sometimes the families cannot cope with them. On balance, however, despite the stresses and strains, it is better to have a family than not. As these family members are actively engaged in trying to help and care for the patient, it is essential that their efforts are taken seriously.

Teams are expected to ensure that families are fully informed about treatment strategies, that their views on treatments are taken into account, and that they are kept fully in the picture in terms of understanding the illness and the full range of possible treatments and care options. Put like that, it sounds a tall order, but in practice it is usually rewarding and welcomed work.

Psycho-education

Teaching patients and their families about the illness they have to contend with is generally referred to by the clumsy term 'psycho-education'. At its most basic, it can comprise meeting the family and explaining what the diagnosis is, giving the best estimate of the prognosis, and explaining what the current treatment entails, with both its benefits and side effects outlined. Involving carers, when the patient agrees, and providing them with a copy of the agreed care plan can be a simple and efficient start to the process.

Psycho-education can be significantly improved by using a more structured approach. The 'knowledge about schizophrenia' interview (Barrowclough et al. 1987) provides a method of assessing the carer's prior knowledge about the illness. Specially prepared leaflets and information sheets, as well as online resources and videos, are useful follow-ups. These allow the family member (and the patient) to read and reread the material—most of us know from personal experience how little we remember of the information our doctors give us. Being able to take away a well-written resource pack, tailored to their needs, means they can study it at leisure. They can also ask about anything they are unclear about when they next meet their key worker or doctor. It is difficult to ascertain how effective psycho-education is, because it is usually studied as part of a more comprehensive intervention (Hogarty et al. 1991; Leff et al. 1990). There is no recommendation for psycho-education on its own for patients or families in NICE guidance (2014).

Clinical experience confirms how essential explanations of illness and treatment are to any intervention that requires family members to work as part of the therapeutic team. It is vital not only to make sure we are all pulling in the same direction, but also to dispel, as much as possible, residual guilt and shame that are so common in parents of the mentally ill. Although we may have moved on from superficial theories blaming them for their offspring's illness (Chapter 14), they will certainly be regularly exposed to such prejudices in their daily life. They need to know that we do not share those views; psycho-education is a very powerful means of emphasizing that fact.

Behavioural family management

Research aimed at understanding why some patients with schizophrenia relapsed despite effective maintenance pharmacotherapy (Hirsch et al. 1973) led to studies of the family environment to which they were discharged. It was found that patients from families who were emotionally intense and generally very involved were more likely to relapse. Work by Leff and colleagues further indicated that relapse was likely when the patient spent a lot of time with family members (the studies used 35 hours per week as the cut-off, although there is nothing magical about this figure), and particularly so if the family members were critical of the patient. These families came to be referred to as 'high expressed emotion' ('high EE') families, and a series of studies showed that family treatments to reduce high EE led to a reduction in relapse rates (Falloon et al. 1982; Leff et al. 1990; Linszen et al. 1996; Tarrier et al. 1989; Vaughan et al. 1992).

Most of these studies used an approach which comprised psycho-education about schizophrenia (usually delivered jointly to patient and family members) followed by regular meetings (weekly or fortnightly) for several months to explore strategies to reduce or avoid critical comments towards the patient and to help the family disengage somewhat from each other. Simple interventions are often remarkably welcome and effective. Pointing out to a concerned mother that her son may need to be left alone when he is aroused and disturbed is quite counter-intuitive (most of us want to comfort and care for distressed relatives). The education helps reduce the emotional charge which many individuals with severe mental health problems (not just those with schizophrenia) find difficult to handle.

Exploration of the family interactions often revealed common, repeated, and undramatic stresses (e.g. lying in bed all day, repetitive questioning, smoking in bed) that families struggle with. Helping find a form of words or action which modifies the behaviour without causing a row can be developed jointly by the therapist and family members, and they can be supported in practising it. Over time, families realize that this less confrontational and slightly more distanced style pays off, and both they and the patient feel better. Family members also really appreciate finding out that their problems are not unique, and that the problem is not so much them as the illness. Indeed, one study has shown better results by engaging in family problem-solving in a group session (McFarlane et al. 1995).

In truth, we find establishing behavioural family interventions very difficult. In the initial series of studies, five courses of treatment were necessary to prevent one relapse, and in later studies (conducted perhaps with less committed families and less expert therapists), seven courses were required to prevent one relapse (Mari and Streiner 1994). NICE (2014b) has provided an updated and more optimistic estimate that the number needed to prevent one relapse within 12 months' follow-up is four. We should not underestimate how difficult it is to remain committed to a treatment which is time-consuming and in which perception of direct improvement is not obvious but supported with a statistical reduction in risk. In one way, we experience what the patient has to tolerate with maintenance medication—no immediate benefit but simply our reassurance that they are less likely to fall ill. Despite these difficulties, this is an effective treatment that can bring significant benefits to both patient and family, and teams need to develop strategies to encourage and support its provision.

Involving social systems

Two approaches have emerged from Scandinavia that emphasize work with social systems and families integrated into their community outreach models. Resource group assertive community treatment prioritizes shared decision-making, utilizing a resource group of the patient and members of their social network together with professionals (Nordén et al. 2012). Within the Swedish context, the model blends aspects of the recovery approach through family interventions, assertive outreach, and empowering the patient. Open dialogue (Aaltonen et al. 2011; Seikkula et al. 2006) is a recovery-oriented psychosocial approach developed in Finland and rooted in psychotherapy traditions. Open dialogue puts less emphasis on medication for people in psychiatric crisis in favour of a rapid response through close collaboration between services and an individual's family and social network. Specifically, the model prioritizes a treatment meeting of the network within 24 hours of the referral in crisis. The open dialogue method assumes meaning to the emergence of the psychosis, conceptualizing its emergence as happening between people, not within a person. Both these approaches have published some evidence for their outcomes, though neither has been incorporated into NICE guidance (2014b).

In the UK, the need to incorporate social systems—particularly carers and families—into decision-making for recovery is typically referred to as the 'triangle of care' (Carers Trust 2013). The triangle refers to the essential three-way relationship between professionals, service users, and their carers and families.

Patient-focused interventions

Two different theoretical approaches are identifiable for most psychosocial interventions (though in practice there is much overlap):

◆ stress-vulnerability model—emphasizes coping strategy enhancement

◆ cognitive model—emphasizes similarity between normal and abnormal thinking, using the patient's beliefs and experiences to explore links between thoughts, feelings, and subsequent actions or behaviour

Both approaches draw heavily on the core principles of CBT:

◆ the central position of the patient as an active agent in the change process

◆ a collaborative rather than prescriptive exercise

◆ scientific method (predicting consequences and testing those predictions)

◆ focus on individual symptoms, not the disorder

The collaborative approach is probably the most important feature of all CBT approaches. Two key concepts often written about are 'collaborative empiricism' and the 'Socratic dialogue'. Collaborative empiricism describes the way the therapist and patient develop and test ideas together. They agree what would be the results of one view (the delusion) and what would happen if the delusion were not true, and then test out what actually does happen. Socratic dialogue refers to the Greek philosopher's habit of instructing his pupils by questioning them, so that eventually they came out with the answers themselves—they discovered what they already knew. In psychotic disorders, it enables the inconsistency or inner doubts about delusions to be aired without a direct assault on them (which we have all learnt from bitter experience rarely works!).

Stress-vulnerability model

This view accepts that the individual with a severe mental illness has some specific vulnerability to stress which manifests itself in the symptoms of the illness (Zubin and Spring 1977). The view lies at the heart of much of community outreach practice described in this book. CBT techniques are aimed at reducing these stressors—whether they are the external stresses of family and friends or the stress of the symptoms themselves. In both cases, it is understood that it is the patient's own appraisal of the event which determines whether or not it is a stress, and if so, how severe.

Coping strategy enhancement

Tarrier and colleagues (Tarrier et al. 1998) consider that patients who have a wide range of coping strategies manage better with their psychotic experiences. They advise identifying as many effective strategies as possible that reduce distress from symptoms and encouraging the patient to use them. Such strategies can be *affective* (relaxation, sleep), *behavioural* (activity, seeking company), or *cognitive* (distracting, challenging). The origins, content, or meaning of persistent symptoms are not critical to this pragmatic approach. The work is more focused on maintaining emotional and physiological well-being despite potentially distressing symptoms such as persecutory delusions.

'Mindfulness' carries a more modern interpretation of this idea and it has been suggested that, in an adapted form, mindfulness can be used safely and effectively in psychosis (Chadwick 2014) and can be delivered in groups. Mindfulness is a meditation approach focusing awareness on the present moment, acknowledging and accepting feelings, thoughts, and bodily sensations. Chadwick recommends that sessions be short and instruction frequent to avoid 'people becoming lost in a struggle with malevolent voices or in paranoid ruminations'.

CBT for psychosis

CBT for psychosis involves challenging delusions and assumptions about hallucinations using the Socratic dialogue outlined previously. It explicitly draws on the evidence from normal psychology that most of us preferentially register information that strengthens our prejudices and ignore information that contradicts them. The approach is one of accessing the patient's inner doubts, often by working with the double awareness that is often so striking in psychotic patients (i.e. patients behave in ways that are totally at variance with their intensely held beliefs). Four components of this 'disputing' approach are distinguished (Chadwick et al. 1996):

- evidence for belief challenged (starting with less important issues first)
- internal logic and plausibility challenged
- reformulate as understandable response, seek meaningful alternative
- assess alternative and delusion against available evidence

NICE guidance (2014) is refreshingly clear on the evidence summarizing well-conducted trials comparing CBT for psychosis with standard care. There is consistent evidence that CBT is effective in reducing rehospitalization rates and days in hospital (8.26 days on average). CBT is also effective in reducing symptom severity and this can still be seen at 12 months' follow-up. The NICE (2014) recommendations are as follows:

- offer CBT to all people with psychosis or schizophrenia during the acute phase or later (including promoting recovery in people with persisting positive and negative symptoms and for people in remission)
- advise people who want to try psychological interventions alone that these are more effective when delivered in conjunction with antipsychotic medication
- deliver CBT on a one-to-one basis over at least 16 planned sessions
- follow a treatment manual that guides the therapist to:
  - establish links between thoughts, feelings, and actions
  - re-evaluate people's perceptions, beliefs, reasoning as they relate to the target symptoms
  - help people monitor their thoughts, feelings, and behaviours with respect to their symptoms, and promote alternative ways of coping

Early warning signs and relapse signatures

Many patients have identifiable relapse signatures—a group of symptoms, experiences, or behaviours that herald an impending breakdown (see Box 25.1).

For some disorders, there are well-recognized warnings that are specific to the disorder rather than individual patients (e.g. poor sleep is very typical in incipient mania; being preoccupied and withdrawn is common in schizophrenia). All mental health workers learn to be alert for such indicators. It is the basis of much of our clinical training.

Early recognition of emerging patterns of breakdown, often before full-blown symptoms are obvious, comes with experience. Monitoring to assess mental state and functioning should take place (whether in depth or, more

---

Box 25.1 Common early warning signs

- tensions, nervousness, irritability, sense of impending doom
- difficulty sleeping; overactivity
- social withdrawal; disengagement from services; self-neglect
- increased positive symptoms: paranoia, thought disorder, auditory hallucinations

often, informally as part of another activity) as an integral part of any contact between a patient and a mental health professional. Monitoring to spot early signs of destabilization or breakdown is one of the primary purposes of any outreach service.

As well as the more general early signs of relapse, there are some patients who have their own unique pattern which precedes breakdown. This is particularly so in bipolar disorder, and teaching patients (and their families) how to recognize such patterns, and what to do, is a valuable intervention. Agreeing what should be done and—most important—writing the agreement down as a contingency plan is increasingly routine practice. The procedures we use are outlined in the chapters on bipolar disorder (Chapter 16) and out-of-hours working (Chapter 6), and will not be repeated here.

Tarrier's work shows that the approach is of value for more patients than just those who have a strikingly obvious relapse signature (Perry et al. 1999). Most bipolar patients and their families can be helped to identify the early stages of relapse, and encouraged and taught what to do. We have been using a similar approach in our CBT with schizophrenia, but have not found making a distinction between relapse signatures and responding to periods of increased stress that valuable. With schizophrenia patients, we focus on identifying indicators of stress and worry, and strategies to use should the need arise, rather than conceptualizing it as relapse prevention.

As with psychosocial interventions generally, early intervention has the added benefit of empowerment, reducing the sense of hopelessness for both patient and family.

Understanding and support

At the beginning of this chapter and at other places in this book, we have warned against the possible downside of being excessively evidence-based in approach. Yes, we do need to make sure that most of our time and effort goes into providing treatments that are known to work—whether these are broadly psychological, social, or medical. On the other hand, we must not forget that this work is about people and relationships. Patients and their families need understanding and support, though not as an alternative to effective psychosocial interventions. They may need understanding and support even more when they are receiving such psychosocial interventions because the treatments are demanding and can, despite our best efforts, be quite stressful.

Time needs to be devoted to simply being nice to patients and their families. If we cannot learn to respect and like them, and they us, then we are unlikely to be able to help them even with the most sophisticated treatments. Expressing sympathy and support, and paying attention to the broader canvas of patients' lives, are necessary foundations for collaborative work. It is not wasted time or a case of 'avoiding the issue'. In a health service with rising demand and limited resources, staff do not actively seek work. Adopting a rather business-like tone has traditionally been one way of managing the pressures. With the severely mentally ill, this approach is probably inefficient in the long term. A welcoming and genuinely supportive approach, which leads to problem-solving early on, will save time in the long run.

Older counselling approaches (whether non-directive or Rogerian or psychodynamic) have a role to play in outreach work. Tragic and difficult events are far from uncommon for our patients, who need the opportunity to talk them through, make sense of them, and come to terms with them. Most mental health workers appreciate the value of such approaches. The trick is to avoid dogma. There is no set number of sessions or length of session that must be followed. What is important is that the sessions are safe, respectful, and supportive.

Received wisdom is that psychodynamic approaches with individuals with severe mental illnesses do more harm than good. When this means attempting to interpret and uncover unconscious material in an individual who has difficulty distinguishing the inner world from the outer at the best of times, we would agree. However, concepts like 'denial', 'unconscious worrying', 'transference', and having a 'complex' about something are all useful ways of understanding experience. The language is intuitive and now easily understood by all involved, and can help make otherwise confusing experiences more understandable.

While we would not encourage psychoanalytic therapy for our patients, we see no harm in using many of the terms and ideas that derive from it. These terms are generally regarded as more respectful and equal than the technical terms we use in formal therapies (e.g. 'automatic thoughts'). Psychodynamic language is that which patients hear on the television (e.g. 'you're just repressing it') and that they know we use about each other—it is no longer associated with illness. It is also a robust conceptual framework which makes some sort of sense of difficult experiences in ways that help us, as therapists, to keep sight of the patient's essential humanity.

Conclusions

In the broad, holistic approach used in community outreach work, patients and their families are seen as complete individuals, in all their complexity. The work ranges from the narrowly prescriptive aspects of medication, to social and personal support, through dramatic life crises. The rather vague concept of 'psychosocial interventions' straddles this range. It consists of a group of disparate treatments with proven efficacy, and which are based on using understanding (and the collaborative relationship that develops from it) to achieve quite specific behavioural changes. They are both effective and conceptually attractive to outreach workers.

Such interventions are, however, often unhelpfully presented as being easy. *Learning* to do them, and do them well, is reasonably easy. They are well described and operationalized. Most of our staff have been able to gain a working ability with the main interventions in a one-year day-release course. But *applying* them, and applying them consistently, is not at all easy. To do so requires effort, sensitivity, and persistence. Time for them needs to be protected in the midst of crises, admissions, and the like. Their results are very real but not immediately obvious, and their success requires continued attention to detail. None of this is easy, and we should not pretend it is.

The real challenge is not to strive endlessly to keep at the cutting edge of practice, but to ensure that established and effective psychosocial interventions are made available to those who can benefit from them. There is a need to monitor and audit to ensure that we deliver the psychosocial interventions that we know work.

Part III

Management and development

Chapter 26

Operational and team management

Introduction

Health care is a complex activity. Managing this activity involves aligning people, processes, and, increasingly, technology towards clear outcomes and standards. It relies on coordination, communication, and a clearly understood policy framework at the team level.

Rummler and Brache (1990) differentiate three levels within organizations for targeting effective performance. The simplest is the *job performer* level, which covers individual role clarity, performance, coaching, development, and training. This chapter starts with job roles and the qualities of leadership. The *process* level is the team and clinical systems level. We look at what team systems and processes in a typical week help ensure a safe, efficient, patient-centred, equitable, and timely service that has effective outcomes (Institute of Medicine 2001). The top level is the *organizational* level of strategic direction and deployment of resources, which is outside the scope of this chapter.

Outreach in community mental health is a labour-intensive activity and it is the human factors that are often the most challenging. We believe that community outreach teams need a clinical team leader who is a mental health professional and capable of combining a small amount of team casework with operational management. Team managers often find themselves propelled from clinical roles without managerial preparation and instruction, so we have included basic management concepts along with the contemporary policy framework.

Role of the team leader

The main tasks carried out by the team leader are summarized in Box 26.1. The role calls for a generalist with clinical experience, sound judgement, and the ability to plan and prioritize the many varied tasks into a week's work. It's like juggling a number of balls at the same time—and some of those balls can cause damage if they are dropped!

Box 26.1 Key tasks of the team leader

- decision-making in conjunction with the consultant psychiatrist
- working clinically with small caseload of patients; stepping in to resolve issues with complex team patients
- coordinating the handovers and meeting schedule
- overseeing the team's caseload size, mix, and priorities; management supervision of team members
- coordinating clinical supervision
- staff recruitment, selection, retention, induction, and training
- managing the team budget
- implementing and protecting the model and policies
- dealing with problems—clinical and operational (e.g. complaints, untoward incidents)
- delivering and managing processes and strategies for change
- representing the team externally
- linking and negotiating with external agencies
- monitoring and evaluating the service; regular audit

Team leader is clearly not a job that suits everyone. The following are some important characteristics to include in the person specification:

- clear communicator
- good interpersonal skills
- able to work under pressure
- able to make key decisions for both day-to-day problem-solving and strategy
- able to lead by example in clinical work
- good presentational skills
- able to work as part of a team
- able to delegate tasks and responsibilities
- able to involve and motivate the team

Role of the consultant psychiatrist

A single consultant for the team provides direction and a consistent approach to patient care. It also simplifies compliance with statutory procedures with accountability. For some large teams with two or more consultant psychiatrists, leadership arrangements can be difficult, and areas of accountability need to be established.

The tasks that make up the consultant's role are as follows:

- direct team vision, model, and priorities
- responsible medical officer for the purposes of the Mental Health Act (Department of Health 1999b)
- primary clinical decision maker
- clinical work across entire team caseload, but focusing on complex cases
- medical input to clinical reviews
- represent the team externally
- line manage medical staff

Structuring a week in community outreach

A flexible team needs a predictable timetable. The timetable shown in Table 26.1 is the one that was used by the Wandsworth assertive outreach team; it is one way of coordinating team activity over a seven-day period. Teams that operate a shift system or are on call may have a handover at the beginning and end of each shift. Our timetable represents a compromise between a team that operates in normal office hours and one that is on call 24 hours a day, seven days a week. The majority of time is unstructured for patient contact and activity. This activity is not predictable, and key workers need to allow time in their diaries for the unexpected.

Monday morning's handover is important for planning the week ahead. Shared care using a team approach (Chapter 5) means that individual visits and tasks can be allocated throughout the week. Different weekdays may have a specific focus—collecting clozapine blood samples on one particular day, attending the ward on another, planning weekend cover and activity on a Friday, etc. Such a weekly schedule accommodates many factors such as consultant availability, postgraduate training, and inpatient unit schedules and shifts.

Balancing coordination with clinical time

Meetings should be just long enough for coordination, cover, communication, and support, allowing the majority of time for patient contact. A 'tight' meeting will limit expansive and overly detailed backgrounds and discussion. A strategy in our team is to bring drifting discussion into line by asking for the 'headline' first, followed by any relevant facts. A more structured framework increasingly

Table 26.1 A weekly timetable for a community outreach team

MONDAY	TUESDAY	WEDNESDAY	THURSDAY	FRIDAY	SATURDAY	SUNDAY
0900–0930 HANDOVER To include team approach planning of visits for week	**0900–1100** COMMUNITY REVIEW MEETING	**0900–0930** HANDOVER	**0900–0930** HANDOVER	**0900–0930** HANDOVER	**0900–1700** ROUTINE VISITS (with capacity for emergency cover)	**0900–1700** ROUTINE VISITS (with capacity for emergency cover)
1000–1100 CLINICAL SUPERVISION (alternate weeks)	**1100–1200** BUSINESS MEETING (monthly)	VISITS AND LIAISON WITH WARD AND HOME TREATMENT TEAMS	VISITS AND LIAISON WITH WARD AND HOME TREATMENT TEAMS	VISITS AND LIAISON WITH WARD AND HOME TREATMENT TEAMS		
1000–1100 DEVELOPMENT MEETING (monthly)	VISITS AND LIAISON WITH WARD AND HOME TREATMENT TEAMS					
VISITS AND LIAISON WITH WARD AND HOME TREATMENT TEAMS						

used in safety-critical environments is provided by the 'SBAR' approach (Kaiser Foundation Health Plan, Inc. 2004):

S=Situation (a concise statement of the problem)

B=Background (pertinent and brief information related to the situation)

A=Assessment (analysis and considerations of options—what you found/think)

R=Recommendation (action requested/recommended—what you want)

For example, the situation may be 'Patrick wants to negotiate a reduction in his medication'; the background might be that there are relevant side effects; mental state assessment shows absence of positive symptoms, and drug history indicates relapse often occurs following negotiation down to subclinical doses. A brief multidisciplinary discussion of options can then be held and a recommendation agreed to see Patrick for shared decision-making.

Handover and briefing

'Handover' is a nursing term for relaying information from shift to shift. With shared caseloads, effective transmission of verbal and written information is essential on a daily basis. Teams in England and Wales use a key worker system (Department of Health 1990), strengthened with a team approach for patients needing more intensive input. When key workers are identified and shift work is not the model, the handover is more of a morning briefing session (see Boxes 26.2–26.3). Even with video conferencing, mobile working, and electronic access to care records from tablets and laptops, we value the physical meeting at the team base each morning. Together with the planning board or digital white board, the planning meeting is also a central feature of the flexible ACT model described in Chapter 4.

Weekly review meeting

Patients with complex needs, such as those cared for by community outreach teams, require regular reviews of their treatment and care. Annual reviews are required as a minimum for all patients on the care programme approach (CPA) (Department of Health 1990) (see Box 26.4). We reviewed in depth every six months.

Whenever possible, all those involved with the care and welfare of the patient are invited to the meeting. This may include the patient, carers, and voluntary sector and day or residential care workers. A balance has to be struck, however, between such inclusiveness and the efficient use of team time. We routinely reviewed five patients each week, allocating 20 minutes to each review.

Box 26.2 Format for handover and briefing

- takes place first thing in the morning (or beginning and end of the day when using a shift system)
- 30 minutes, depending on caseload size
- prioritization framework drawing upon zoning or flexible ACT model
- visual management of information and actions ('patient status at a glance' or FACT board)
- discussion only if there has been a change, development, or concern; if advice is needed, or when visit allocation or cover is needed
- chairperson to curtail lengthy discussion or refer to clinical supervision or weekly review meeting
- Monday handover may be more involved with allocation of work for the week (e.g. which patients to be visited each day; tasks for the support worker)
- Friday handover may include time for planning support over the weekend if cover is limited

By providing such practical assistance as transport, reminders, and reassurance, it is possible to facilitate the presence of the patient and their carers routinely at the review. Sometimes patients do not want to be present to hear all their history, and prefer to come into the review for input to the

Box 26.3 Functions of handover and briefing

- structured exchange of information on every patient, in a time-efficient forum
- allocation of tasks and visits
- organization of cover for staff on leave, training, or away sick
- organization of joint visits either for safety or specific input
- group support and multidisciplinary problem-solving
- prioritization of resources for the day
- regular access to a doctor for advice, prescriptions, medicine titration, or changes
- reinforce 'teamness' through face-to-face planning and discussion

Box 26.4 Functions of care programme approach (CPA) review meeting

- forum for involving users, carers, and other agencies in care planning and review process
- opportunity for extended discussion with full multidisciplinary team and all relevant parties to current and long-term management
- statutory requirement (Care Programme Approach—Department of Health 1990)
- agreement and completion of full documentation—CPA, care plan, risk and contingency plans, treatment plan, review of aftercare under supervision, etc.

discussion of the care plan. The format described in Box 26.5 is one we evolved in our team.

If the patient is attending, it will be necessary to adjust the style and content of the review to allow for sensitivity to potential embarrassment, denial, and third-party information. With this caveat, the information summarized in Box 26.6 should be covered.

Box 26.5 Preparations for CPA review

- Put reviews in your diary.
- Arrange joint visit with psychiatrist.
- Repeat HoNOS, side effects, or any other relevant structured assessment and outcome scales.
- Invite the patient and carer and relevant others. Book a time slot and arrange transport if necessary. An alternative is to conduct CPA in the patient's home or hostel involving only key multidisciplinary team representatives if this is more acceptable or appropriate.
- Prepare the patient well; explain the purpose and procedure. Explain the time limitations. Agree on whether they wish to hear all their history or only wish to attend care planning.
- Plan what you and your patient each need to get out of the review.

Box 26.6 Content of review

- name and age
- length of time with team
- diagnosis
- summary of relevant family/social history
- summary of psychiatric history:
  - number and frequency of admissions
  - relapse signature
  - untoward events
  - risks associated with relapse
  - treatment responses
  - medication summary
- social circumstances
- medical history
- current situation and problems:
  - current BPRS and mental health
  - current medication
  - side-effect assessment
  - Mental Health Act status: supervision register/supervised discharge/Section 17 leave
  - prioritize other problems from physical health, housing, finance, occupation, daily living skills
  - risks
- discussion
- formulation of new care plan
- presentation of risk documentation
- review crisis and contingency plan (see Chapter 6)

There is currently such an emphasis on completing paperwork in reviews that it is easy to forget that their main purpose is to plan treatment. Key workers need to schedule in 'post-review' time (and energy) to make sure the paperwork is completed that day. Leaving it for a day or so risks confusion and the possibility of forgetting important issues.

During this post-review time, the care plan, contingency plan, and risk documentation should be completed *fully*, with copies to the GP and other agencies as necessary and agreed.

Business meetings, team days, and development meetings

Business meetings

A rolling programme of business and development meetings ensures regularity and helps team members to organize their time. Business meetings provide a structured space for senior staff to inform others of changes affecting the team or external agencies (e.g. information on new community groups, changes in arrangements for accessing meals on wheels, pharmacy opening times over bank holidays, forthcoming conferences, deadlines for returning monitoring information). Consultation on strategic changes and discussion of operational policies can take place. Business meetings are not entirely focused on high-flying strategy. They provide an essential opportunity to resolve practical issues that team members find themselves dealing with day to day. Such issues—ranging from parking changes to heating and cleaning grumbles—are usually not important or big enough to wait for team days. At one early stage, we called this our 'moans and groans' forum. If there is no formalized place to ensure these issues are addressed, they leak into clinical meetings and undermine staff morale.

Generation of new working practices or ideas is encouraged from individual team members. A single team leader cannot resolve and contain all aspects of team dynamics, individual anxieties, organizational change, or team direction and adaptation. Nor should they attempt to. All teams have a wealth of professional and personal experience. Solutions are usually readily found through collective effort.

Team days

Business meetings should be backed up by regular team days (once or twice a year) which can focus on major, non-clinical decision-making. Team days are generally best arranged away from the base. They provide additional 'thinking time' and need an agenda that will allow both brainstorming and detailed constructive problem-solving. A typical agenda might include a mix of specific topics that have filtered through from business meetings, reorganization, and specific incidents, as well as issues from clinical supervision.

Team days can be stressful when conflicts are confronted so it is good to finish with some unstructured time and team building.

Facilitators

The decision to have a professional outside facilitator is best decided by the team as a whole. There are quite strongly divided opinions on this issue. Structured, business parts of the day will not generally require an outside facilitator, but the team may choose to have one for that part of the programme which is more personal and more to do with team dynamics.

Development meetings

Development meetings are part of the team training and audit cycle (Chapter 27). Team members can take it in turns to facilitate or present a training topic, or external speakers can be invited. Group training in the use of routine assessment and outcome tools (e.g. HoNOS-Health of the Nation Outcome Scale; Wing et al. 1999) generates greater inter-rater reliability and team understanding, plus it reinforces a common language used to discuss change. Specific topics can be introduced in development sessions by external speakers. A relevant new publication or research paper can be presented. In this way, the development meeting becomes a learning aid, helping staff to keep up to date and encouraging evidence-based practice by developing the necessary skills to interpret the often confusing evidence around us.

Development meetings can also generate audit ideas or standards, or even be used to conduct an audit. For example, to audit compliance with risk assessment documentation standards, the team can scan ten sets of randomly selected electronic care records in the meeting and determine key gaps or quality markers. Team members also get to understand how and why audits are performed.

Operational policy

The team's purpose, objectives, and working protocols should be defined in a written operational policy. This should include local criteria for accepting referrals, discharge, and team structure. Operational policies can also include specific team-level priorities and targets on measurable and achievable activities such as frequency of contact and interventions offered. Operational policies give a concise overview of the functions and structure of the team to new and existing staff, other clinical colleagues, and to managers and commissioners (see Box 26.7).

Using the operational policy to set team priorities, goals, and targets allows for management by objectives. For example, the organization's mission statement may be: 'To provide the best mental health services for people in the locality'. This lacks any specific information on how to achieve or measure it. What

---

Box 26.7 Key areas for operational policy

- model and purpose of the team
- team aims and objectives
- target patient group
- referral criteria
- discharge criteria
- team-level priorities and targets
- relationships with other parts of the service
- team staffing, composition, and accountability
- operating hours and cover arrangements
- training and staff support
- research and outcome measures

---

would 'good' look like? At the team level, targets must be more realistic and performance must be visible to staff. Providing regular visual dashboards of performance metrics to team managers and clinicians at their desktop is one useful approach. A small number of graphs or charts summarizing the recent key team data—perhaps with a comparison with a previous month or with the service average—gives staff the tools and data to self-evaluate and to observe measureable improvement or emerging problems.

In community outreach, typical shared goals are the avoidance of psychiatric hospitalization, housing stability, independent living, and competitive employment. Monitoring and charting rates of actual bed use over time and observing trends and blips (while being alert to other external factors) helps staff understand the impact of any recent quality improvement initiatives or staffing problems. Much of this information will be provided through 'contractual performance data' at the organizational level—i.e. what the Trust or hospital has to extract and report on. When accurate electronic data is lacking, teams can ask themselves questions that may lead to improved processes. For this it is important to use simple ratings rather than the complicated ones more suitable for research studies. The Substance Abuse and Mental Health Services Administration (SAMHSA) (2008) gives the positive example of 'Did the consumer hold a competitive job in this quarter?' rather than the more challenging 'How many hours during this quarter did the consumer work competitively?'

Management approaches

Leadership style should be that of an accessible and supportive facilitator rather than a remote and supervisory manager. There is enough of that elsewhere in the system! Team leadership implies inspiring a group of people towards a common set of objectives rather than simply getting things done through instructing them.

Autocratic leadership may evolve where an experienced and confident senior clinician leads an inexperienced team with a number of unqualified support workers. The advantages are that such a leadership is clear and decisions made quickly, maximizing time available for patients. The disadvantages of concentrating responsibility around one person include an inhibition of learning, growth, and ownership within the group. The team may function poorly in the absence of the leader, who in turn is bombarded with requests from staff to sanction each decision.

The style generally favoured for effective team functioning is more democratic. The advantages are that commitment and responsibility are fostered in all team members. The potential disadvantages are delay, or even paralysis, in decision-making. This can slow down the flexible, rapid response to both patient need and organizational change. Meetings become longer and less efficient, delegation negotiated, and difficulties achieving goals or time pressures cause frustrations.

In practice, consultation and involvement of all staff as a cohesive but multidisciplinary team are essential. Leadership style is not fixed and invariable—a shift to a more autocratic style is common when there are crises or the workload is excessive.

Accountability and responsibility

An individual team member has responsibilities to patients and their families, to other team members, and to the team as a whole. They are also accountable to their line manager, to their professional body, and, under the law, to society. Associated responsibilities are shown in Fig 26.1.

Management supervision

Most team leaders from a clinical background find managing staff the hardest new skill to master. Regular, structured, one-to-one supervision with team members, together with handovers and team meetings, are the mechanisms to shape and lead the team. Management supervision creates a formal time in which staff can raise specific questions and requests with their line manager

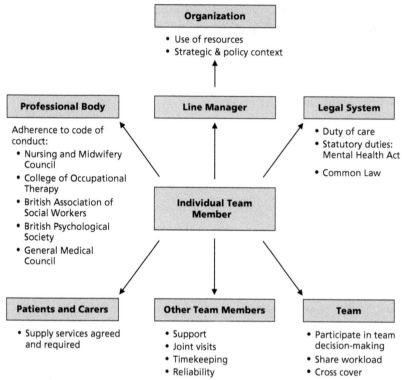

Fig 26.1 An individual team member's responsibilities and accountabilities
Data from NHS Training Authority (1990) Effective team working in the community, MacMillan Intek Ltd, Hove.

relating to their work. This uses a hierarchical system of monitoring individual staff performances, standards, and development.

Difficulties can arise with supervision arrangements because of the multidisciplinary nature of the team. Cross-disciplinary supervision requires an understanding and acceptance of the different styles of working that create a dynamic multidisciplinary team. For the same objective of helping a patient find work, the social worker may use the language of 'discrimination'; an occupational therapist, 'activity analysis'; and a psychologist, 'graded exposure'. While the use of these varied styles is to be welcomed, it should not be at the expense of the common purpose defined by the model and operational policy (see Box 26.8).

Documentation

The content of management supervision sessions needs to be recorded in a suitable and consistent format to provide continuity and for purposes of appraisal.

Box 26.8 Content of management supervision

- provide feedback and check performance of individual staff
- encourage, recognize, and develop strengths of staff
- help identify and problem-solve weaknesses
- individual performance review (annual)
- monitor activity and documentation standards
- monitor sickness and annual leave
- help identify training needs and delivery of training
- negotiate and agree on goals and targets with staff member
- allocate and delegate tasks, projects, and caseload

The form should record the date, areas covered, action agreed, and timescale for implementation. Sometimes forms require signing by the line manager and the supervisee to record agreement on content and outcomes. Should changes fail to take place and disciplinary action is indicated, these records provide the necessary evidence. That the documentation can be used for such different purposes as professional development and possible disciplinary action requires sensitivity and clear thinking in their use. Documents should be stored safely and securely.

New staff and staff experiencing difficulties will need management supervision every few weeks. Experienced and more autonomous staff may require only periodic supervision every few months. The frequency needs to be negotiated with each individual and not just assumed.

Personal issues

One-to-one management supervision will inevitably uncover and have to deal with personal and interpersonal matters that have a bearing on a team member's ability to do their job. Domestic problems and family commitments will impact periodically, for example, on timekeeping, concentration, and motivation. Being able to acknowledge and discuss such problems reduces the stress on the staff member and the level of frustration and risk of misinterpretation at under-performance for the manager. It is the manager's responsibility, however, to deal with such feelings and circumstances without the process slipping into a counselling session.

Clinical supervision

How does clinical supervision differ from management supervision? Is it appropriate for a line manager to also give clinical supervision to their staff?

These are difficult questions, and it is worth making a clear distinction between the two activities.

The Care Quality Commission (2013), which monitors registration and quality in English health and social care providers, describes clinical supervision as

> provid[ing] a safe and confidential environment for staff to reflect on and discuss their work and their personal and professional responses to their work. The focus is on supporting staff in their personal and professional development and in reflecting on their practice.

They acknowledge that clinical and professional supervision can be synonymous when supervision is carried out by another member of the same profession.

A good use of clinical supervision in community outreach is to support staff in the use of the skills they have learnt. For example, staff sent on training courses such as CBT or family interventions have often failed to employ these interventions with patients when there is no post-course supervision (see Box 26.9).

Practice varies as to whether it is the role of the team leader to provide clinical supervision as well as management supervision for each case manager. Doing both can develop the relationship between the key worker and manager through a two-way process of feedback. Clinical supervision is focused on individual patients and is more likely to result in the development of therapeutic skills. Combining the two functions can, however, carry risks. The clinical supervisor's other role as line manager may inhibit the supervisee from expressing concerns.

One model is to set up regular group clinical supervision, perhaps for one hour every two weeks. This session has a facilitator who may be a senior, experienced member of the team—but is not the team leader. The role of the facilitator is to avoid the development of a cosy peer supervision format, which can lack the rigour to confront poor practice. It is arguably a more effective use of time than one-to-one supervision because of the generic approach to patient care.

Box 26.9 Content of clinical supervision

- reflection on complex or difficult cases
- evaluation to improve clinical practice
- support of developing skills such as the use of sophisticated psychosocial interventions
- consideration of professional issues
- sharing of new ideas and practice

A drawback of the team leader's absence from group clinical supervision is that it can insulate them from the real anxieties and concerns of their staff. Group clinical supervision needs to retain confidentiality within the group to allow free expression. Feedback by the facilitator to the team leader is not an option, unless sanctioned by the group.

Recruitment and selection of staff

Our experience has shown that working collaboratively with patients in their own homes requires specific personal qualities which are only partially amenable to training and development. For example, staff who attempt to control patients do not generally achieve long-term solutions. Patients also quickly understand staff and their underlying motives and values. Staff who harbour negative stereotypes of patients, or have overly rigid ideas of what is appropriate behaviour, will not be able to establish an authentic therapeutic relationship (see Box 26.10).

Patients can be demoralized and pessimistic, having often experienced failure in important areas of their lives in the past. The community outreach worker has to be able to contribute his or her own optimism to the joint effort. There are always a million reasons why something may not be possible. What is needed from the outreach worker is a desire to make it happen, perhaps in very small steps. A 'can do' attitude is an essential care quality (see Box 26.11).

Specific interview questions and scenarios can elicit the types of responses that might indicate desirable or undesirable characteristics and attributes. For example: 'During the course of building up a relationship with a patient, they ask if you are married and how many children you have. How would you respond?' Our view would be that unless there is a likelihood from the presentation or history of stalking or similar pathological risks, then limited self-disclosure is harmless and helpful in establishing rapport and team attachment. This is not

Box 26.10 Undesirable personal characteristics

◆ over-controlling
◆ needing to do for others
◆ pessimistic approach to patients' motives and behaviours; 'seen it all' attitude
◆ protective of professional boundaries
◆ unwilling to use self-disclosure as part of engagement process

Box 26.11 Desirable personal characteristics

- flexible
- pragmatic
- practical problem-solving ability
- patient-centred approach
- nurturing and supportive style
- gentle firmness
- non-judgemental
- 'can do' attitude

psychotherapy but an altogether more social undertaking 'symbolized' by the encounter taking place in the person's home.

The traditional person specification summarizes skills and personal qualities into essential and desirable. Communication skills and the ability to cope with pressure sit alongside more formally acquired knowledge and qualifications. In our mental health Trust, 'personal experience of mental health problems' is entered into all clinical person specifications as desirable (unless specific exemptions are agreed by the chief executive). US experience has shown that 'consumer workers' are a valuable resource in outreach, particularly in relation to engagement. In recent years, UK 'service users' have become fully paid employees in many aspects of mental health services, including outreach teams.

Community outreach is labour-intensive, with skilled labour accounting for the majority of the team's budget. The ability to develop a long-term, therapeutic relationship with difficult patients is vital to the success of the undertaking. For all these reasons and more, the investment of time and energy in recruitment and selection will pay dividends in the long term. Short-term approaches to filling vacancies with relocated internal staff who do not go through full selection procedures and filters can be a costly mistake.

New technologies

For community outreach services, some of the challenges around missed appointments, travel time, and geography are starting to be addressed by technology. Staff can access and write up electronic care records in the field. Some situations have proved amenable to intelligent text (SMS) prompts. These are widely used with patients struggling to maintain abstinence from drugs or alcohol. Patient experience, complaints, and opinion feedback can also be given in real time via the Internet and smartphone applications.

Many patients have smartphones and can be offered simple remote consultations using systems like Skype. When combined with home visits, video consultations have proved a convenient and flexible alternative to face-to-face appointments. Indeed, a systematic review of telepsychiatry trials (García-Lizana and Muñoz-Mayorga 2010) came to the following conclusions:

- Videoconference seems to be a useful tool for diagnosis, treatment, and follow-up of patients in remote areas.
- Telepsychiatry improves symptoms in various mental disorders.
- The main barrier to successful telepsychiatry implementation is professional acceptance.

Conclusions

In this chapter we have tried to set out basic operational management activities and apply them to a typical week in community outreach. More generic tasks—managing budgets, strategic planning, managing change, and service review—have been omitted. The following chapters of this book also examine team training, service planning, and service evaluation.

The central resource is people. Successful teams rely on the skills and commitment of individual staff members. The managerial role is to harness these skills in a clear, meaningful, and effective operational framework. In the NHS, we are used to management activities that divert clinicians from patient care. Such external forces are usually about servicing the organization. A team-based manager is in a position to have a dual perspective, in which promoting patient care remains dominant.

Chapter 27

Training

Introduction

A comprehensive approach to the care of the severely mentally ill through community outreach means utilizing a wide range of skills and knowledge as reflected in the breadth of chapters in this book. Here we set out training frameworks and key skills and competencies that underpin comprehensive care. The list is too long to replicate in full, so we have chosen to illustrate how competencies and training can be applied to a number of common functions.

In the previous chapter we introduced the three levels within organizations for thinking about effective performance (Rummler and Brache 1990). Training is often thought of as simply concerning the *job performer level* which covers role clarity, performance, coaching, development, and training for individuals. However, community outreach is also about teams, and requires us to pay attention to the *process level* of team development, team culture, and standards. The multidisciplinary team provides a sound basis for a flexible and creative workforce. We often talk about the skill mix of staff in multidisciplinary teams. We refer to staff as trained and untrained, professionals and non-professionals, qualified and unqualified. It is probably more helpful to view the objective as creating a team that has staff with a suite of core, generalist, and specialist skills and competencies rather than a pick list of qualifications. Staff such as support workers, aides, and peer workers have high levels of patient contact compared to many specialist staff, and consequently their training and development are as important as producing advanced practitioners.

Changing needs and roles

All health care services must now be responsive to patient and carer involvement, choice, shared decision-making, and to work towards promoting self-management in long-term conditions. In mental health and addictions, the blurring of roles across traditional health and social care boundaries is well established. Where appropriate, we need to be comfortable in flexing our roles within the team to cross-cover and in support of shared team care approaches. In community outreach, we work with several partner agencies—both statutory agencies, such as social welfare and benefits agencies, and non-statutory agencies in housing and addictions.

Can we be sure that the statements from a review 20 years ago of roles and training for staff working with the severely mentally ill are not still true today? (Sainsbury Centre for Mental Health 1997):

- Rigid professional demarcations increasingly fail to reflect current workload requirements and current practice.
- Professional staff roles overlap considerably between the various disciplines and with support staff.
- The demands of purchasers of services and of training consortia are forcing a reconsideration of the skill mix required in mental health services.
- There is increasing emphasis on competent performance of role rather than qualification and status.

Core and advanced competencies for community outreach

Competence combines the general attributes of knowledge, skill, and attitudes, but also incorporates professional and personal judgement. A competence describes what is important for the workforce and provides performance indicators for assessment. The National Occupational Standards (Skills for Health 2010) and the NHS Knowledge and Skills Framework (Department of Health 2004) offer complementary standard frameworks covering roles and functions in the NHS. The NHS Knowledge and Skills Framework is about the *application* of knowledge and skills in the workplace, not just having the knowledge. Competencies enable job descriptions to show standard descriptors and skill levels for the job to support the effective learning and development of individuals and teams. Advanced skills including a range of psychosocial interventions are integral components in the management of schizophrenia rather than just worthy extras (Burns 1997). Each step forward increases knowledge and carries training implications, as do new requirements from regulatory changes.

Let us consider as an example some competencies for different members of team staff when it comes to conducting assessments. A support worker would be required to be competent in maintaining confidentiality when dealing with health information in assessments and when responding to enquiries. In the main, however, they would be engaged in providing care according to accepted practices and undertaking well-defined tasks as indicated from the assessment, and not tasks requiring very skilled judgements. A clinician conducting assessments, however, would need to show advanced competences, including the following (Skills for Health 2010):

♦ question and observe the individual in sufficient depth to justify and support the evaluation of their mental disorder, and identify sufficient characteristics and symptoms to form a justifiable diagnosis or formulation of the problem

♦ use a recognized assessment and diagnostic system (e.g. DSM-IV, ICD-10) and validated psychometric measures when possible

♦ provide and record for audit information, evidence, and reasoning about:

  • the nature and severity of the individual's mental disorder

  • risks posed by the individual to themselves, specific persons, and the public, using a recognized measure of risk

  • the individual's vulnerability to harm from others

  • a recommendation as to medical and psychological treatment, environment, support, and the individual's likely contribution to their recovery

  • whether the individual is detainable under relevant mental health legislation

  • the influence of co-morbidities (e.g. substance misuse, personality or developmental disorders)

  • contextualized formulation of the biological, psychological, and social factors influencing the clinical presentation

Other assessment skills (e.g. for the approved mental health professional role or an occupational therapist's functional assessment) are part of routine professional training and practice, and need no special mention here. Condition-specific assessment tools should not just be the preserve of individual professions. We would strongly advocate training in—and, more importantly, the use of—a limited number of assessment and outcome instruments by the whole team in routine practice. Training the whole team, together, in the use of structured assessment tools helps to build a shared language and structure around which to discuss patient care and progress at team meetings. All team members will then be able to articulate and quantify changes in functioning, symptoms, and behaviour. When patients are seen frequently in outreach, it can be difficult to perceive gradual improvements or deteriorations in mental state without such structured assessments. Comparing assessment scores at six-month intervals can often highlight otherwise insidious changes.

Inter-rater reliability is improved by training together as a team, which yields common understandings of terminology and the anchor points used in assessment and outcomes scales. Training to use these scales is brief and can be easily accommodated within the team's induction and development time. Common training and the use of common instruments also reinforces team culture and solidarity.

One commonly provided advanced training relevant to outreach is the psychosocial interventions course (Gournay and Birley 1998), with modules in case management for the severely mentally ill, schizophrenia family work, and psychological interventions such as CBT for psychosis. The course demonstrates a commitment to evidence-based practice and is the most obvious 'off-the-peg' diploma-level course for this work. Courses run on a day-release basis, over an academic year, with 40–50 study days. There are practice as well as theory assessments and supervision is built into the course. Practice involves the conducting and writing up of interventions with patients in the student's workplace. For example, the student is expected to conduct a formal programme of schizophrenia family work with a suitable family, including assessments, delivery, and evaluation. The theoretical assignment might be to write an essay reviewing the evidence base for family interventions.

As a result of an audit in our outreach team, we identified the need to increase the number of patients assessed for and offered treatment with clozapine. To do this it became necessary to train team members to take blood from patients in their homes. Venepuncture clinics and clozapine clinics were not an option for some of our more disabled patients. The facility to have blood taken at home by their key worker or a member of the team reduced the fragmentation of services and increased our ability to maintain people on this treatment. We trained nurses and support workers to perform this activity.

Operational training

Operational training describes the skills and knowledge required to enable a team to function safely, sensitively, and effectively as a unit. For example, during staff induction we stress the importance of early exposure to team- and organizational-level policies and procedures on safety, communication, and managing risk. Both qualified and unqualified staff must be aware of certain basics before they enter a patient's home alone. Our first-day induction checklist requires completion to show that the new member of staff has read and discussed the policy on dealing with violence, aggression, and risk. This includes communication procedures for home visits, such as daily diaries, to ensure that the team knows where staff are and how to contact them. Reporting in safe at the end of the day is an essential procedure.

Box 27.1 outlines the subjects in the Core Skills Training Framework (Skills for Health 2014), which reflect minimum standards expected. Many of the

Box 27.1 Statutory or mandatory subjects in the UK Core Skills Training Framework

- ◆ equality, diversity, and human rights
- ◆ health, safety, and welfare
- ◆ conflict resolution and de-escalation
- ◆ fire safety
- ◆ infection prevention and control
- ◆ moving and handling
- ◆ safeguarding adults
- ◆ safeguarding children
- ◆ resuscitation
- ◆ information governance

skills are provided through online training. Staff are required to work through an online course, often including videos and case scenarios, and then complete an assessment of knowledge. Pass or fail scores and record of completion are all captured by the online system. Whilst this affirms a snapshot of knowledge and provides the organization with an ability to track training compliance, online learning is less effective at confirming competence—the application of that knowledge. A good team manager will pick this up through supervision, appraisal, and observation.

Monitoring training needs, outcomes, and competencies

It is good practice to keep a 'live list' of the training received by each member of the team. Most organizations monitor this closely with electronic centralized records because it is simply not defensible to have patients exposed to risk from untrained staff or staff overdue for refresher training. Management supervision and appraisal is the mechanism for identifying training needs beyond the core skills. Appraisal is also an opportunity to ensure that skills learnt on training courses are being incorporated into practice. Further training needs for the whole team are often required by changes, such as the introduction of new risk assessment protocols or in response to critical incidents.

Outcomes of training are often overlooked. What matters is that the training translates to practice and influences patient outcomes. Price et al. (2015)

reviewed the evidence for improvements in learning and performance outcomes for training in de-escalation techniques by mental health staff for the management of violence and aggression. Reviewing 38 studies, they could not find any good-quality evidence of the impact of training on assaults, injuries, or organizational outcomes, and indeed some studies produced contradictory results. They could, however, see some impact on knowledge, confidence in managing aggression, and performance in artificial de-escalation training scenarios.

Barriers often exist to the use of learnt skills, and there is considerable inertia in the system, with staff allowing their acquired skills to lie dormant on return to routine clinical practice. Fadden (1997) surveyed 86 trainees in the UK who had completed a behavioural family therapy course for work with patients with schizophrenia. At between nine months and three-and-a-half years after training, 70 per cent reported that they had used the approach with families. However, this use was modest—equating to 1.7 families seen per therapist, and 8 per cent of the therapists accounting for 40 per cent of the interventions. A significant number of staff from all disciplines had simply not implemented their new skills. This is not an isolated finding. Audits and informatics on agreed standards provide useful information to quantify the effect of training on local practice. How many patients in your current service have been assessed using the agreed outcome scale, or have had the required physical health assessment? We would suggest a standard of more than 95 per cent is needed for such an audit to drive compliance where the goal is best practice. We audited the number of our patients who had significant contact with a carer. A surprisingly low figure of 27 per cent demonstrated the degree of isolation experienced by many of our patients. We then audited how many of those had been offered or received family intervention. The majority had received intervention to at least the psycho-education stage, demonstrating utilization of learning, but few had been engaged in extended problem-solving sessions.

Conclusions

Throughout this book, there is a recurring theme of investing in people, in what is a low-tech but demanding, skilled, and labour-intensive activity. The team contains individual and multidisciplinary knowledge, skills, and experience in abundance. Organizing the team so that these can be passed on through clinical supervision, handover meetings, review meetings, and development meetings is as important as the provision of formal training and induction.

Developing key staff with advanced knowledge and skills conforming to best practice and evidence—through, for example, diploma-level psychosocial intervention courses—should be encouraged. These courses require a large investment of time and resources. The team must facilitate and audit the routine implementation of these skills acquired to justify such an investment. A focus on competencies provides a framework for unqualified support staff and trained professionals alike to judge training needs and performance.

Chapter 28

Service planning

Introduction

This chapter aims to guide practitioners and managers in setting up and reviewing community outreach services for people with severe mental illness from a non-technical, service planning perspective. Examples of different service configurations within a comprehensive local system will be given, with some observations on their relative merits and drawbacks. Service models and structures are important for providing a framework for delivering quality care. However, the importance of the detail of quite small differences has often been overstated by inward-looking service providers and ardent model adherents. From the perspective of the service user, many of these details (e.g. team or key worker caseload size, staffing mix, ownership of beds, degree of shared caseload) are invisible. We know this because they tell us. They also tell us what is important to them: local access, responsiveness, consistency of individuals and care, and other more human aspects of the service. The original ACT model components and subsequent arguments of model fidelity are discussed in detail in Chapter 4. Evaluation of services is covered in the following chapter on research and development (Chapter 29).

The expansion of assertive outreach in England was mandated by central policy together with the establishment of crisis resolution home treatment teams and early intervention in psychosis services. By 2005, the government's *NHS Plan* (Department of Health 2000) saw over 250 assertive outreach teams established, serving nearly 20,000 people with severe and enduring mental health problems. By contrast, the North American experience saw assertive outreach develop through a 'franchising' process (Bond 1991). Model assertive outreach programmes were replicated in other parts of the country over a relatively long time period. Using a particularly American metaphor, Bond suggests that service planners may be able to learn something from the fast food industry in its successful transmission of standards to new locations!

In both countries, these highly specialized and relatively expensive services have been gradually dissolved, diluted, or dismantled over the last eight years (Firn et al. 2013). The Netherlands has seen the emergence and widespread adoption of the hybrid model of flexible ACT (Van Veldhuizen 2007; Van Veldhuizen and Bähler 2015). Norway has seen a programme implementing ACT teams from 2009 and now its first flexible ACT teams (Ruud and Landheim 2015).

Much has been learnt along the way, as outlined in Chapter 4. We continue to learn about the design of care services and the importance of context deriving from specific historical, geographic, demographic, political, legislative, and financial factors.

Principles of good community-based care for people with severe mental health problems

It is worth reminding ourselves of some fundamental questions on what we are trying to achieve through community outreach services. At a higher level, the triple aim articulated by the Institute of Healthcare Improvement (Stiefel and Nolan 2012) gives us some goals:

1. improve health outcomes for your given population
2. provide good-quality care as experienced by individuals
3. do this affordably

So how do you achieve this triple aim for people with severe mental health problems? If we go the route of highly specialized teams with low caseloads (ACT), then we increase costs and improve some aspects of quality, such as engagement, but many now accept that actual health outcomes of relapse and hospitalization are measurably unaffected. We might also exclude some people from an intensive service when they need it through the application of rigid referral criteria and we will fragment the service into separate 'silos'. At the other extreme lies a completely general service organized predominantly from primary care for a wide range of mental health needs. Indeed, this was tested with community psychiatric nurses in general practice in the late 1980s, when nearly a quarter of community psychiatric nurses were based in primary care away from mental health providers. It was generally acknowledged that the more severe psychiatric population was neglected as mild to moderate mental illness prevailed with a primary care and counselling focus (Gournay and Brooking 1994). Worse still, outcomes for non-psychotic patients were generally no better than people just seeing their GP.

So, consensus now favours a range of forms of community-based case management, delivered by multidisciplinary mental health services as the best approach for patients with more severe psychotic disorders (Van Os and Kapur 2009). In the UK, this is founded on the CMHT model (Burns 2007).

How does assertive and community outreach fit into the whole system?

The cornerstones of mental health service provision in the UK are GPs and CMHTs. These services reach and treat the vast majority of people. Fig 28.1 shows the range of core mental health services for adults in a typical locality for a population of 250,000 or so. The size of each service 'bubble' approximates the number of people served. We have included assertive outreach on our schematic as a separate service, but, as we will see, assertive outreach and forensic services for offenders are increasingly being subsumed into the remit of the CMHT. The generic CMHT accepts referrals from GPs for people with mental health problems with few explicit exclusions. Specialized teams, sometimes referred to as functional teams—such as forensic, assertive outreach, crisis, and early onset services—have explicit criteria which can protect their workload as well as focus treatment and support on their target function or groups. For example, the crisis teams' function is to act as a short-term alternative to hospital admission.

Problems occur in the wider system when there are boundary confusions or disputes between specialist services in their response to particular patients with challenging needs and when the arrangements for transferring care and responsibility between teams is slow or unclear. This movement between teams according to need is why such arrangements are often called care pathways.

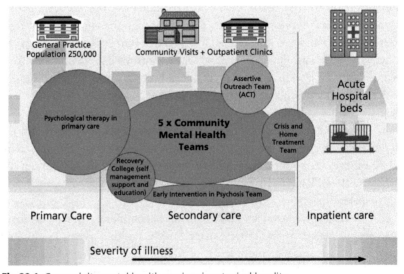

Fig 28.1 Core adult mental health services in a typical locality

---

Case study

A CMHT has been struggling with a psychotic patient who is poorly compliant with medication and abuses crack cocaine regularly. His offending behaviour is escalating and he has a forensic history of dangerous behaviour.

The CMHT knows that the local forensic service only takes people with very serious index offences—usually those who have been through the courts. They are not sure how such seriousness is measured. Will their patient be taken on by the community forensic team or will they only offer an opinion? The local drug and alcohol service has difficulty engaging psychotic patients who are poorly motivated to change their drug-taking behaviour.

Finally, they consider a referral to assertive outreach, but know that the local team is under review, and in any case has a waiting list. How are the current needs of the patient to be met?

In Chapter 4, we introduced the flexible ACT (FACT) model as a response to providing periods of more intensive and ongoing standard case management care through the coordination of a single team. Proponents of FACT regard this approach as an affordable and integrated adaptation. Even early advocates of high-fidelity ACT have supported this rethinking of the original ACT model. Bond and Drake (2007) state that Stein and Test's notion that ACT should be time unlimited appears impractical and unnecessary given that many individuals don't need ACT most of the time. Highly specialized ACT teams are unworkable in dispersed rural populations, and the flexibility of intensity offered by FACT is an appealing alternative.

The planning process

Service planning and adoption is made easier when the evidence base is clear and when treatment models and service structures are codified or manualized. Such was the case with assertive outreach. Stein and Test provided the evidence, and subsequent manuals added the team blueprint, complete with staffing arrangements and indicative caseload numbers (Stein and Test 1980; Allness and Knoedler 1998). All that was required was fitting to the local system with agreement and funding. When a restructure is required by government agencies, as happened in the UK, the drivers are complete. The FACT model has been similarly manualized (van Veldhuizen and Bähler 2013), in several languages, with fidelity scales and even certification arrangements. Other configurations and adaptations have been implemented in a piecemeal fashion and rarely evaluated. These tend to follow financial necessity, fashion, and imitation rather than evidence.

An example of such a development is where some secondary care services have tried to separate community teams working with people with psychosis from those working with non-psychotic diagnoses. In England and the

Netherlands, this has been fostered in part by considering what skills and competencies are required for working with these diagnostic groups, and partly by this categorization in funding arrangements. Some division and specialization is uncontroversial. Clearly, brain surgery requires a discrete surgical service staffed by people with rigorous training and a set of competencies and professional controls. We take the view that in general psychiatry you should seek to specialize only where there is a good case that a special skill set and team structure brings benefits to patients. Otherwise, pooling and integrating teams makes good sense from the perspective of simple pathways of care, affordability, and having a team which is diverse and large enough to support itself.

Steering group

The diversity of stakeholders in health care and the need for input and consultation requires, in most cases, a cumbersome but ultimately effective planning process based on the framework described as follows.

The steering group is responsible for leading the change process, prioritizing the resources, defining the broad policy framework, and setting the values and principles of the proposed service. Local politics will determine the profile and power of service user and carer representation, primary care input, and perspectives from local minority groups or voluntary agencies. The steering group includes senior members of the major professions, senior managers who will be responsible for the service, and representatives from the major agencies of health and social care.

Stakeholder conference or focus groups

A large stakeholder conference may be more appropriate for wholesale changes in the provision of community services. Focus groups are an alternative way of defining needs and demands across a range of perspectives. Open individual and group questions to service users and staff should elicit responses to the following questions:

1. What is particularly good about the current service?
2. What concerns do you have about the way the service is currently delivered?
3. What do you think could be improved?
4. What have you tried in the past? Did it work? If not, why not?
5. How do you think it could be improved now?

By capturing multiple responses from individuals and groups, themes will develop as target areas for correction and improvement. Starting with closed questions and predefined options generates resistance to change and takes away from ownership and co-production of the change process. Equally important is not to close your mind to people who object strongly: they may have useful insights.

> It is important to keep in mind that those placing obstacles in the path of change are doing so for heartfelt and legitimate reasons. It is too easy to become overly cynical, imputing the worst motives. (Onyett 1992)

Local needs profile

Estimating population needs is a complex task. Data from needs assessments exists at the national level and from local commissioners, public health authorities, and social service departments. You will find data on socio-economic and age profiles for the locality. Benchmarking and public health data will give prevalence rates (proportion of cases in the population at a given time) for common conditions and indicate future trends. For example, longer life expectancy will reliably increase the prevalence of dementia and cancer over time. Converting data to something manageable that can inform decision-making is not simple, but a job for a small project group.

Writing the service proposal or option appraisal

The next step is for the steering group to agree on options within which one approach is finally to be recommended, having been appraised against a set of risk and benefit criteria. This will outline at least three options; typically option one is the base case of 'do nothing'. Of the two possible change options, the relevant benefits are compared with costs or savings against the base case. Ideally, one course of action outscores the others and is recommended by the group and ultimately the executive decision-making committee. The proposal can then be used to secure the funding and as a consultation document for further feedback.

Service change example

Rathod et al. (2014) describe a whole systems service change for a population of 1.3 million in one region of the UK involving a reduction of adult mental health beds supported by a reconfiguration of community mental health team functions.

Case study

The baseline service consisted of four management units in the east, west, north, and south of the region comprising services similar to Fig 28.1. There were six inpatient units for adults.
Key changes to the system components resulted in the following:

♦ Reduction in numbers of beds and inpatient units.

+ Strengthening of the hospital-at-home function.

+ Establishment of a new access and assessment team functioning as a single point of access in each area to provide a core assessment for new referrals and allocate appropriate follow-up care.

+ Closure of the assertive outreach teams with the caseload integrated into six local community treatment teams.

+ The six local services were extended to 8 p.m. in the evenings and included weekend working; the term 'shared care' was adopted in preference to 'FACT'. A common electronic FACT board was developed which helped embed and standardize practice. The teams adopted daily planning (shared care) meetings typically lasting 30 minutes each morning.

+ Incorporation of the early intervention in psychosis (EIP) function into the local teams was tried initially. Following evaluation at 18 months, the EIP function was reformed as a specialist, stand-alone team.

This sort of complex service redesign is challenging to evaluate. Qualitative evaluation based on surveys of service users, staff, GPs, and carer focus groups concluded that the integrated pathway improved access to the right level of care for severely mentally ill patients.

Conclusions

Service planning and evaluation is a continuous process. By involvement of key stakeholders, a local needs analysis, and careful attention to the impact of the whole system, many mistakes can be avoided. Change can be stepwise in relatively small elements, or change can be large scale, as described in the previous case study. It will not, however, be possible to have full consensus at the outset or to establish an effective, smooth-running service immediately. Fine-tuning and problem-solving is needed, and teams evolve through testing towards their optimum. Lessons can be learnt from the literature, from visits, and from demonstration sites, but ultimately you need to evaluate the impact of your change in your context. Community outreach must compete for funding with other critical services. The better you can describe your service model and the more evidence you have for the impact and outcomes of your service, the stronger your case.

Chapter 29

Research and development

Introduction

This is a handbook primarily for practitioners and not for academics or researchers. However, assertive outreach has been one of the models, par excellence, of evidence-based practice (Chapters 1 and 4). It has been responsible for introducing a more critical approach to the organization of mental health care. We now strive to provide treatment and care based when possible on research evidence rather than 'because we have always done it that way'.

As outlined in Chapter 1, ACT became one of the most intensively researched mental health care systems. At the last count, there were over 90 published studies. This has established a healthy scepticism about unfounded claims for the superiority of various services—practitioners now want to be able to check if such claims are true. To accomplish this we have to gain some basic understanding of how different types of evaluation and research are conducted and how much trust can be placed in their results.

As the range of possible interventions has increased within finite resources, we also need to be sure we use those resources in the most effective way. This is an ethical as much as an economic issue—we owe it to our patients to ensure that they get the best out of what is available.

As outlined in Box 29.1, several types of evaluation tend to get bundled together as 'doing research'. These can, and should, be disentangled. There are four broad categories. Of these, three should be part of routine practice for all teams and one—research proper—engaged in only after considerable thought. Each of these methodologies can be used to explore and measure any one of the three key features of mental health provision: outcomes, processes, and inputs.

Outcomes

The most commonly reported outcomes for outreach services at a patient level are symptom severity, social functioning, hospitalization, and loss to follow-up. Framing these measures as positive targets is often considered more constructive so we can report these traditional outcomes as symptom *reduction*, community *tenure*, and successful *engagement*. It is important to remember, however, that patients and their families may not necessarily view these

---

Box 29.1 Types of evaluation

- **Monitoring**: routine or special collection of data (e.g. caseload demographics, occupied bed days, referrals, untoward incidents).

- **Clinical audit**: the systematic analysis of the quality of clinical care assessed against known quality standards.

- **Service development**: the considered and evaluated introduction of changes in practice to improve outcomes.

- **Formal research**: using defined patient populations to test a clearly stated hypothesis, often related to some innovation.

---

outcome measures as particularly important to them. They will usually stress social and vocational outcomes and quality of life (Chapter 23).

Aggregated outcomes (e.g. the average of various outcomes for all patients in a service) provide the information at a service level. This can be used to compare against a known standard in audit or compared with outcomes in a comparator group when conducting a more formal research study.

Processes

Thornicroft and Tansella (1999) define process as 'those activities which take place to deliver mental health services'.

An audit of the frequency of contact with patients is an evaluation of process. Monitoring caseload sizes or the rate of use of clozapine or compulsory treatment orders are examples of measuring processes. Process evaluation is a fundamental question in the decision about establishing a specific service such as providing an outreach service. What do we hope to achieve by having the outreach service (or a crisis team, or a recovery team)? What will it do differently? What evidence-based treatments and care can we provide with such a team that we cannot provide without it? It is with such identified processes that we can achieve better outcomes for patients.

Inputs

Inputs are the resources that are used by mental health services. All individual treatments which carry specific cost implications, such as newer drugs, are inputs as well as having process and outcome implications. At the service level, the obvious inputs are staffing, training, hospital beds, equipment, and buildings. For example, the investment required to train a member of staff to diploma level in the use of psychosocial interventions for psychosis is considerable. Comparing inputs and outcomes is how the efficiency of a service is judged. Stein and Test's study (1980) was so influential because it demonstrated both improved outcomes *and* reduced costs.

Routine monitoring of care

All professionals have to keep records. The most important records are the patients' clinical case notes and, in any legal process, it is these which will be examined most closely. We have learnt over the last decades just how important it is to keep up-to-date, high-quality notes. For community outreach work, recording 'failed visits' (visits where the patient was not in or we were unable to make contact with them) is of particular importance. The legal profession assumes that if it was not recorded, then it did not happen, so keeping good notes is not only essential for good care and coordination—it is good for your professional security. As discussed later, good-quality notes are also essential for audit.

In addition to clinical case notes, we are also required to return various 'statistics' on our work. Originally this was simply a record of the number of contacts with patients. As we have moved to electronic records, the detail captured in these statistics has increased exponentially. Now the NHS collects treatment details approaching the level captured in systems developed for billing and insurance purposes. Time spent, location, content, and seniority of outreach workers are now routinely monitored. Luckily there is, as yet, no external interference on what types of activity are permitted. In insurance-based systems, some of the routine practices of outreach workers can be classified as 'nonbillable' and this can subtly distort practice. For instance, in one US state, case managers cannot bill time spent picking up groceries provided free for mentally ill individuals if they do it alone, whereas if the patient comes along and sits outside in the car, then it suddenly becomes billable time.

Regular inputting of contact data is generally considered one of the less enjoyable parts of the job. This is especially so where the IT systems are complex or slow. Certainly, early IT systems—still sadly in use in many services, as many were purchased with binding contracts—required soul-destroying hours importing into computers. The increasing use of portable technology— smartphones and tablets, and even voice recognition software—means that notes can be updated quickly in real time. However, this very ease brings its own challenges. It is important to exercise discretion and be succinct. Voluminous notes with excessive detail help nobody and can obscure what is important.

Making routine monitoring more acceptable

Part of the resistance to routine monitoring is that it often appears to be imposed from above and to have little clinical relevance. However, it is not going to go away. So it is worth considering how it can be used to serve the team's purposes and, consequently, be more worthwhile. Using such data to actively monitor and review current practice is one way to accomplish this; specifically:

1. emphasize the 'professionalism' of data returns
2. use routine data for individual supervision
3. use routine data for monitoring team targets

Emphasize the 'professionalism' of data returns

The work we do is worthwhile, so it is worth recording. The increased insistence that nursing and community activity be comprehensively recorded is evidence that it is taken seriously. Instead of focusing on the 'big brother' aspect of being checked on, focus on the importance that the activity is clearly being accorded. This emphasis can be strengthened by taking the business of making returns seriously and setting proper time aside for it. In the Wandsworth assertive outreach team in the late 1990s, we encouraged all members to timetable an hour or two a week for doing their returns. This meant we had some chance of doing them accurately—not rushed at the end of a month when the Trust is demanding them and memory has faded. That was then! Most staff now spend much, much more time on record-keeping. Whether this has gone too far is endlessly debated; it certainly seems so to us. However, there are some enduring benefits. It is, at the very least, 'thinking time'. Inevitably, when entering data, there is stimulus to think about where one is going with a specific patient. A protected session in the office once a week—when statistics can be done, notes reviewed, and some paperwork completed—should be part of any outreach worker's timetable.

Use routine data for individual supervision

Routine data can often highlight patterns of practice for individuals that need attention. We aimed in the Wandsworth assertive outreach team for around 20 contacts a week, but this inevitably included considerable variation. Depending on their needs, some patients will require frequent short visits, such as daily meds, and some require fewer but more extensive visits. For example, a well-established patient may need complex negotiations to help him get a flat or job. However, even allowing for variation, if an individual's contact frequency is very different from the team average, it may indicate problems to be taken up in supervision. It can be just as concerning if the rate is too high as too low.

Case study

Anne is a new outreach worker who had wanted to join the team for some time. She contributed extensively in review meetings and was optimistic and enthusiastic for her patients. Six months into the job, her statistics still averaged nearly 35 visits a week, including seeing four of her patients daily, five days a week. In supervision, her enthusiasm was recognized and praised. The high visit frequency was used as a way into discussing her anxiety levels about her new patients and the need to let herself trust them more.

Robert's contact frequency fell from a steady 20 or so per week to a month when it averaged about 12 a week. This included more failed visits than usual. In supervision, he did not comment on any difficulties. When the downturn was highlighted, it became clear that this occurred after an unfounded accusation from a female patient, when he had felt let down by the organization. He had hardly been aware of the impact himself until the change in visit pattern was discussed.

Obviously, this use of statistical returns needs to be sensitive and collaborative. It has an enormous potential to seem persecutory, which can interfere with good data collection.

Use routine data for monitoring team targets

Just as routine monitoring data can be used for individual supervision, so it can also be used for team supervision. This is often referred to as monitoring fidelity to the model of care and is covered in detail in Chapter 4. However, here we have broadened it to include all team targets. It is remarkably easy, for even the most committed team, to 'drift' in its practice. Getting an overview of how well the team is meeting its target of weekly visits for each high-risk patient (if that is what is agreed) is quickly obvious from such data. Similarly, it becomes obvious how these visits vary between different patients and different outreach workers. Comparing clinical impression against routinely collected data can be a sobering experience! It is remarkable how different reality and rhetoric can become without anyone noticing. Recognizing the difference can help formulate more realistic expectations—most teams set far too high goals for contact frequency. This monitoring of team targets is a form of audit to be dealt with later. More sophisticated team assessments will require more detailed recording of contacts.

Audit

Audit does not involve discovering new ways to provide care, but examining how well established and accepted standards of care are being applied locally. It consists of a cycle of setting standards of care that one would expect to provide, and then testing whether these are being met. If they are not, then efforts have to be made to improve practice, and then the audit repeated after an agreed interval. If they are then being met, then a decision can be made whether the achieved standards should be raised for a further cycle, or whether that is fine and a different target is chosen for the next audit. The audit cycle is now well described with clinical audit a requirement for all services in the UK. As with routine data collection, one can either suffer audit as a necessary evil or embrace it as an opportunity to reflect on, improve, and celebrate good practice. We would encourage the latter!

Although most organizations provide extensive help with audit, the real value is in doing it yourself. Increasingly, the expanding prescribed audit agenda concerns routine monitoring of bureaucratic and administrative targets, such as compliance with the care programme approach, physical health monitoring, and smoking cessation, or discharge procedures and follow-up. To avoid bad feeling, it is worth spending time together as a team to understand the benefits of such non-negotiable activities. There is usually a requirement for a set number of internal audits, with some discretion on the topics. It is important that the team is involved as much as possible in the selection of topics, that it discusses the rationale for each of them, and is interested in the answers. We have chosen to conduct audits on out-of-hours contacts and the proportion of family contacts, and a series of paper-based audits on the content of individual care plans. We have been surprised by some of our results (e.g. the low level of contact with relatives despite consistent efforts) and heartened by others (e.g. the extremely low rate of out-of-hours emergency contacts with services).

Audits get increasingly sophisticated as teams get more settled and teething problems are resolved. They may even influence the way data is recorded, either temporarily or permanently. No matter how skilful or sophisticated an audit is, however, it will be a wasted opportunity if the topic is not 'owned' by the team and results reported back and even displayed prominently to reinforce behaviour. The team may even want to display audit results in outpatient waiting rooms or web pages. Examples are when work has been done on improving waiting times for referral, responses to complaints, or results of smoking cessation initiatives. We prioritized audits when the complete team could be involved in the whole process. An example was auditing ten sets of notes each to identify frequency of vocational activity recorded. When possible, we did this all in the room together and made 'an event' of it. If this is not possible, aim for a rapid turnaround so that the results are available fairly soon after the question has been set. Usually one member of the team takes responsibility for ensuring that the audit is conducted and for timetabling it. This person is responsible for 'seeing it happens'—not for doing it. The practice in many teams of simply dumping the responsibility for audit on the junior doctor is pretty much a waste of everyone's time (especially the doctor's).

Service developments and quality improvement

It is not just hospital services that can become rigid and inward-looking. Community teams can become institutionalized, too. Paradoxically, assertive outreach, early intervention, and crisis teams may be at more risk of this because they are often set up with such a detailed service model and a commitment to model fidelity. While we have regularly stressed the value of an explicit model for a service, it does carry with it a risk of becoming fossilized. This is especially so if the focus centres on structure rather than on treatments and quality of care. Service development through quality improvement is an essential, ongoing aspect of service planning and innovation.

CMHTs need to have a mechanism for overviewing their practice and making sure that it adapts to changes around them. This may be as basic as responding to an influx of refugees to the local area or reorganizing liaison meetings with primary care following a service restructuring. Developments may, however, have to be more substantial and reflect new techniques or treatments. For instance, the Wandsworth team reorganized considerably to accommodate an increased use of clozapine in our resistant schizophrenia patients (Chapter 15). This was one of the major drivers for a move to a seven-day a week service, but it has also had knock-on effects because of the increased volume of daily supervised medicines. Two examples of service developments stemming from this were the formalization of an early-evening drug round and the training of all staff in venepuncture.

Service developments should be thought through carefully at events such as team away days (Chapter 26), and we would strongly advise that a review date should be set for any innovation. Current thinking is that virtually all change is innovation, and all innovation is good. Indeed, 'innovative' is routinely used as a term of approval of services and taken to imply 'improvement'. Not all changes are improvements. Whether they are improvements is a judgement that can only be made in retrospect. Innovations need to be rigorously reviewed with at least three questions in mind:

1. Is the change sustainable?
2. Does it bring demonstrable benefits?
3. What price is paid to achieve it?

The value of introducing any major change in practice on an explicitly time-limited, 'pilot' basis is that it is then impossible to neglect these questions. It is no use introducing a change that only lasts as long as it has novelty value. A good test is how much support it receives from those who have to provide the input over sustained periods. The enthusiast who comes up with the idea is not the one to judge it. We had a series of safety-reporting systems that have all seemed brilliant when first launched (e.g. detailed diaries for each member, with complex ringing-in obligations), but none persisted, apart from a simple, efficient notification of risky visits. A predetermined review after a set interval is vital in such circumstances because it avoids complacency. It can also reveal a mistaken belief that a system is in place when it has in fact fallen into disuse.

That an idea seems good does not necessarily mean that it makes any real difference. Providing an out-of-hours service both reflected received wisdom for assertive outreach and had an impelling logic. After several years of providing only flexible evening work, we undertook to introduce extended-hours availability to the Wandsworth assertive outreach team on a routine basis. Although there were no complaints from the staff about it, a review of the use of the provision showed that it simply was not used (Chapter 6). On the other hand, the review of our extension to seven days' working showed that the contact frequency was high, targeted, and effective in improving medication compliance. That innovation continued.

Even if an innovation is effective, careful thought must be given to its cost-effectiveness. Putting extra resources into any new provision must mean stopping something else. The benefits of the new treatment should be weighed against the alternative activities that could otherwise be provided with the staff time now devoted to it. The economic concept of 'opportunity cost' examines alternative uses of the varied inputs within a system. For every use of resources, there is an alternative lost opportunity. There are formal methods of estimating added health value for different treatments (e.g. quality-adjusted life years, life years saved, number of relapses averted). Their use is complex, very time-consuming, and rarely feasible outside of research projects involving expert health economists.

The simplest and most pragmatic method for a basic evaluation of an intervention is to use a cost-consequence analysis. This is similar in some respects to a business case comparing direct and indirect costs, with a range of different consequences from the chosen interventions. Or, it can be phrased as a question: 'What are the comparative costs and consequences of two or more alternative courses of action?' This allows the freedom to measure and compare multiple clinically relevant costs and savings from new ways of working (e.g. the direct costs of buying new technology, clinician time saved or added in the first and subsequent years).

Increasingly, these difficult decisions are being made in the UK by the National Institute for Health and Care Excellence. NICE evaluates all new treatments before authorizing their use in the NHS, using a standard benchmark of a specific monetary sum per improved quality-adjusted life years (£30,000 in 2015). This works well with new drugs, but is clearly less straightforward in mental health. Despite this, NICE has been enormously successful in sifting through mountains of evidence to provide clinical guidance on most areas of mental health care (NICE 2014a, 2014b, 2015a). These summaries are particularly helpful in summarizing the status of knowledge about interventions—whether they are clearly beneficial and essential, likely to be helpful, or promising but unproven. NICE relies on high-quality research, but this broad approach of reflecting on changes in services with a critical, open mind is one any team needs.

Being open to innovation is, despite all the problems outlined here, an essential virtue in community mental health practice. Not only does it allow teams to adopt new and more effective treatments more quickly, it also keeps our perspective fresh. Even the most evidence-based interventions will be of limited effect if they are delivered in a stale, mechanistic manner. A culture of enquiry and flexibility is an asset in its own right.

Research

Research is a process by which new knowledge is acquired. It is not the only way. New knowledge can be obtained by careful clinical observation and even by pure chance. What is special about scientific research is that it uses well-tested methods to resolve difficult questions; its methods are transparent and repeatable; and it strives actively to reduce bias, both conscious and unconscious. Typically research uses an *experiment* to test which of one or more outcomes is associated with an intervention. There are a number of experimental (and 'quasi-experimental') research approaches to answering difficult questions.

Research is distinguished from audit by its aim to derive new knowledge about its subject matter rather than test how well current knowledge is being used. It is distinguished from local surveys and needs assessments by the generalizability of its findings. Research questions are framed so that their answers are as independent as possible of local conditions and, therefore, applicable in a wide range of settings. For instance, demonstrating the successful outcome of an operation simply by examining the results obtained by an outstandingly good surgeon does not tell us how successful that operation is. It tells us how successful *that* surgeon is with that operation with particular patients. To research the success of the operation as such, we would need to have it carried out by a group of ordinary surgeons and ensure that the patients receiving it are also those likely to need it, not a selected (good prognosis) group. We easily recognize these issues in other fields of endeavour. For example, a school's outstanding exam results do not automatically prove the superiority of its teachers—we need to know about its area and what sort of pupils it gets in the first place.

Why are research methods important?

Why do academics seem to spend so much time arguing about methodology? Are research methods that important in mental health? Surely it is often quite obvious when a treatment works. Sometimes, of course, it is, and there is no need for a careful research study. The first heart transplants are a good example. All the patients would have died in a few days or weeks without a transplant, and many of them lived for a long time with their new hearts. However, as transplants became more common, the point at which the clinical decision to undertake one changed. No longer is immediate death the inevitable alternative: transplants are undertaken to relieve disabling heart failure, and, in addition, there are different techniques for the operation. Individual surgeons are unlikely to be able to make careful and convincing comparisons; they will stick to the method they know best and feel safest with. This is the point at which more careful scientific research needs to be employed.

Attention to detail is particularly essential to resolve long-running controversies where, despite extensive experience, experts continue to disagree. How can trained people continue to have strongly held differences of opinion despite accumulating evidence? The reasons are twofold. First, there is our own enthusiasm and natural tendency to be optimistic for the treatments we use. This is not surprising—we use them because they have worked in the past but also because they reflect our understanding of the task. For example, enthusiasts for family work will persist longer with a difficult family and are more likely to judge the outcome successful than a sceptic. Similarly, an enthusiast for aggressive psychopharmacology would persist longer with various drug changes and be more likely to attribute any improvements to that intervention.

Few outcomes in individual patients in mental health practice are a simple yes/no—recovered/not recovered—so there is enormous scope for the interpretation of results. In psychotherapy research, professionals consistently rate more change in their patients than either the patients or an external observer would. The healthy optimism that therapists need to make a success of their treatments makes judging outcomes difficult.

Bias in research

The second difficulty is bias. Most research methods are aimed at reducing bias. Bias refers to all those extraneous factors (other than the intervention whose effect is to be judged) which can affect the outcome. We have already mentioned the therapist's bias. This is not wilful or deliberate, not some form of dishonesty, but normal human behaviour ('giving people the benefit of the doubt', 'hoping for the best for them'). For this reason, one of the commonest features of research is that 'independent' researchers, rather than the doctors or nurses treating the patient, should assess the outcome and collect the data.

Bias can also come from a number of other sources.

Sampling bias and regression to the mean

How the patients are recruited may exert a powerful influence on the outcome. Two examples are particularly relevant to assertive outreach studies. Patients were recruited into the experimental service in some early studies at the point of intended admission to hospital (e.g. Muijen et al. 1992; Stein and Test 1980). There is thus an in-built bias in these 'diversion' studies. If hospital admission is the outcome (it generally was), then you can only find that the experimental group is equal to or better than the control. The admission rate cannot be higher in the experimental group as all the control patients in an admission diversion study are admitted.

If we select patients for a study because they have been very ill and repeatedly in hospital, the natural pattern is for them to be comparatively better over the following years. This is called 'regression to the mean'. Psychoses and severe mental illness are fluctuating disorders. There is a natural tendency for people to improve going forward if we select them at their worst, and, similarly, if we select them in good periods, they are likely to become worse. It is simply a reflection of the natural fluctuations in the illness. For this reason, pre-post studies (i.e. comparing hospital usage for the same patients for a period before and after the introduction of a new service) can be misleading. Such studies should be interpreted cautiously. If you look closely, you will see there is often also a significant improvement over time in the control patients in RCTs!

If a clinic can choose its patients, then it may attract either less ill or possibly more ill patients. This is one reason why outcome in specialist clinics may be much worse than in routine ones. For instance, modern research into the outcome in anorexia nervosa arose because psychiatrists (who saw the most difficult cases) thought it was a very serious disease, whereas physicians (who treated younger easier cases) thought it was a brief, relatively mild disorder.

Another form of sampling bias in clinical practice is to base opinions on patients you can follow up and neglect to account for those who do not come back or you cannot find. Many of us have a much gloomier view of the long-term prognosis for schizophrenia than is probably warranted because we work long term with those who do not get better. Similarly, some of the oft-quoted long-term follow-up studies (Ciompi 1988; Harding et al. 1987) report an exaggeratedly good outcome because they based it on those they could follow up after 20 or so years, ignoring those who died early or were lost.

Hawthorne effect

One of the most important sources of bias in mental health research is the Hawthorne effect (Grufferman 1999). This describes the improvement in outcome in behavioural studies resulting from the extra interest and enthusiasm the study generates. It is generally recognized that patients do better in research trials than in routine practice and, while there are several practical reasons for this (sampling, better adherence by both patient and doctor to proper procedures, etc.), the Hawthorne effect plays its part.

The Hawthorne effect is the overall sense of well-being and optimism that a trial generates. After all, patients with long-term disorders may be fairly demoralized, and the sense that 'something new is being done' can boost morale, producing a direct improvement in outcome, reported or real. The same holds for the staff involved. Possibly the most striking example of this in psychiatry was the continued use of modified insulin coma therapy for schizophrenia. This dominated practice from 1934–54 despite serious doubts about its effect and with no coherent theoretical explanation for its action. A very careful RCT in 1954 demonstrated that equally improved outcome was achieved simply by transfer to a specialist unit and the increased nursing care, even when the insulin was not given. It was the extra attention and hope that made the difference. Clinical observation alone could not have identified this distinction, but a careful clinical research trial has saved countless patients from what was a potentially risky and ineffective procedure.

All of us involved in new and exciting service developments need to be aware of the potential for bias in interpreting our success. We may select easier patients (or have them selected for us). We may attribute to the new way of working benefits that really come from having more motivated, enthusiastic, or better-trained staff. Research increasingly attempts to control for these factors. In themselves they are not bad things—a team that can foster and attract great staff may have a real story to tell about improving care. What careful research aims to achieve is clarity about exactly what is achieving what.

The hierarchy of research methods

This is not the book to discuss individual study methods and research practice in great detail. As will be obvious from the foregoing, it is more important for us to understand the purpose of having such tightly defined methodologies in research so that conclusions can be drawn with confidence and be generalizable. If you agree to become involved in research, it will have an impact on your work. No matter what approach is used—even pragmatic trials (see later)—it will inevitably involve more careful recording of activity and data collection. It does not, however, necessarily mean that there will have to be that most demanding method, the RCT.

The randomized controlled trial (RCT)

The RCT has come to dominate research practice since its first use in medicine in the late 1930s. It is often referred to as the 'gold standard' in research and is certainly the most powerful format to test specific questions of effect. It reduces bias at the start of the trial by randomly allocating patients to either the experimental arm (in which they receive the treatment under scrutiny) or the control (in which they receive no treatment) or a comparator (in which they receive another standard, accepted treatment) arm. In drug trials when the control is no treatment, a dummy pill is used, and this is called a placebo-controlled trial. Neither patient nor clinician (nor researcher) has any say in which treatment is given—usually a sealed envelope is opened for each patient which simply has A or B printed on it.

This is the only trial design which can really answer questions about causality—whether or not the experimental treatment is responsible for the outcome. To do so it needs to be designed as closely as possible to have a single variable differing between the experimental and control arms; everything else needs to be the same. This is not easy to achieve in community psychiatry studies where the interventions are often complex. When it is achieved (e.g. the UK700 study; UK700 Group: Burns et al. 1999b; Burns et al. 2013), it may be criticized for being too narrow or for distorting practice.

Other designs can only tell us about association (i.e. that patients who have had one or other treatment also tend to have a specific outcome). Non-randomized controlled studies are often used when randomization seems too difficult. A group receiving a treatment is matched with patients who are otherwise as similar as possible (e.g. same age, diagnosis, duration of illness) and their outcomes compared over an agreed period. These are examples of cohort studies, as described later. They often use a before-and-after design (e.g. comparing outcomes such as admissions in the two groups during a period of years before and after the intervention) (Maughan et al. 2014). Obviously, the matching cannot be perfect—there is usually a reason that the intervention was used with one patient and not with another, which is why these types of studies are less convincing than RCTs.

Blinding

Because of rater bias and patient expectations, the optimal aim is to make RCTs 'double blind'. This means that neither the patient nor the research or clinical staff know if the patient is receiving the experimental treatment or the control. Their expectations thus cannot affect the outcome. This avoids a possible Hawthorne effect. For instance, in antidepressant trials, both patients and staff would expect those getting the drug to do better and, if they knew who was getting them, would probably rate them higher.

It is rarely possible to achieve blinding in studies of complex mental health interventions such as assertive outreach. The alternative approach is to try to make the outcome measures as concrete as possible, reducing the scope for bias by defining outcomes very carefully and training and retraining the raters. In severe mental illness RCTs (particularly for psychosis), hospital readmission is the most widely used outcome measure. It is not subject to rater bias, and is clinically meaningful and readily accessible (Burns 2007).

Statistics

The results of most research trials are interpreted 'probabilistically'. This means that statistics are used to estimate the likelihood of any difference found being due to the treatment rather than to chance. Results are often presented as 'statistically significant', but it is important to remember that this is not a statement of absolute fact but of the *likelihood* that the study results represent reality. Given that people vary and few results are black and white, most studies have to compare the range of outcomes in the experimental group with that in the control group. To be able to draw conclusions from this difference requires a calculation (and this needs to be done *before* the study is started) about whether the sample is big enough to draw such conclusions. This is called a 'power calculation'.

It is also important to bear in mind that a result can be highly statistically significant while not being at all *clinically* significant. This is especially so in very large studies of thousands of patients. For example, a reduction in blood pressure by, say, 2 mm/Hg may be demonstrated with statistical significance for a new drug. But is a reduction of 2 mm/Hg clinically meaningful? Is it worth taking the drug to achieve? This is clearly a different question.

Although RCTs have to be designed very carefully (otherwise they would not get funding, and they are expensive to conduct), they are sometimes reported without the same care. A key feature of an RCT is that it has a *primary outcome*. This is the single outcome which motivates the study (see later) and which hopefully should yield the yes/no answer to the question, 'Does it work?'. Of course, researchers collect and publish lots more data than just this. However, it is the primary outcome that matters. Community psychiatry research has been particularly poor in this area—often obscuring a negative primary outcome result (i.e. no difference in outcome) by reporting lots of secondary, less important positive results. Always ensure when you read an RCT that you understand which is the primary outcome, and draw your conclusions from that.

Power

If there is a lot of natural variation between individual patients, and the expected treatment differences are modest, then studies need to be large. This is invariably the case for community mental health research. However, we persist with a tradition of conducting 'underpowered' studies. This is a serious failing in our discipline (Coid 1994; Burns 2000b) and needs to be grappled with and resolved. It is particularly important for community outreach workers because of the likelihood of being asked to take part in local evaluations that drift into research projects. It is very unlikely indeed that a study of 50–100 patients can really 'prove' anything even if the questions are posed carefully. Certainly the commonest question, namely that of testing whether a team reduces bed usage, is not answerable with small samples for all the reasons outlined earlier. And yet such studies are still being regularly conducted, soaking up time and energy to produce results that do not have any real substance. A multi-centre study of the same question but employing several teams can, however, achieve adequate power. It will also reduce local Hawthorne effects and probably include a more representative patient sample.

Non-experimental studies

An RCT, with its attendant costs and disruption, is indicated only if an important question cannot be resolved by simpler research methods. In order of decreasing rigour—the degree to which we can place confidence in their results—these simpler methods are usually classed as follows: cohort studies, case series, and individual case histories.

Cohort studies consist of following up a defined group ('cohort') of patients over a defined period and recording their outcomes. By having detailed descriptions of them at baseline, we can draw conclusions about outcomes in different subgroups (e.g. women, younger patients, shorter histories). Long-term follow-up studies in schizophrenia are an example. There is no experimental intervention, but at the end we may know more about the predictors of outcome, such as the influence of gender or family history, than if these have been recorded (Ciompi 1988; Harding et al. 1987).

Exposure to treatment may be one of the characteristics included in a cohort study, and in some cases (where the exposure or non-exposure has been in a relatively consistent manner), this can be called a 'quasi-experimental' study.

Although the patients have not been randomly allocated to two treatments, such allocations may have arisen in the form of a 'natural experiment'. Examples are when a service is available in one area but not in another and the outcomes are then compared (Thornicroft et al. 1998a; Maughan et al. 2014). There are real risks in such studies; often the treatment is reported as 'causing' the outcome when technically this is not justified. How carefully the study is conducted can make up for many of these limitations. Enormous nationwide databases are now making such studies very powerful. This is particularly so in Scandinavia where the health care records of the whole population can be interrogated.

Case control studies are a type of cohort study where for each subject followed up there is a control patient, matched as closely as possible on all measures apart from the one under examination. Thus, the control patient is usually about the same age and same gender, and perhaps has other similarities, such as length of illness. Very careful matching in case control trials (Thornicroft et al. 1998a) can bring them close to RCTs in explanatory power, but they do remain open to much greater risks of bias.

Case series and individual case histories are often dismissed in research, but are essential for very rare conditions. They can be helpful in relatively neglected areas or for reporting new variations in treatment patterns (e.g. our experience with establishing patients on clozapine at home) (O'Brien and Firn 2002).

Clinical effectiveness and pragmatic trials

The complexity and cost of RCTs has led to concerns that simpler, yet important questions are often overlooked in research and that results are poorly transferable to 'the real world' of day-to-day clinical practice (Thornley and Adams 1998). In particular, the contrast is drawn between 'therapeutic efficacy', which tells us how well a treatment works under optimal conditions, and 'clinical effectiveness' (Thornicroft et al. 1998b), which indicates what we can expect under normal clinical conditions, when doctors are imperfect and patients sometimes forget to take their drugs and miss appointments.

Pragmatic trials are an attempt to address this. These trials are designed to be easy to conduct in routine clinical practice, with no onerous extra data collection (Thornley and Adams 1998). They are RCTs, but have few exclusion criteria and have simple randomization procedures with tightly defined and unequivocal outcome measures. To allow for the extensive variation within them, they aim for very large samples—sometimes several thousand patients. The establishment of bodies such as NICE has accelerated improvements in RCT methodology and the prominence of pragmatic trials investigating real-world clinical effectiveness.

Systematic reviews and meta-analyses

The main challenge in medical research is not so much an absence of evidence but rather the sheer volume of published studies and how to weigh them up against each other. A whole industry of 'evidence-based medicine' has grown up around how to draw confident conclusions from studies which may have contradictory results. The hierarchy of evidence presented later is a summary of the overall conclusions.

One of the most important results of this movement has been the Cochrane Collaboration. This collects together all the relevant studies on a given topic in a systematic review and presents their results in a comprehensive manner—identifying and grading them by quality.

Meta-analysis is one step further. In meta-analysis, all high-quality RCTs of the same question with similar outcome measures are added together—effectively becoming one much larger, more powerful RCT. Some of the early successes of meta-analysis were to combine a series of underpowered studies and detect real therapeutic effects that had not been obvious—the most dramatic example of which was the demonstration of the benefits of clot-busting drugs for heart attacks and strokes. The meta-analysis of ACT studies in 1998 (Marshall and Lockwood 1998), and its contrast with that for case management (Marshall et al. 2001), were instrumental in rolling out assertive outreach in the UK.

Meta-analyses are regularly updated as new studies are added and the results of all the accumulated studies can yield a different final answer. In 2007, the same meta-analysis of ACT as conducted by Marshall and Lockwood in 1998 no longer showed a clear superiority (Burns et al. 2007). Luckily, the variation in these studies and the quality of data allowed for a more refined analysis (meta-regression), which helped identify the effective ingredients within the 'black box' of assertive outreach (Wright et al. 2004). These procedures are highly technical, but luckily the Cochrane Collaboration and NICE regularly update and summarize them in a readable, reliable, and unbiased manner. The RCTs are graded for quality of work (including how well randomization was conducted, how complete the follow-up was, etc.). All the studies are subject to the same analysis against a limited and well-defined group of outcome measures. Repeating meta-analyses involves re-analysing from scratch all the data together so that a total effect can be deduced.

Hierarchy of evidence

NICE continually revises the current state of knowledge in the different fields of medical research. In our era of evidence-based medicine with so much to read and sift through, their guidelines are invaluable. However, they don't produce guidelines on everything, and it is important for us to have a useable system of trying to interpret the flood of research. Over the last 30 years, systems have been developed—first in the US with three levels, but since expanded in the UK to five levels—to rank evidence and give a framework for comparing the strength of different studies. This is often referred to as the 'hierarchy of evidence' and is represented as a pyramid with meta-analyses at the top. NICE bases its decisions for the availability of new treatments very firmly according to this pyramid (see Fig 29.1 and Table 29.1).

Qualitative research

This chapter has concentrated on research designs based on measuring processes and outcomes as accurately as possible, and then subjecting these results to statistical analysis. This is often referred to as 'quantitative' research to emphasize its numerical aspect. Quantitative research is usually employed to test hypotheses (beliefs about the nature of the subject) which are stated as precisely as possible right at the beginning. Where do all these hypotheses come from? For the most part they come from clinical impressions. We work with a group of patients over time and gradually the idea emerges that, say, 'Men benefit more from daily supervised meds'. If we want to be certain whether this is the truth or not (we doubt it!), then we propose it as a hypothesis and design a study to test it.

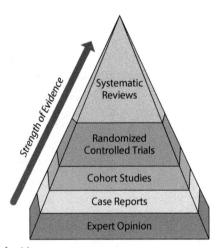

Fig 29.1 Hierarchy of evidence

Adapted from *Evidence-based medicine: how to practice and teach it*, second edition, Sackett D.L., Straus S.E., Richardson W.S. et al, 2000. Copyright 2000 with permission by Churchill Livingstone, published by Elsevier Inc.

Table 29.1 Hierarchy of evidence and recommendations grading scheme

Level	Type of evidence (NHS Executive)	Grade	Evidence (US Agency for Healthcare Policy)
I	Evidence obtained from a single RCT or a meta-analysis of RCTs	A	At least one RCT as part of a body of literature of overall good quality and consistency addressing the specific recommendation (evidence level I) without extrapolation
IIa	Evidence obtained from at least one well-designed controlled study without randomization	B	Well-conducted clinical studies but no randomized clinical trials on the topic of recommendation (evidence levels II or III); or extrapolated from level I evidence
IIb	Evidence obtained from at least one well-designed quasi-experimental study		
III	Evidence obtained from well-designed non-experimental descriptive studies, such as comparative studies, correlation studies, and case studies		
IV	Evidence obtained from expert committee reports or opinions and/or clinical experiences of respected authorities	C	Expert committee reports or opinions and/or clinical experiences of respected authorities (evidence level IV) or extrapolated from level I or II evidence; this grading indicates that directly applicable clinical studies of good quality are absent or not readily available
		GPP	Recommended good practice based on clinical experience

Data from *Health Technology Assessment*, 5, 16, Eccles M. and Mason J., 'How to develop cost conscious guidelines', 2001. Data from Clinical Guidelines: Using Clinical Guidelines to Improve Patient Care within the NHS, Mann T., 1996, Department of Health.

Sometimes qualitative research is used to generate hypotheses. Qualitative research is an emerging branch of science with increasing credibility. It arises more from social sciences, where it is much more difficult to conduct controlled experiments. Qualitative methods generally study complex processes and the experiences and perceptions of the people involved, with particular attention to contextual issues (e.g. timing, leadership, nature or size of the team or institution involved) that may influence the effectiveness of the intervention. They draw on a number of techniques from both social sciences and anthropology to refine the process of understanding what is going on. It encompasses a whole range of approaches from focus groups to participant observation.

There is an ongoing debate about whether qualitative work is purely 'hypothesis generating' or whether it can give definitive answers in its own right. The argument is muddied by an unfortunate practice of sometimes calling poorly thought-out or underpowered research 'qualitative'. It is clear that high-quality qualitative research is not just a matter of collecting a series of opinions, but requires as much (if not more) rigour than quantitative research. It is beyond our personal competences to advise on it other than to point out that it should not be undertaken without highly skilled supervision.

Conclusions

Assertive outreach came to prominence at the same time as a rising interest in evidence-based practice. It is also an unusually well-defined form of care, and earlier examples were subjected to research studies that produced remarkable results which became internationally famous. Not surprisingly then, outreach staff have been involved in much more clinical research than most mental health teams (Mueser et al. 1998; Catty et al. 2002). All of us are likely to be increasingly involved in audit, research, and development. The benefits in keeping us critical and reflective in our thinking are enormous if we take it seriously and do not simply collect data.

We owe it to ourselves to make sure that research in this area is conducted ethically and sensibly. Questions have to mean something. Clinicians, patients, and carers have much to contribute in both the setting of the questions and the design and conduct of the research. Only if there is a rich dialogue between all stakeholders will research deliver the results we need. We can also ensure that time and energy are not wasted on small-scale, underpowered studies whose results will not advance our understanding or practice. We should be particularly sceptical of research conducted to 'prove' that some treatment is better. Research should be to test *if* a treatment is better. We must always be open to the possibility (sadly a frequent outcome!) that it will not be better. There is a whole range of new questions to ask (not just effects on hospital use), and who better to raise them than the people who receive or work in the services?

References

Aaltonen, J., Seikkula, J., and Lehtinen, K. (2011) Comprehensive open-dialogue approach. I: Developing a comprehensive culture of need-adapted approach in a psychiatric public health catchment area the Western Lapland Project. *Psychosis*, **3**, 179–91.

Allness, D., and Knoedler, W. (1998) *The PACT model of community-based treatment for persons with severe and persistent mental illness: a manual for PACT start-up*, National Alliance for the Mentally Ill Anti-Stigma Campaign, Arlington, VA.

Álvarez-Jiménez, M., Hetrick, S.E., González-Blanch, C., Gleeson, J.F., and McGorry, P.D. (2008) Non-pharmacological management of antipsychotic-induced weight gain: systematic review and meta-analysis of randomised controlled trials. *The British Journal of Psychiatry*, **193**(2), 101–7.

American Psychiatric Association (1994) *Diagnostic and statistical manual of mental disorders* (4th ed.), American Psychiatric Association, Washington, DC.

American Psychiatric Association (2015) *Diagnostic and statistical manual of mental disorders* (5th ed.), American Psychiatric Association, Washington, DC.

Angermeyer, M.C., Loffler, W., Muller, P., Schulze, B., and Priebe, S. (2001) Patients' and relatives' assessment of clozapine treatment. *Psychological Medicine*, **31**(3), 509–17.

Appleby, L., Morriss, R., Gask, L., Roland, M., Perry, B., Lewis, A., et al. (2000) An educational intervention for front-line health professionals in the assessment and management of suicidal patients (the STORM Project). *Psychological Medicine*, **30**(4), 805–12.

Appleby, L., Shaw, J., Amos, T., McDonnell, R., Kiernan, K. and Davies, S. (1999) *Safer services. Report of the National Confidential Inquiry into Suicide and Homicide by People with Mental Illness*, HMSO, London.

Audit Commission (1994) *Finding a place: a review of mental health services for adults*, HMSO, London.

Bak, M., van Os, J., Delespaul, P., de Bie, A., á Campo, J., Poddighe, G., et al. (2007) An observational 'real life' trial of the introduction of assertive community treatment in a geographically defined area using clinical rather than service use outcome data. *Social Psychiatry and Psychiatric Epidemiology*, **42**(2), 125–30.

Barrowclough, C., Tarrier, N., Watts, S., Vaughn, C., Bamrah, J.S., and Freeman, H.L. (1987) Assessing the functional value of relatives' knowledge about schizophrenia: a preliminary report. *British Journal of Psychiatry*, **151**, 1–8.

Bartels, S.J. (2015) Can behavioral health organizations change health behaviors? The STRIDE study and lifestyle interventions for obesity in serious mental illness. *The American Journal of Psychiatry*, **172**(1), 9–11.

Bartels, S.J., Teague, G.B., and Drake, R.E. (1993) Service utilisation and costs associated with substance use disorder among severely mentally ill patients. *Journal of Nervous & Mental Disease*, **177**, 400–7.

Barton, R. (1959) *Institutional neurosis*, John Wright, Bristol.

Bateman, A., and Fonagy, P. (1999) Effectiveness of partial hospitalization in the treatment of borderline personality disorder: a randomized controlled trial. *American Journal of Psychiatry*, **156**, 1563–9.

Bateman, A.W., Gunderson, J., and Mulder, R. (2015) Treatment of personality disorder. *The Lancet*, **385**, 735–43.

Bateson, G., Jackson, D., Haley, J., and Weakland, J. (1956) Towards a theory of schizophrenia. *Behavioral Science*, **1**, 251–64.

Beard, J.H., Propst, R.N., and Malamud, T.J. (1982) The Fountain House model of rehabilitation. *Psychosocial Rehabilitation Journal*, **5**(1), 47–53.

Beauchamp, T.L. and Childress, J.F. (2013) *Principles of medical ethics* (7th ed.), Oxford University Press, Oxford.

Bebbington, P.E., Angermeyer, M., Azorin, J., Brugha, T., Kilian, R., Johnson, S., et al. (2005) The European Schizophrenia Cohort: a naturalistic prognostic and economic study. *Social Psychiatry and Psychiatric Epidemiology*, **40**, 707–17.

Bech, P., Allerup, P., Gram, L.F., Reisby, N., Rosenberg, R., Jacobsen, O., et al. (1981) The Hamilton Depression Scale: evaluation of objectivity using logistic models. *Acta Psychiatrica Scandinavica*, **63**(3), 290–9.

Beck, A.T., Ward, C.H., Mendelson, M., Mock, J.E., and Erbaugh, J.K. (1961) An inventory for measuring depression. *Archives of General Psychiatry*, **4**, 561–71.

Beynon, S., Soares-Weiser, K., Woolacott, N., Duffy, S., and Geddes, J.R. (2008) Psychosocial interventions for the prevention of relapse in bipolar disorder: systematic review of controlled trials. *The British Journal of Psychiatry*, **192**(1), 5–11.

Bhugra, D. and Bhui, K. (2001) *Cross cultural psychiatry: a practical guide*, Edward Arnold, London.

Bhugra, D., Ayonrinde, O., Butler, G., Leese, M., and Thornicroft, G. (2011) A randomised controlled trial of assertive outreach vs. treatment as usual for black people with severe mental illness. *Epidemiology and Psychiatric Sciences*, **20**, 83–9.

Bindman, J., Beck, A., Thornicroft, G., Knapp, M., and Szmukler, G. (2000) Psychiatric patients at greatest risk and in greatest need. Impact of the supervision register policy. *British Journal of Psychiatry*, **177**, 33–7.

Birchwood, M. and Iqbal, Z. (1998) Depression and suicide thinking in psychosis: a cognitive approach. In: *Outcome and innovation in psychological management of schizophrenia*, (ed. T. Wykes, N. Tarrier, and S. Lewis), Wiley, Chichester, 81–100.

Birchwood, M., Connor, C., Lester, H., Patterson, P., Freemantle, N., Marshall, M., et al. (2013) Reducing duration of untreated psychosis: care pathways to early intervention in psychosis services. *The British Journal of Psychiatry*, **203**, 58–64.

Birchwood, M., Smith, J., Cochrane, R., Wetton, S., and Copestake, S. (1990) The Social Functioning Scale: the development and validation of a new scale of social adjustment for use in family intervention programmes with schizophrenic patients. *British Journal of Psychiatry*, **157**, 853–9.

Birchwood, M., Smith, J., Drury, V., Healy, J., MacMillan, F., and Slade, M. (1994) A self-report insight scale for psychosis: reliability, validity and sensitivity to change. *Acta Psychiatrica Scandinavica*, **89**(1), 62–7.

Bleuler, E. (1950) *Dementia praecox or the group of schizophrenias* (transl. J. Zinkin), International Universities Press, New York.

Bond, G.R. (1991) Variations in an assertive outreach model. *New Directions for Mental Health Services*, **52**, 65–80.

Bond, G.R. (1992) Vocational rehabilitation. In: *Handbook of psychiatric rehabilitation* (ed. R.P. Liberman), Macmillan, New York.

Bond, G.R. and Dincin, J. (1986) Accelerating entry into transitional employment in a psychosocial agency. *Rehabilitation Psychology*, **31**, 135–45.

Bond, G.R. and Drake, R.E. (2007) Should we adopt the Dutch version of ACT? Commentary on 'FACT: a Dutch version of ACT'. *Community Mental Health Journal*, **43**(4), 435–8.

Bond, G.R., Drake, R.E., and Becker, D.R. (2008) An update on randomized controlled trials of evidence-based supported employment. *Psychiatric Rehabilitation Journal*, **31**(4), 280–9.

Bond, G.R., Drake, R.E., Mueser, K.T., and Becker, D.R. (1997) An update on supported employment for people with severe mental illness. *Psychiatric Services*, **48**(3), 335–46.

Bond, G.R., Witheridge, T.F., Dincin, J., Wasmer, D., de Webb, J., and Graaf-Kaser, R. (1990) Assertive community treatment for frequent users of psychiatric hospitals in a large city: a controlled study. *American Journal of Community Psychology*, **18**(6), 865–91.

Bowlby, J. (1961) Process of mourning. *International Journal of Psychoanalysis*, **42**, 317–40.

Braun, P., Kochansky, G., Shapiro, R., Greenberg, S., Gudeman, J.E., Johnson, S., et al. (1981) Overview: deinstitutionalization of psychiatric patients, a critical review of outcome studies. *American Journal of Psychiatry*, **138**(6), 736–49.

Brayne, H.A. and Martin, G. (1990) *Law for social workers*, Blackstone Press Limited, London.

Brooker, C., Falloon, I., Butterworth, A., Goldberg, D., Graham–Hole, V., and Hillier, V. (1994) The outcome of training community psychiatric nurses to deliver psychosocial intervention. *British Journal of Psychiatry*, **165**(2), 222–30.

Brown, G.W., Birley, J.L., and Wing, J.K. (1972) Influence of family life on the course of schizophrenic disorders: a replication. *British Journal of Psychiatry*, **121**(562), 241–58.

Burns, T. (1997) Psychosocial interventions. *Current Opinion in Psychiatry*, **10**, 36–9.

Burns, T. (2000a) Maxwell Jones lecture: the legacy of therapeutic community practice in modern community mental health services. *Therapeutic Communities*, **21**(3), 165–74.

Burns, T. (2000b) Psychiatric home treatment: vigorous, well designed trials are needed. *BMJ*, **321**(7254), 177.

Burns, T. (2000c) Supervised discharge orders. *Psychiatric Bulletin*, **24**(401), 402.

Burns, T. (2007) Community mental health teams. *Psychiatry*, **6**, 325–28.

Burns, T. (2007) Hospitalisation as an outcome measure in schizophrenia. *The British Journal of Psychiatry*, **191**(50), 37–41.

Burns, T. (2016) Psychiatric services. In: *Shorter Oxford textbook of psychiatry* (7th ed.), Oxford University Press, Oxford.

Burns, T. and Bale, R. (1997) Establishing a mental health liaison attachment with primary care. *Advances in Psychiatric Treatment*, **3**, 219–24.

Burns, T., Beadsmoore, A., Bhat, A.V., Oliver, A., and Mathers, C. (1993) A controlled trial of home-based acute psychiatric services. I: clinical and social outcome. *British Journal of Psychiatry*, **163**, 49–54.

Burns, T., Catty, J., Becker, T., Drake, R.E., Fioritti, A., Knapp, M., et al. (2007) The effectiveness of supported employment for people with severe mental illness: a randomised controlled trial. *The Lancet*, **370**(9593), 1146–52.

Burns, T., Catty, J., Dash, M., Roberts, C., Lockwood, A., and Marshall, M. (2007) Use of intensive case management to reduce time in hospital in people with severe mental illness: systematic review and meta-regression. *BMJ*, **335**(7615), 336.

Burns, T. and Cohen, A. (1998) Item-of-service payments for general practitioner care of severely mentally ill persons: does the money matter? *British Journal of General Practice*, **48**, 1415–16.

Burns, T., Creed, F., Fahy, T., Thompson, S., Tyrer, P., and White, I. (1999) Intensive versus standard case management for severe psychotic illness: a randomised trial. *The Lancet*, **353**, 2185–9.

Burns, T., Fiander, M., Kent, A., Ukoumunne, O.C., Byford, S., Fahy, T., & Kumar, K.R. (2000) Effects of case-load size on the process of care of patients with severe psychotic illness: report from the UK700 trial. *British Journal of Psychiatry*, **177**(5), 427–33.

Burns, T. and Molodynski, A. (2014) Community treatment orders: background and implications of the OCTET trial. *Psychiatric Bulletin*, doi:10.1192/pb.bp.113.044628

Burns, T. and Priebe, S. (1996) Mental health care systems and their characteristics: a proposal. *Acta Psychiatrica Scandinavica*, **94**(6), 381–5.

Burns, T., Rugkåsa, J., Molodynski, A., Dawson, J., Yeeles, K., Vasquez-Montez, M., et al. (2013) Community treatment orders for patients with psychosis (OCTET): a randomised controlled trial. *The Lancet*, **381**(9878),1627–33.

Burns, T., Yeeles, K., Koshiaris, C., Vasquez-Montez, M., Molodynski, A., Puntis, S., et al. (2015) Effect of increased compulsion on readmission to hospital or disengagement from community services for patients with psychosis: follow-up of a cohort from the OCTET trial. *Lancet Psychiatry*, http://cs.doi.org/10.1016/S2215-0366(15)00364-8.

Burns, T., Yeeles, K., Langford, O., Vazquez-Montes, M., Burgess, J., Anderson, C., et al. (2015) A randomised controlled trial of time-limited individual placement and support: IPS-LITE trial. *The British Journal of Psychiatry*, **207**(4), 351–6. doi:10.1192/bjp.bp.114.152082

Burns, T., Yeeles, K., Molodynski, A., Nightingale, H., Vasquez-Montez, M., et al. (2011) Pressures to adhere to treatment ('leverage') in English mental health care. *British Journal of Psychiatry*, **199**, 145–50.

Burns, T., Yiend, J., Doll, H., Fahy, T., Fiander, M., and Tyrer, P. (2007) Using activity data to explore the influence of case-load size on care patterns. *British Journal of Psychiatry*, **190**, 217–22.

Byrne, D.L., Asmussen, T., and Freeman. Descriptive terms for women attending antenatal clinics: mother knows best? *British Journal of Obstetrics and Gynaecology*, **107**, 1233–6.

Caplan, G. (1964) *Principles of preventive psychiatry*, Basic Books, New York.

Care Quality Commission (2013) *Supporting information and guidance: Supporting effective clinical supervision*. https://www.cqc.org.uk/sites/default/files/documents/20130625_800734_v1_00_supporting_information-effective_clinical_supervision_for_publication.pdf

Care Quality Commission (2015) *Community mental health survey*, CQC: London.

Carers Trust (2013) *The triangle of care, carers included: a guide to best practice in mental health care in England* (2nd ed.), Carers Trust, London.

Carey, K.B. (1995) Treatment of substance use disorders and schizophrenia. In: *Double jeopardy: chronic mental illness and substance abuse* (ed. A.F. Lehman and L.B. Dixon), Harwood Academic Publishers, Baltimore.

Catty, J., Burns, T., Knapp, M., Watt, H., Wright, C., Henderson, J., et al. (2002) Home treatment for mental health problems: a systematic review. *Psychological Medicine*, 32(3), 383–401.

Catty, J., Cowan, N., Poole, Z., Ellis, G., Geyer, C., Lissouba, P., et al. (2011) Attachment to the clinical team and its association with therapeutic relationships, social networks, and clinical well-being. *Psychology and Psychotherapy: Theory, Research and Practice*, 85, 17–35.

Chadwick, P. (2014) Mindfulness for psychosis. *The British Journal of Psychiatry*, 204(5), 333–4. doi: 10.1192/bjp.bp.113.136044

Chadwick, P.D., Birchwood, M., and Grower, P. (1996) *Cognitive therapy for delusions, voices and paranoia*, John Wiley, Chichester.

Chaplin, R., Gordon, J., and Burns, T. (1999) Early detection of antipsychotic side-effects. *Psychiatric Bulletin*, 23, 657–60.

Chaplin, R. and Kent, A. (1998) Informing patients about tardive dyskinesia. Controlled trial of patient education. *British Journal of Psychiatry*, 172, 78–81.

Charlton, J., Kelly, S., Dunnell, K., Evans, B., and Jenkins, R. (1994) Suicide deaths in England and Wales: trends in factors associated with suicide deaths. In: *The prevention of suicide* (ed. R. Jenkins et al.), HMSO, London.

Ciompi, L. (1988) Learning from outcome studies toward a comprehensive biological-psychosocial understanding of schizophrenia. *Schizophrenia Research*, 1, 373–84.

Cipriani, A., Hawton, K., Stockton, S., and Geddes, J.R. (2013) Lithium in the prevention of suicide in mood disorders: updated systematic review and meta-analysis. *BMJ*, 346, f3646.

Clark, D. (2011) Implementing NICE guidelines for the psychological treatment of depression and anxiety disorders: the IAPT experience. *International Review of Psychiatry*, 23, 375–84.

Coid, J.W. (1994) Failure in community care: psychiatry's dilemma. *BMJ*, 308(6932), 805–6.

Coid, J.W. (1996) Dangerous patients with mental illness: increased risks warrant new policies, adequate resources, and appropriate legislation. *BMJ*, 312(7036), 965–6.

Committee of Inquiry (1969) *Report of the Committee of Inquiry into allegations of ill-treatment of patients and other irregularities at the Ely Hospital, Cardiff, presented to Parliament by the Secretary of State of the Department of Health and Social Security*, HMSO, London.

Cooper, J.E. (1979) Crisis admission units and emergency psychiatric services. In: *Public health in Europe, No. 2*, WHO, Copenhagen.

Craig, T. and Timms, P.W. (1992) Out of the wards and onto the streets? Deinstitutionalization and homelessness in Britain. *Journal of Mental Health*, 1, 265–75.

Crow, T.J. (1980) Molecular pathology of schizophrenia: more than one disease process? *BMJ*, 280(6207), 66–8.

Crow, T.J., MacMillan, J.F., Johnson, A.L., and Johnstone, E.C. (1986) A randomised controlled trial of prophylactic neuroleptic treatment. *British Journal of Psychiatry*, 148, 120–7.

Crowther, R.E., Marshall, M., Bond, G.R., and Huxley, P. (2001) Helping people with severe mental illness to obtain work: systematic review. *BMJ*, **322**, 204–8.

Cunningham-Owens, D.G. (1999) *A guide to the extrapyramidal side effects of antipsychotic drugs*, Cambridge University Press, Cambridge.

Curson, D.A., Barnes, T.R., Bamber, R.W., Platt, S.D., Hirsch, S.R., and Duffy, J.C. (1985) Long-term depot maintenance of chronic schizophrenic out-patients: the seven year follow-up of the Medical Research Council fluphenazine/placebo trial. III. Relapse postponement or relapse prevention? The implications for long-term outcome. *British Journal of Psychiatry*, **146**, 474–80.

Curtis, J.L., Millman, E.J., Struening, E., & D'Ercole, A. (1992). Effect of case management on rehospitalization and utilization of ambulatory care services. *Hospital & Community Psychiatry*, **43**(9), 895–9.

David, A., Buchanan, A., Reed, A., and Almeida, O. (1992) The assessment of insight in psychosis. *British Journal of Psychiatry*, **161**, 599–602.

David, A.S. (1990) Insight and psychosis. *British Journal of Psychiatry*, **156**, 798–808.

Davies, W. and Frude, N. (1993) *Preventing face-to-face violence: the T-PIP programme*, The Association of Psychological Therapies, Leicester, England.

Davis, S.M., Scott Stroup, T., Koch, G.G., Davis, C.E., Rosenheck, R.A., and Lieberman, J.A. (2011) Time to all-cause treatment discontinuation as the primary outcome in the Clinical Antipsychotic Trials of Intervention Effectiveness (CATIE) Schizophrenia Study. *Statistics in Biopharmaceutical Research*, **3**, 253–65.

Dawson, J. and Burns, T. (2016) Reducing legal barriers to smooth transition between forensic and general mental health care. In: *Care of the mentally disordered offender in the community* (ed. L. Wooton and A. Buchanan), Oxford University Press, Oxford.

Degen, K., Cole, N., Tamayo, L., and Dzerovych, G. (1990) Intensive case management for the seriously ill. *Administration and Policy in Mental Health*, **17**(4), 265–9.

Department of Health (1959) *The Mental Health Act: England and Wales*, Department of Health, London.

Department of Health (1990) *The Care Programme Approach for people with a mental illness referred to the Special Psychiatric Services*, Joint Health/Social Services Circular HC (90)23/LASS(90)11, Department of Health, London.

Department of Health (1995) *Patients in the Community Mental Health Act 1995*, HMSO, London.

Department of Health (1998a) *Modernising mental health services, safe, sound and supportive*, HSC 1998/233/LAC(98)25, Department of Health, London.

Department of Health (1999a) *Modern standards and service models: National Service Framework for Mental Health*, Department of Health, London.

Department of Health (1999b) *Code of practice: Mental Health Act 1983*, HMSO, London.

Department of Health (2000) *The NHS plan—a plan for investment, a plan for reform*, Department of Health, London.

Department of Health (2001) *The mental health policy implementation guide*, Department of Health, London.

Department of Health, National Institute for Mental Health in England (2003) *Personality disorder: no longer a diagnosis of exclusion. Policy implementation guidance for the development of services for people with personality disorder*. Department of Health, London.

Department of Health (2002) *Dual diagnosis good practice guide*, Department of Health, London.

Department of Health (2004) *The NHS Knowledge and Skills Framework (NHS KSF) and the development review process*. Department of Health, London.

Department of Health (2008) *Mental Health Act: code of practice*, Department of Health, London.

Department of Health. (2010) *Prioritising need in the context of* Putting People First: *a whole system approach to eligibility for social care*, Department of Health, London.

Department of Health (2013) *No health without mental health*, Department of Health. HMSO London.

Di Forte, M., Morgan, C., Dazzan, P., Pariante, C., Mondelli, V., Marques, T.R., et al. (2009) High-potency cannabis and the risk of psychosis. *The British Journal of Psychiatry*, **195**(6), 488–91.

Diamond, D.M., Campbell, A.M., Park, C.R., Halonen, J., and Zoladz, P.R. (2007) The temporal dynamics model of emotional memory processing: a synthesis on the neurobiological basis of stress-induced amnesia, flashbulb and traumatic memories, and the Yerkes-Dodson law. *Neural Plasticity*, **3007**:60803. doi: 10.1155/2007/60803

Dixon, L., Turner, J., Krauss, N., Scott, J., and McNary, S. (1999) Case managers' and clients' perspectives on a representative payee program. *Psychiatric Services*, **50**(6), 781–6. doi: http://dx.doi.org/10.1016/j.schres.2004.09.009

Drake, R.E. and Becker, D.R. (1996) The individual placement and support (IPS) model of supported employment. *Psychiatric Services*, **47**(5), 473–5.

Drake, R.E. and Mercer-McFadden, C. (1995) Assessment of substance use among persons with chronic mental illnesses. In: *Double jeopardy: chronic mental illness and substance abuse* (ed. A.F. Lehman and L.B. Dixon), Harwood Academic Publishers, Baltimore.

Drake, R.E., Becker, D.R., Clark, R.E., and Mueser, K.T. (1999b) Research on the individual placement and support model of supported employment. *Psychiatric Quarterly*, **70**(4), 289–301.

Drake, R.E., McHugo, G.J., Bebout, R.R., Becker, D.R., Harris, M., Bond, G.R., et al. (1999a) A randomized clinical trial of supported employment for inner-city patients with severe mental disorders. *Archives of General Psychiatry*, **56**(7), 627–33.

Drake, R.E., McHugo, G.J., Clark, R.E., Teague, G.B., Xie, H., Miles, K., et al. (1998) Assertive community treatment for patients with co-occurring severe mental illness and substance use disorder: a clinical trial. *American Journal of Orthopsychiatry*, **68**(2), 201–15.

Drake, R.E., Noordsy, D.L., and Ackerson, T. (1995) Integrating mental health and substance abuse treatments for persons with chronic mental disorders: a model. In: *Double jeopardy: chronic mental illness and substance abuse* (ed. A.F. Lehman and L.B. Dixon), Harwood Academic Publishers, Baltimore.

Drake, R.E., Yovetich, N.A., Bebout, R.R., Harris, M., and McHugo, G.J. (1997) Integrated treatment for dually diagnosed homeless adults. *Journal of Nervous & Mental Disease*, **185**(5), 298–305.

Drukker, M., Maarschalkerweerd, M., Bak, M., Driessen, G., à Campo, J., de Bie, A., et al. (2008) A real-life observational study of the effectiveness of FACT in a Dutch mental health region. *BMC Psychiatry*, **8**(93), 1–10.

Eastman, N. (1994) Mental health law: civil liberties and the principle of reciprocity. *British Medical Journal*, **308**(6920), 43–45.

English National Board (1996) *Working in partnership: a collaborative approach to care. Report of the mental health nursing review team. Progress two years on*, English National Board, London.

Equality Act 2010. HMSO, London.

Essock, S., Mueser K.T., Drake, R.E., Covell, N.H., McHugo, G.J., Frisman, L.K., et al. (2006) Comparison of ACT and standard case management for delivering integrated treatment for co-occurring disorders. *Psychiatric Services*, **57**, 186–96.

Fadden, G. (1997) Implementation of family interventions in routine clinical practice following staff training programs: a major cause for concern. *Journal of Mental Health*, **6**(6), 599–612.

Falloon, I.R., Boyd, J.L., McGill, C.W., Razani, J., Moss, H.B., and Gilderman, A.M. (1982) Family management in the prevention of exacerbations of schizophrenia: a controlled study. *New England Journal of Medicine*, **306**(24), 1437–40.

Falret, J. (1854) Memoire sur la folie circulaire. *Bulletin de la Acadamie Imperiale de Medicin, Paris*, **19**, 382–400.

Farkas, M. and Anthony, W.A. (2010) Psychiatric rehabilitation interventions: a review. *International Review of Psychiatry*, **22**, 114–29.

Faulkner, G., Cohn, T., and Remington, G. (2007) Interventions to reduce weight gain in schizophrenia. *Cochrane Schizophrenia Group, The Cochrane Collaboration*, Wiley & Sons Ltd. doi: 10.1002/14651858.CD005148.pub2.

Fazel, S., Långström, N., Hjern, A., Grann, M., Lichtenstein, P. (2009) Schizophrenia, substance abuse, and violent crime. *JAMA*, **301**, 2016–23.

Fazel, S., Singh, J.P., Doll, H., and Grann, M. (2012) Use of risk assessment instruments to predict violence and antisocial behaviour in 73 samples involving 24 827 people: systematic review and meta-analysis. *BMJ*, **345**, e4692.

Feeley, M., DeRubeis, R.J., and Gelfand, L.A. (1999) The temporal relation of adherence and alliance to symptom change in cognitive therapy for depression. *Journal of Consulting and Clinical Psychology*, **67**, 578–82.

Fervaha, G., Foussias, G., Agid, O., and Remington, G. (2014) Motivational and neurocognitive deficits are central to the prediction of longitudinal functional outcome in schizophrenia. *Acta Psychiatrica Scandinavica*, **130**(4), 290–9. doi: 10.1111/acps.12289. Epub 22 May 2014.

Fiander, M. et al. (2001) Process of care under intensive case management (ICM): changes over time. *British Journal of Psychiatry*.

Fiander, M., Burns, T., Ukoumunne, O.C., Fahy, T., Creed, F., Tyrer, P., et al. (2006) Do care patterns change over time in a newly established mental health service? A report from the UK700 trial. *European Psychiatry*, **21**(5), 300–6.

Firn, M., Hindhaugh, K., Hubbeling, D., Davies, G., Jones, B., and White, S.J. (2013) A dismantling study of assertive outreach services: comparing activity and outcomes following replacement with the FACT model. *Social Psychiatry and Psychiatric Epidemiology*, **48**, 997–1003.

Firn, M., White, S.J., Hubbeling, D., and Jones, B. (2016) The replacement of assertive outreach services by reinforcing local community teams: a four-year observational study. *Journal of Mental Health*. doi: 10.3109/09638237.2016.1139073.

Fleischhacker, W.W., Roth, S.D., and Kane, J.M. (1990) The pharmacologic treatment of neuroleptic-induced akathisia. *Journal of Clinical Psychopharmacology*, **10**(1), 12–21.

Frank, A.F. and Gunderson, J.G. (1990) The role of the therapeutic alliance in the treatment of schizophrenia. Relationship to course and outcome. *Archives of General Psychiatry*, 47(3), 228–36.

Franklin, J.L., Solovitz, B., Mason, M., Clemons, J.R., and Miller, G.E. (1987) An evaluation of case management. *American Journal of Public Health*, 77(6), 674–8.

Freeman, D., Waite, F., Startup, H., Myers, E., Lister, R., McInerney, J., et al. (2015) Efficacy of cognitive behavioural therapy for sleep improvement in patients with persistent delusions and hallucinations (BEST): a prospective, assessor-blind, randomised controlled pilot trial. *The Lancet*, 2, 975–83.

Fromm-Reichmann, F. (1948) Notes on the development of treatment of schizophrenics by psychoanalytic psychotherapy. *Psychiatry*, 11, 263–70.

Gabbard, G. (2007) *Personality disorders: Gabbard's treatment of psychiatric disorders* (4th ed.), APPI, Washington, DC.

García-Lizana, F. and Muñoz-Mayorga, I. (2010) What about telepsychiatry? A systematic review. *Primary Care Companion –Journal of Clinical Psychiatry*, 12(2), e1–e5.

Gardner, W., Hoge, S.K., Bennett, N., Roth, L.H., Lidz, C.W., Monahan, J., et al. (1993) Two scales for measuring patients' perceptions for coercion during mental hospital admission. *Behavioural Sciences and the Law*, 11(3), 307–21.

Geddes, J., Freemantle, N., Harrison, P., and Bebbington, P. (2000) Atypical antipsychotics in the treatment of schizophrenia: systematic overview and meta-regression analysis. *BMJ*, 321(7273), 1371–6.

Geddes, J.R. and Miklowitz, D.J. (2013) Treatment of bipolar disorder. *The Lancet*, 381, 1672–82.

Gelenberg, A.J., de Leon, J., Eden Evins, A., Parks, J.J., and Rigotti, N.A., (2008) Smoking cessation in patients with psychiatric disorders. *Primary Care Companion –Journal of Clinical Psychiatry*, 10(1), 52–58.

Glover, G., Arts, G. and Babu, K.S. (2006) Crisis resolution/home treatment teams and psychiatric admission rates in England. *British Journal of Psychiatry*, 189, 441–5.

Goffman, E. (1960) *Asylums: essays on the social situation of mental patients and other inmates.* Penguin Books, Harmondsworth, Middlesex.

Goldstein, R.B., Black, D.W., Nasrallah, A., and Winokur, G. (1991) The prediction of suicide. Sensitivity, specificity, and predictive value of a multivariate model applied to suicide among 1906 patients with affective disorders. *Archives of General Psychiatry*, 48(5), 418–22.

Goodwin, I., Holmes, G., Cochrane, R. and Mason, O. (2003) The ability of adult mental health services to meet clients' attachment needs: the development and implementation of the Service Attachment Questionnaire. *Psychology and Psychotherapy: Theory, Research and Practice*, 76, 145–61.

Gournay, K. and Birley, J. (1998) Thorn: a new approach to mental health training. *Nursing Times*, 94(49), 54–5.

Gournay, K. and Brooking, J. (1994) Community Psychiatric Nurses in Primary Care. *British Journal of Psychiatry*, 165, 231–8.

Graham, J.H. (2006) Community care or therapeutic stalking: two sides of the same coin? *Journal of Psychosocial Nursing and Mental Health Services*, 44(8), 41–7.

Gray, S., Taylor, J., and Snowden, R.J. (2008) Predicting violent reconvictions using the HCR-20. *The British Journal of Psychiatry.* 192, 384–387. doi: 10.1192/bjp.bp.107.044065

Green, B., Young, R., and Kavanagh, D. (2005) Cannabis use and misuse prevalence among people with psychosis. *The British Journal of Psychiatry*, **187**(4) 306–13.

Green, M.F. (1996) What are the functional consequences of neurocognitive deficits in schizophrenia? *American Journal of Psychiatry*, **153**(3), 321–30.

Green, M.F., Kern, R.S., Heaton, R.K. (2004) Longitudinal studies of cognition and functional outcome in schizophrenia: implications for MATRICS. *Schizophrenia Research*, **72**, 41–51.

Greenwood, N., Hussain, F., Burns, T., and Raphael, F. (2000) Asian in-patient and carer views of mental health care. Asian views of mental health care. *Journal of Mental Health*, **9**(4), 397–408.

Grove, B. (1999) Mental health and employment: shaping a new agenda. *Journal of Mental Health*, **8**, 131–40.

Grove, B. (2000) *Work and employment*, Health Advisory Service, London.

Grufferman, S. (1999) Complexity and the Hawthorne effect in community trials. *Epidemiology*, **10**(3), 209–10.

Harding, C.M., Brooks, G.W., Ashikaga, T., Strauss, J.S., and Breier, A. (1987) The Vermont longitudinal study of persons with severe mental illness. II: Long-term outcome of subjects who retrospectively met DSM-III criteria for schizophrenia. *American Journal of Psychiatry*, **144**(6), 727–35.

Harris, E.C. and Barraclough, B. (1998) Excess mortality of mental disorder. *British Journal of Psychiatry*, **173**, 11–53.

Harrison, G., Hopper, K., Craig, T., Laska, E., Siegel, C., Wanderling, J., et al. (2001) Recovery from psychotic illness: a 15- and 25-year international follow-up study. *The British Journal of Psychiatry*, **178**(6) 506–17.

Hawton, K., Sutton, L., Haw, C., Sinclair, J., Deeks, J.J. (2005) Schizophrenia and suicide: systematic review of risk factors. *The British Journal of Psychiatry*, **187**(1), 9–20. doi: 10.1192/bjp.187.1.9

Hegarty, J.D., Baldessarini, R.J., Tohen, M., Waternaux, C., and Oepen, G. (1994) One hundred years of schizophrenia: a meta-analysis of the outcome literature. *American Journal of Psychiatry*, **151**, 1409–16.

Henquet, C., Murray, R., Linszen, D., and van Os, J. (2005) The environment and schizophrenia: the role of cannabis use. *Schizophrenia Bulletin*, **31**, 608–12.

Hinton, J. (1967) *Dying*, Penguin Books, Middlesex, England.

Hirsch, S. (1988) *Psychiatric beds and resources: factors influencing bed use and service planning*, Gaskell Press (Royal College of Psychiatrists), London.

Hirsch, S.R., Gaind, R., Rohde, P.D., Stevens, B.C., and Wing, J.K. (1973) Outpatient maintenance of chronic schizophrenic patients with long-acting fluphenazine: double-blind placebo trial. Report to the Medical Research Council Committee on clinical trials in psychiatry. *BMJ*, **1**(854), 633–7.

Hogarty, G.E., Anderson, C.M., Reiss, D.J., Kornblith, S.J., Greenwald, D.P., Ulrich, R.F., et al. (1991) Family psychoeducation, social skills training, and maintenance chemotherapy in the aftercare treatment of schizophrenia. II. Two-year effects of a controlled study on relapse and adjustment. Environmental–Personal Indicators in the Course of Schizophrenia (EPICS) Research Group. *Archives of General Psychiatry*, **48**(4), 340–7.

Hogarty, G.E., Kornblith, S.J., Greenwald, D., DiBarry, A.L., Cooley, S., Flesher, S., et al. (1995) Personal therapy: a disorder-relevant psychotherapy for schizophrenia. *Schizophrenia Bulletin*, 21(3), 379–93.

Holloway, F. (2005) The forgotten need for rehabilitation in contemporary mental health services: a position statement from the executive committee of the Faculty of Rehabilitation and Social Psychiatry. *Royal College of Psychiatrists*, www.rcpsych.ac.uk/pdf/frankholloway_oct05.pdf.

Holloway, F. and Carson, J. (1998) Intensive case management for the severely mentally ill: controlled trial. *British Journal of Psychiatry*, 172, 19–22.

Holloway, F., Oliver, N., Collins, E., and Carson, J. (1995) Case management: a critical review of the outcome literature. *European Psychiatry*, 10, 113–28.

Hoult, J. (1986) Community care of the acutely mentally ill. *British Journal of Psychiatry*, 149, 137–44.

Hoult, J., Rosen, A., and Reynolds, I. (1984) Community orientated treatment compared to psychiatric hospital orientated treatment. *Social Science and Medicine*, 18(11), 1005–10.

HQIP and The Royal College of Psychiatrists (2014) *Report of the Second Round of the National Audit of Schizophrenia (NAS)*. London: Healthcare Quality Improvement Partnership.

Hunt, G.E., Bergen, J. and Bashir, M. (2002) Medication compliance and comorbid substance abuse in Schizophrenia. Impact on community survival 4 years after relapse. *Schizophrenia Research*, 54, 253–64.

Hwang, S.W. and Burns, T. (2014) Health interventions for people who are homeless. *The Lancet*, 384, 1541–7.

Institute of Medicine (2001) *Crossing the quality chasm: a new health system for the 21st century*, National Academy Press, Washington, DC.

Intagliata, J. (1982) Improving the quality of community care for the chronically mentally disabled: the role of case management. *Schizophrenia Bulletin*, 8(4), 655–74.

Jääskeläinen, E., Juola, P., Hirvonen, N., McGrath, J., Saha, S., Isohanni, M., et al. (2013) A Systematic Review and Meta-Analysis of Recovery in Schizophrenia. *Schizophrenia Bulletin*, 39, 1296–1306. doi: 10.1093/schbul/sbs130.

Jaeger, M. and Rössler, W. (2010) Enhancement of outpatient treatment adherence: patients' perceptions of coercion, fairness and effectiveness. *Psychiatry Research*, 180(1), 48–53.

Johnson, M.J., Williams, M., and Marshall, E.S. (1999) Adherent and non-adherent medication—taking in elderly hypertensive patients. *Clinical Nursing Research*, 8(4), 318–35.

Johnson, S. and Thornicroft, G. (1993) The sectorisation of psychiatric services in England and Wales. *Social Psychiatry & Psychiatric Epidemiology*, 28(1), 45–7.

Johnson, S. and Thornicroft, G. (1995) Service models in emergency psychiatry: an international review. In: *Emergency mental health services in the community* (ed. M. Phelan, G. Strathdee, and G. Thornicroft), Cambridge University Press, Cambridge.

Johnson, S., Needle, J., Bindman, J.P., and Thornicroft, G. (eds) (2008) *Crisis resolution and home treatment in mental health*. Cambridge: Cambridge University Press.

Jolley, S., Garety, P.A., Ellett, L., Kuipers, E., Freeman, D., Bebbington, P.E., et al. (2006) A validation of a new measure of activity in psychosis. *Schizophrenia Research*, 85, 288–95.

Jones, D. (1982) The Borders mental health service. *British Journal of Clinical & Social Psychiatry*, 2, 8–12.

Jones, M. (1952) *Social Psychiatry: a study of therapeutic communities*, Tavistock, London.

Jorm, A.F., Korten, A.E., Jacomb, P.A., Rodgers, B., Pollitt, P., Christensen, H., et al. (1997) Helpfulness of interventions for mental disorders: beliefs of health professionals compared with the general public. *British Journal of Psychiatry*, 171, 233–7.

Kaiser Foundation Health Plan, Inc. (2004) Available at http://www.ihi.org/resources/pages/tools/sbartoolkit.aspx

Kaltiala-Heino, R. (1996). Involuntary psychiatric treatment: a range of patients' attitudes. *Nordic Journal of Psychiatry*, 50, 27–34.

Kaltialo-Heino, R., Välimäki, M., Korkeila, J., Tuohimäki, C., and Lehtinen, V. (2003) Involuntary medication in psychiatric inpatient treatment. *European Psychiatry*, 18(6), 290–5.

Kamali, M., Kelly, L., Gervin, M., Browne, S., Larkin, C., and O'Callaghan, E. (2001) Psychopharmacology: insight and comorbid substance misuse and medication compliance among patients with schizophrenia. *Psychiatric Services*, 52, 161–6.

Kane, J., Honigfeld, G., Singer, J., and Meltzer, H. (1988) Clozapine for the treatment-resistant schizophrenic. A double-blind comparison with chlorpromazine. *Archives of General Psychiatry*, 45(9), 789–96.

Kane, J.M. and McGlashan, T.H. (1995) Treatment of schizophrenia. *Lancet*, 346(8978), 820–5.

Katsakou, C. and Priebe, S. (2006) Outcomes of involuntary hospital admission—a review. *Acta Psychiatrica Scandinavica*, 114(4), 232–41.

Kay, S.R., Fiszbein, A., Opler, L.A. (1987) The positive and negative syndrome scale (PANSS) for schizophrenia. *Schizophrenia Bulletin*, 13, 261–71.

Kemp, R., Hayward, P., and David, A. (1997) *Compliance therapy manual*, King's College School of Medicine and Dentistry and Institute of Psychiatry, London.

Kemp, R., Hayward, P., Applewhaite, G., Everitt, B., and David, A. (1996) Compliance therapy in psychotic patients: randomised controlled trial. *BMJ*, 312(7027), 345–9.

Kendrick, T. (1996) Cardiovascular and respiratory risk factors and symptoms among general practice patients with long-term mental illness. *British Journal of Psychiatry*, 169(6), 733–9.

Kendrick, T., Burns, T., Freeling, P., and Sibbald, B. (1994) Provision of care to general practice patients with disabling long-term mental illness: a survey in 16 practices. *British Journal of General Practice*, 44(384), 301–5.

Kendrick, T., Millar, E., Burns, T., and Ross, F. (1998) Practice nurse involvement in giving depot neuroleptic injections: development of a patient assessment and monitoring checklist. *Primary Care Psychiatry*, 4, 149–54.

Keown, P., Weich, S., Bhui, K.S., and Scott, J. (2011) Association between provision of mental illness beds and rate of involuntary admissions in the NHS in England 1988–2008: ecological study. *BMJ*, 343. doi: http://dx.doi.org/10.1136/bmj.d3736.

Kernberg, O.F. (1984) *Severe personality disorders: psychotherapeutic strategies*, Yale University Press, New Haven, CT.

Killaspy, H. (2014) The ongoing need for local services for people with complex mental health problems. *Psychiatric Bulletin*, 38, 257–9. doi: 10.1192/pb.bp.114.048470.

Killaspy, H. (2016) Supported accommodation for people with mental health problems. *World Psychiatry*, **15**(1), 74–5.

Killaspy, H., Bebbington, P., Blizard, R., Johnson, S., Nolan, F., Pilling, S., et al. (2006) The REACT study: Randomised Evaluation of Assertive Community Treatment in north London. *British Medical Journal*, **332**, 815–18.

Killaspy, H., Johnson, S., Pierce, B., Bebbington, P., Pilling, S., Nolan, F., King, M. (2009) Successful engagement: a mixed methods study of the approaches of assertive community treatment and community mental health teams in the REACT trial. *Social Psychiatry and Psychiatric Epidemiology*, **44**, 532–40.

Kingdon, D.G. and Turkington, D. (1994) *Cognitive-behavioural therapy for schizophrenia*, Guildford Press, New York.

Kinzel, A.F. (1970) Body-buffer zone in violent prisoners. *American Journal of Psychiatry*, **127**(1), 59–64.

Kirkbride, J.B., Barker, D., Cowden, F., Stamps, R., Yang, M., Jones, P.B., et al. (2008) Psychoses, ethnicity and socio-economic status. *The British Journal of Psychiatry*, **193**(1), 18–24.

Kisely, S. and Hall, K. (2014) An updated meta-analysis of randomized controlled evidence for the effectiveness of community treatment orders. *Canadian Journal of Psychiatry*. **59**(10), 561–4.

Kissling, W., Kane, J.M., Barnes, T.R.E., Dencker, S J., Fleischhacker, W.W., Goldstein, M.J., et al. (1991) Guidelines for neuroleptic relapse prevention in schizophrenia: towards a consensus view. In: *Guidelines for neuroleptic relapse prevention in schizophrenia* (ed. W. Kissling), Springer-Verlag, Berlin, pp. 155–63.

Kleinman, A. (1980) *Patients and healers in the context of culture*, California Press, California.

Kosky, N. and Burns, T. (1995) Patient access to psychiatric records: experience in an in-patient unit. *Psychiatric Bulletin*, **19**, 87–90.

Kovess, V., Boisguerin, B., Antoine, D., and Reynauld, M. (1995) Has the sectorization of psychiatric services in France really been effective? *Social Psychiatry & Psychiatric Epidemiology*, **30**(3), 132–8.

Kraepelin, E. (1919) *Dementia praecox and paraphrenia* (transl. R.M. Barclay), facsimile ed. (1971), Kreiger, New York.

Kübler-Ross, E. (1969) *On death and dying*, Scribner, New York.

La Grenade, J. (1999) The National Health Service and ethnicity: services for black patients. In: *Ethnicity: an agenda for mental health* (ed. D. Bhugra and K. Bahl), Gaskell, London.

Laing, R.D. (1960) *The divided self*, Tavistock, London.

Laugharne, R. (1999) Evidence-based medicine, user involvement and the post-modern paradigm. *Psychiatric Bulletin*, **23**, 641–3.

Leamy, M., Bird, V., Le Boutillier, C., Williams, J., and Slade, M. (2011) Conceptual framework for personal recovery in mental health: systematic review and narrative synthesis. *The British Journal of Psychiatry*, **199**(6), 445–52.

Lees, J., Manning, N., and Rawlings, B. (1999) *Therapeutic community effectiveness. A systematic international review of therapeutic community treatment for people with personality disorders and mentally disordered offenders.* CRD Report 17 NHS, Centre for Reviews and Dissemination, University of York, York.

Leff, J. (1993) All the homeless people—where do they all come from? *BMJ*, **306**(6879), 669–70.

Leff, J. and Vaughn, C. (1981) The role of maintenance therapy and relatives' expressed emotion in relapse of schizophrenia: a two-year follow-up. *British Journal of Psychiatry*, **139**, 102–4.

Leff, J., Berkowitz, R., Shavit, N., Strachan, A., Glass, I., and Vaughn, C. (1990) A trial of family therapy versus a relatives' group for schizophrenia: two-year follow-up. *British Journal of Psychiatry*, **157**, 571–7.

Lehman, A.F. and Dixon, L.B. (1995) *Double jeopardy: chronic mental illness and substance abuse*, Harwood Academic Publishers, Baltimore.

Lehman, A.F., Dixon, L., Hoch, J.S., DeForge, B., Kernan, E., and Frank, R. (1999) Cost-effectiveness of assertive community treatment for homeless persons with severe mental illness. *British Journal of Psychiatry*, **174**, 346–52.

Lehman, A.F., Dixon, L.B., Kernan, E., DeForge, B.R., and Postrado, L.T. (1997) A randomized trial of assertive community treatment for homeless persons with severe mental illness. *Archives of General Psychiatry*, **54**(11), 1038–43.

Lehman, A.F., Myers, C.P., Thompson, J.W., and Corty, E. (1993) Implications of mental and substance use disorders. A comparison of single and dual diagnosis patients. *Journal of Nervous & Mental Disease*, **181**(6), 365–70.

Lidz, C.W., Hoge, S.K., Gardner, W., Bennett, N.S., Monahan, J., Mulvey, E.P., et al. (1995) Perceived coercion in mental hospital admission: pressures and process. *Archives of General Psychiatry*, **52**(12), 1034–9.

Lidz, R.W. and Lidz, T. (1949) The family environment of schizophrenic patients. *American Journal of Psychiatry*, **106**, 332–45.

Lieberman, J.A., Stroup, T.S., McEvoy, J.P., Swartz, M.S., Rosenheck, R.A., Perkins, D.O., et al. (2005) Effectiveness of antipsychotic drugs in patients with chronic schizophrenia. *New England Journal of Medicine*, 353,1209–23.

Linehan, M.M., Armstrong, H.E., Suarez, A., Allmon, D., and Heard, H.L. (1991) Cognitive-behavioral treatment of chronically parasuicidal borderline patients. *Archives of General Psychiatry*, **48**(12), 1060–4.

Linszen, D., Dingemans, P., Van der Does, J.W., Nugter, A., Scholte, P., Lenior, R., et al. (1996) Treatment, expressed emotion and relapse in recent onset schizophrenic disorders. *Psychological Medicine*, **26**(2), 333–42.

Littlewood, R. and Lipsedge, M. (1997) *Aliens and alienists: ethnic minorities and psychiatry*, Routledge, London.

Mari, J.J. and Streiner, D.L. (1994) An overview of family interventions and relapse on schizophrenia: meta-analysis of research findings. *Psychological Medicine*, **24**(3), 565–78.

Marmot, M. (2005) Social determinants of health inequalities. *The Lancet*, **365**, 1099–1104.

Marshall, M. (1996) Case management: a dubious practice. *BMJ*, **312**(7030), 523–4.

Marshall, M. and Lockwood, A. (1998) Assertive community treatment for people with severe mental disorders. *Cochrane Database of Systematic Reviews*, Issue 2, CD001089.

Marshall, M. and Lockwood, A. (1998) Assertive community treatment for people with severe mental disorders. *Cochrane Database of Systematic Reviews*, CD001089.

Marshall, M., Crowther, R., Almaraz-Serrano, A.M., and Tyrer, P. (2001) Day hospital versus outpatient care for psychiatric disorders. *Cochrane Database of Systematic Reviews*, Issue 3, CD003240.

Marshall, M., Bond, G., Stein, L.I., Shepherd, G., McGrew, J., Hoult, J., et al. (1999) PRiSM psychosis study: design limitations, questionable conclusions. *British Journal of Psychiatry*, **175**, 501–3.

Maslow, A.H. (1954) *Motivation and personality*, Harper and Row, New York.

Maughan, D., Molodynski, A., Rugkåsa, J., and Burns, T. (2014) A systematic review of the effect of community treatment orders on service use. *Social Psychiatry and Psychiatric Epidemiology*, **49**(4), 651–63.

Mayou, R.A., Ehlers, A., and Hobbs, M. (2000) Psychological debriefing for road traffic accident victims. Three-year follow-up of a randomised controlled trial. *British Journal of Psychiatry*, **176**, 589–93.

McCrone, P., Menezes, P.R., Johnson, S., Scott, H., Thornicroft, G., Marshall, J., et al. (2000) Service use and costs of people with dual diagnosis in South London. *Acta Psychiatrica Scandinavica*, **101**(6), 464–72.

McFarlane, W.R., Dushay, R.A., Deakins, S.M., Stasny, P., Lukens, E.P., and Toran, J. (2000) Employment outcomes in family-aided assertive community treatment. *American Journal of Orthopsychiatry*, **70**(2), 203–14.

McFarlane, W.R., Lukens, E., Link, B., Dushay, R., Deakins, S.A., Newmark, M., et al. (1995) Multiple-family groups and psychoeducation in the treatment of schizophrenia. *Archives of General Psychiatry*, **52**(8), 679–87.

McGorry, P.D., Edwards, J., Mihalopoulos, C., Harrigan, S.M., and Jackson, H.J. (1996) EPPIC: an evolving system of early detection and optimal management. *Schizophrenia Bulletin*, **22**(2), 305–26.

McGrew, J.H., Bond, G.R., Dietzen, L., and Salyers, M. (1994) Measuring the fidelity of implementation of a mental health program model. *Journal of Consulting & Clinical Psychology*, **62**(4), 670–8.

McGrew, J.H., Bond, G.R., Dietzen, L., McKasson, M., and Miller, L.D. (1995) A multisite study of client outcomes in assertive community treatment. *Psychiatric Services*, **46**(7), 696–701.

McHugo, G.J., Drake, R.E., Teague, G.B., and Xie, H. (1999) Fidelity to assertive community treatment and client outcomes in the New Hampshire dual disorders study. *Psychiatric Services*, **50**(6), 818–24.

McKnight, R.F., Adida, M., Budge, K., Stockton, S., Goodwin, G.M, and Geddes, J.R. (2012) Lithium toxicity profile: a systematic review and meta-analysis. *The Lancet*, **379**, 721–8.

Meissen, G., Powell, T.J., Wituk, S.A., Girrens, K., and Arteaga, S. (1999) Attitudes of AA contact persons toward group participation by persons with a mental illness. *Psychiatric Services*, **50**(8), 1079–81.

Menezes, N.M., Arenovich, T., and Zipursky, R.B. (2006) A systematic review of longitudinal outcome studies of first-episode psychosis. *Psychological Medicine*, **36**, 1349–62.

Menezes, P., Johnson, S., Thornicroft, G., Marshall, J., Prosser, D., Bebbington, P., et al. (1996) Drug and alcohol problems among individuals with severe mental illness in South London. *British Journal of Psychiatry*, **168**, 612–19.

Mental Health Foundation (1996) *Mental health and housing (MHF briefing no. 3)*, Mental Health Foundation, London.

Menzies, R., Rocher, I., and Vissandjee, B. (1993) Factors associated with compliance in treatment of tuberculosis. *Tubercle & Lung Disease*, **74**(1), 32–7.

Milgram, S. (1963) Behavioural study of obedience. *Journal of Abnormal & Social Psychology*, **67**, 371–8.

Miller, W.R. and Rollinick, S. (1991) *Motivational interviewing: preparing people to change addictive behavior*, Guildford Press, New York.

Minghella, E., Ford, R., Freeman, T., Hoult, J., McGlynn, P., and O'Halloran, P. (1998) *Open all hours: 24 hour response for people with mental health emergencies*, Sainsbury Centre for Mental Health, London.

Maughan, D., Molodynski, A., Rugkåsa, J., and Burns, T. (2013) A systematic review of the effect of community treatment orders on service use. *Social Psychiatry and Psychiatric Epidemiology*, doi: 10.1007/s00127-013-0781-0.

Monahan, J., Redlich, A.D., Swanson, J., Robbins, P.C., Appelbaum, P.S., Petrila, J., et al. (2005) Use of leverage to improve adherence to psychiatric treatment in the community. *Psychiatric Services*, **56**, 37–44.

Monahan, J., Steadman, H.J., Silver, E., Appelbaum, P.S., Clark Robbins, P., Mulvey, E.P., et al. (2001) *Rethinking risk assessment: the MacArthur study of mental disorder and violence*. Oxford University Press, Oxford.

Monroe-DeVita, M., Teague, G.B., Moser, L.L. (2011) The TMACT: a new tool for measuring fidelity to assertive community treatment. *Journal of the American Psychiatric Nurses Association*, **17**, 17–29.

Moore, S. (1961) A psychiatric out-patient nursing service. *Mental Health*, **20**, 51–5.

Morgan, G. (1994) Assessment of risk. In: *The prevention of suicide* (ed. R. Jenkins et al.), Department of Health, HMSO, London.

Morgan, S. (1993) *Community mental health: practical approaches to long-term problems*, Chapman Hall, London.

Morosini, P., Magliano, L., Brambilla, L., Ugolini, S., and Pioli, R. (2000) Development, reliability and acceptability of a new version of the DSM-IV Social and Occupational Functioning Assessment Scale (SOFAS) to assess routine social functioning. *Acta Psychiatrica Scandinavica*, **101**, 1–7.

Mueser, K.T., Bennett, M., and Kushner, M.G. (1995) Epidemiology of substance abuse disorders among persons with chronic mental illness. In: *Double jeopardy: chronic mental illness and substance abuse* (ed. A.F. Lehman and L.B. Dixon), Harwood Academic Publishers, Baltimore.

Mueser, K.T., Bond, G.R., Drake, R.E., and Resnick, S.G. (1998) Models of community care for severe mental illness: a review of research on case management. *Schizophrenia Bulletin*, **24**(1), 37–74.

Muijen, M., Cooney, M., Strathdee, G., Bell, R., Hudson, A., (1994) Community psychiatric nurse teams: intensive support versus genetic case. *British Journal of Psychiatry*, **165**, 211–17.

Muijen, M., Marks, I.M., Connolly, J., Audini, B., and McNamee, G. (1992) The daily living programme: preliminary comparison of community versus hospital-based treatment for the seriously mentally ill facing emergency admission. *British Journal of Psychiatry*, **160**, 379–84.

Mulder, R. and Chanen, A.M. (2013) Effectiveness of cognitive analytic therapy for personality disorders. *The British Journal of Psychiatry*, **202**(2), 89–90.

Munro, E. and Rumgay, J. (2000) Role of risk assessment in reducing homicides by people with mental illness. *British Journal of Psychiatry*, **176**, 116–20.

National Institute for Health and Care Excellence (NICE) (2009) *Borderline personality disorder: treatment and management.* https://www.nice.org.uk/guidance/cg78/resources/guidance-borderline-personality-disorder-pdf.

National Institute for Health and Care Excellence (NICE) (2014a) *Bipolar disorder: assessment and management.* NICE Guidance [CG185]. Department of Health, London.

National Institute for Health and Care Excellence (NICE) (2014b) *Psychosis and schizophrenia in adults: prevention and management.* NICE Guidance [CG178]. Department of Health, London.

National Institute for Health and Care Excellence (NICE) (2015a) *Psychosis and schizophrenia in adults.* NICE Quality Standard [QS80]. Department of Health, London.

National Institute for Health and Care Excellence (NICE) (2015b) *Violence and aggression: short-term management in mental health, health and community settings.* NICE Guidance [NG10]. Department of Health, London.

National Institute for Health and Clinical Excellence (NICE) (2011) *Self-harm in over 8s: long-term management.* Clinical guideline [CG133]. Department of Health, London.

National Institute for Health and Clinical Excellence (NICE) (2011) *Psychosis with coexisting substance misuse: assessment and management in adults and young people.* Clinical guideline [CG120]. Department of Health, London.

National Institute for Health and Clinical Excellence (NICE) (2011) Psychosis with coexisting substance misuse. Assessment and management in adults and young people. Department of Health, London.

National Institute for Health and Clinical Excellence (NICE) (2011) *Service user experience in adult mental health: improving the experience of care for people using adult NHS mental health services.* Clinical guideline [CG136]. Manchester: NICE.

National Institute for Mental Health for England (2003) *Personality Disorder: no Longer a Diagnosis of Exclusion. Policy Implementation Guidance for the Development of Services for People with Personality Disorder, Gateway Reference 1055.* London: NIMH(E).

National Patient Safety Agency (2009) *Preventing suicide: a toolkit for mental health services.* NHS, London.

National Services Framework (1999) *Better act now! NSF's views on the Mental Health Act Review,* NSF, London.

NHS Training Authority (1990) *Effective team working in the community,* MacMillan Intek Ltd, Hove.

Nicola Davies (1995) *The report of the inquiry into the circumstances leading to the death of Jonathan Newby,* Oxfordshire Health, Oxford.

Noffsinger, S.G. and Resnick, P.J. (1999) Violence and mental illness. *Current Opinion in Psychiatry,* **12**(6), 683–7.

Nordén, T., Malm, U., Norlander, T. (2012) Resource group assertive community treatment (RACT) as a tool of empowerment for clients with severe mental illness: a meta-analysis. *Clinical Practice and Epidemiology in Mental Health,* **8**, 144–51.

Nursing Times (2000) Open learning: clinical supervision: make your experience work: cross-disciplinary supervision. *Nursing Times,* **96**(7), 47–50, 17–23 Feb.

O'Brien, J.G., Thibault, J.M., Turner, L.C., and Laird-Fick, H.S. (2000) Self-neglect: an overview. *Journal of Elder Abuse & Neglect,* **11**(2), 1–9.

O'Brien, A. and Firn, M. (2002) Clozapine initiation in the community. *Psychiatric Bulletin*, 26, 339–41.

O'Callaghan, E., Turner, N., Renwick, L., Jackson, D., Sutton, M., Foley S.D., et al. (2010) First episode psychosis and the trail to secondary care: help-seeking and health-system delays. *Social Psychiatry and Psychiatric Epidemiology*, 45(3), 381–91.

O'Donnell, C., Donohoe, G., Sharkey, L., Owens, N., Migone, M., Harries, R., et al. (2003) Compliance therapy: a randomised controlled trial in schizophrenia. *British Medical Journal*, 327–84.

O'Donnell, I. and Farmer, R. (1995) The limitations of official suicide statistics. *British Journal of Psychiatry*, 166(4), 458–61.

O'Donoghue, B., Lyne, J., Hill, M., Larkin, C., Feeney, L., and O'Callaghan, E. (2011). Physical coercion, perceived pressures and procedural justice in the involuntary admission and future engagement with mental health services. *European Psychiatry*, 26(4), 208–14.

Onyett, S. (1992) *Case management in mental health*, Chapman Hall, London.

Osborn, D.P.J, Nazareth, I., and King, M.B. (2007) Physical activity, dietary habits and coronary heart disease risk factor knowledge amongst people with severe mental illness. *Social Psychiatry and Psychiatric Epidemiology*, 42(10), 787–93.

Osher, F.C. and Kofoed, L.L. (1989) Treatment of patients with psychiatric and psychoactive substance abuse disorders. *Hospital & Community Psychiatry*, 40(10), 1025–30.

Overall, J.E. and Gorham, D.R. (1962) The Brief Psychiatric Rating Scale. *Psychological Reports*, 10, 799–812.

Owen, R.R., Fischer, E.P., Booth, B.M., and Cuffel, B.J. (1996) Medication noncompliance and substance abuse among patients with schizophrenia. *Psychiatric Services*, 47(8), 853–8.

Pantelis, C., Velakoulis, D., McGorry, P.D., Wood, S.J., Suckling, J., Pilling, L.J., et al. (2003) Neuroanatomical abnormalities before and after onset of psychosis: a cross-sectional and longitudinal MRI comparison. *The Lancet*, 361, 281–8.

Parnas, J. (2011) A disappearing heritage: the clinical core of schizophrenia. *Schizophrenia Bulletin*, 37(6), 1121–30.

Pasamanick, B., Scarpitti, F.R., and Leyton, M. (1964) Home versus hospital care for schizophrenics. *Journal of the American Medical Association*, 187, 177–81.

Patel, M.X., Nikolaou, V., and David, A.S. (2003) Psychiatrists' attitudes to maintenance medication for patients with schizophrenia. *Psychological Medicine*, 1, 83–89.

Paykel, E.S., Myers, J.K., Lindenthal, J.J., and Tanner, J. (1974) Suicidal feelings in the general population: a prevalence study. *British Journal of Psychiatry*, 124, 460–9.

Pelosi, A.J. and Jackson, G.A. (2000) Home treatment—enigmas and fantasies. *BMJ*, 320(7230), 308–9.

Perkins, R. and Burns, T. (2001) Home treatment. *International Journal of Social Psychiatry*, 47(3), 55–66.

Perkins, R., Evanson, E.A., and Davidson, B. (2000) *The Pathfinder User Employment Programme*, South West London and St George's Mental Health NHS Trust, London.

Perris, C. 1969, The separation of bipolar (manic-depressive) from unipolar recurrent depressive psychoses. *Behavioural Neuropsychiatry*, 1(8), 17–24.

Perry, A., Tarrier, N., Morriss, R., McCarthy, E., and Limb, K. 1999, Randomised controlled trial of efficacy of teaching patients with bipolar disorder to identify early symptoms of relapse and obtain treatment. *BMJ*, 318, 149–53.

Phelan, M., Stradins, L., and Morrison, S. (2001) Physical health of people with severe mental illness: can be improved if primary care and mental health professionals pay attention to it. *British Medical Journal*, 322(7284), 443–4.

Picket, K., Oliver, J., and Wilkinson, R. (2006) Income inequality and the prevalence of mental illness: a preliminary international analysis. *Journal of Epidemiology and Community Health*, 60, 646–7.

Powell, E. (1961) Opening speech, annual conference, National Association for Mental Health, London.

Prance, N. (1993) Travelling companions. *Nursing Times*, 89(5), 28–30.

Price, O., Baker, J., Bee, P., and Lovell, K. (2015) Learning and performance outcomes of mental health staff training in de-escalation techniques for the management of violence and aggression. *British Journal of Psychiatry*, 206(6), 447–55. doi: 10.1192/bjp. bp.114.144576.

Priebe, S. and Gruyters, T. (1995) Patients' assessment of treatment predicting outcome. *Schizophrenia Bulletin*, 21(1), 87–94.

Priebe, S., Fakhoury, W., Watts, J., Bebbington, P., Burns, T., Johnson, S., et al. (2003) Assertive outreach teams in London: patient characteristics and outcomes. Pan-London Assertive Outreach Study Part 3. *The British Journal of Psychiatry*, 183 (2) 148–54.

Priebe, S., Badesconyi, A., Fioritti, A., Hansson, L., Kilian, R., Torres-Gonzales, F., et al. (2005) Reinstitutionalisation in mental health care: comparison of data on service provision from six European countries. *BMJ*, 330, 123.

Priebe, S., Yeeles, K., Bremner, S., Lauber, C., Eldridge, S., Ashby, D., et al. (2013) Effectiveness of financial incentives to improve adherence to maintenance treatment with antipsychotics: cluster randomised controlled trial. *BMJ*, 347.

Priebe, S., Watts, J., Chase, M., and Matanov, A. (2005) Processes of disengagement and engagement in assertive outreach patients: qualitative study. *British Journal of Psychiatry*, 187(5), 438–43. doi: 10.1192/bjp.187.5.438.

Prochaska, J.O. and DiClemente, C.C. (1992) Stages of change in the modification of problem behaviors. *Progress in Behaviour Modification*, 28, 183–218.

Querido, A. (1968) *The development of socio-medical care in the Netherlands*, Routledge and Kegan Paul, London.

Rapp, C.A. (1992) The strengths perspective of case management with persons suffering from severe mental illness. In: *The strength model of social work: power in the people* (ed. D. Saleebey), Longman, New York.

Rapp, C.A. (1998) The active ingredients of effective case management: a research synthesis. *Community Mental Health Journal*, 34(4), 363–80.

Rapp, C.A. and Wintersteen, R. (1989) The strengths model of case management: results from 12 demonstrations. *Psychosocial Rehabilitation Journal*, 13(1), 23–32.

Rathod, S., Lloyd, A., Asher, C., Baird, J., Leishman, J., Kingdon, D. (2014) Lessons from an evaluation of major change in adult mental health services: effects on quality. *Journal of Mental Health*, 23(5), 271–5.

Razali, M.S. and Yahya, H. (1995) Compliance with treatment in schizophrenia: a drug intervention program in a developing country. *Acta Psychiatrica Scandinavica*, 91, 331–5.

Reed, J.L. (1992) *Review of health and social services for mentally disordered offenders and others requiring similar services—final summary report*, Department of Health, London.

Reed, P.G. and Leonard, V.E. (1989) An analysis of the concept of self-neglect. *Advances in Nursing Science*, **12**(1), 39–53.

Rees, S. (2009) *Mental ill health in the adult single homeless population: a review of the literature*. Public Health Resource Unit. London: Crisis.

Regier, D.A., Farmer, M.E., Rae, D.S., Locke, B.Z., Keith, S.J., Judd, L.L., et al. (1990) Comorbidity of mental disorders with alcohol and other drug abuse: results from the Epidemiologic Catchment Area (ECA) Study. *Journal of the American Medical Association*, **264**(19), 2511–18.

Rethink Mental Illness (2015) *Welfare benefits and mental illness factsheet*. https://www.rethink.org/resources/w

Rinaldi, M. and Hill, R. (2000) *Insufficient concern*, Merton Mind, London.

Rinaldi, M. and Perkins, R. (2007) Implementing evidence-based supported employment. *Psychiatric Bulletin*, **31**, 244–9.

Rinaldi, M., Perkins, R., Glynn, E., Montibeller, T., Clenaghan, M., Rutherford, J., et al. (2007) Individual placement and support: from research to practice. *Advances in Psychiatric Treatment*, **14**(1), 50–60. doi 10.1192/apt.bp.107.003509.

Ritchie, C.W., Hayes, D., and Ames, D.J. (2000) Patient or client? The opinions of people attending a psychiatric clinic. *British Journal of Psychiatry Bulletin*, **24**, 447–50.

Ritchie, J.H. (1994) *The report of the inquiry into the care and treatment of Christopher Clunis presented to the chairman of the North East Thames and South East Thames Regional Health Authorities*, HMSO, London.

Robson, D. and Gray, R. (2007) Serious mental illness and physical health problems: a discussion paper. *Nursing Studies*, **444**(3), 457–66.

Rollinick, S., Heather, N., and Bell, A. (1992) Negotiating behaviour change in medical settings: the development of brief motivational interviewing. *Journal of Mental Health*, **1**, 25–37.

Rorstad, P. and Checinski, K. (1996) *Dual diagnosis: facing the challenge*, Wynne House Publishing, Guildford.

Rosenthal, D., Wender, P.H., Kety, S.S., Welner, J., and Schulsinger, F. (1971) The adopted-away offspring of schizophrenics. *American Journal of Psychiatry*, **128**(3), 307–11.

Rounsaville, B.J., O'Malley, S., Foley, S., and Weissman, M.M. (1988) Role of manual-guided training in the conduct and efficacy of interpersonal psychotherapy for depression. *Journal of Consulting & Clinical Psychology*, **56**(5), 681–8.

Royal College of Psychiatrists (2014) *Report of the Second Round of the National Audit of Schizophrenia (NAS) 2014*. London: Healthcare Quality Improvement Partnership.

Rummler, G. and Brache, A. (1990) *Improving performance: how to manage the white space on the organization chart*. San Francisco: Jossey-Bass

Ruud, T. and Landheim, A. (2015) Assertive outreach in Norway in handbook (flexible) ACT. Van Veldhuizen R, Polhuis D, Bähler M, Mulder N, Kroon H (Eds.) De Tijdstroom, Utrecht.

Ryan, P. and Morgan, S. (2004) *Assertive outreach: a strengths approach to policy and practice*. Churchill Livingstone, London.

Ryle, A. (1997) The structure and development of borderline personality disorder: a proposed model. *British Journal of Psychiatry*, **170**, 82–7.

Sackett, D.L., Straus, S.E., Richardson, W.S., Rosenberg, W., and Haynes, R.B. (1997) *Evidence-based medicine—how to practice and teach EBM*, Churchill Livingstone, Harcourt, London.

Sainsbury Centre for Mental Health (1997) *Pulling together: the future roles and training of mental health staff*, Sainsbury Centre for Mental Health, London.

Sainsbury Centre for Mental Health (1998) *Keys to engagement: a review of care for people with serious mental illness who are hard to engage with services*, Sainsbury Centre for Mental Health, London.

Sainsbury Centre for Mental Health (2001) *Capable practitioner: a framework and list of practitioner capabilities required to implement the National Service Framework for mental health*, Sainsbury Centre for Mental Health, London.

Sainsbury Centre for Mental Health (2008) Making recovery a reality. *Sainsbury Centre for Mental Health*, London.

Sanz, M., Constable, G., Lopez-Ibor, I., Kemp, R., and David, A.S. (1998) A comparative study of insight scales and their relationship to psychopathological and clinical variables. *Psychological Medicine*, **28**(2), 437–46.

Schneider, K. (1923) *Die psychopathischen personalichkeiten*, Springer, Berlin.

Schneider, K. (1959) *Clinical psychopathology* (translated by M.W. Hamilton), Grone and Stratton, New York.

Schwartz, R. and Lehman, A.F. (1995) Overview of treatment principles. In: *Double jeopardy: chronic mental illness and substance abuse* (ed. A.F. Lehman and L.B. Dixon), Harwood Academic Publishers, Baltimore.

Scott, H., Johnson, S., Menezes, P., Thornicroft, G., Marshall, J., Bindman, J., et al. (1998) Substance misuse and risk of aggression and offending among the severely mentally ill. *British Journal of Psychiatry*, **172**, 345–50.

Segal, H. (1983) Some clinical implications of Melanie Klein's work. Emergence from narcissism. *International Journal of Psychoanalysis*, **64**(3), 269–80.

Segal, S.P. and Burgess, P.M. (2006) Effect of conditional release from hospitalization on mortality risk. *Psychiatric Services*, **57**(11), 1607–13.

Sheehan, K.A. and Burns, T. (2011) Perceived coercion and the therapeutic relationship: a neglected association? *Psychiatric Services*, **62**(5), 471–6.

Shiers, D.E., Lester, H., Rafi, I., Holt, R., and Cooper, S. (2014) *Positive cardiometabolic health resource: an intervention framework for patients with psychosis and schizophrenia. 2014 update. Royal College of Psychiatrists*, London.

Singh, S. and Fisher, H. (2007) Early Intervention Services. *Psychiatry*, **6**, 333–8.

Singh, S.P. (2009) Shooting the messenger: the science and politics of ethnicity research. *The British Journal of Psychiatry*, **195**, 1–2.

Singh, S.P. and Burns, T. (2006) Race and mental health: there is more to race than racism. *BMJ*, **333**, 648–51.

Singh, S.P., Burns, T., Tyrer, P., Islam, Z., Parsons, H., and Crawford, M.J. (2014) Ethnicity as a predictor of detention under the Mental Health Act. *Psychological Medicine*, **44**, 997–1004. doi:10.1017/S003329171300086X.

Siris, S.G. (2000) Depression in schizophrenia: perspective in the era of atypical antipsychotic agents. *American Journal of Psychiatry*, **157**(9), 1379–89.

Slade, M., Longden, E. (2015) *The empirical evidence about mental health and recovery: how likely, how long, what helps?* MI Fellowship, Victoria, Australia.

Smyth, M.G. and Hoult, J. (2000) The home treatment enigma. *BMJ*, **320**(7230), 305–9.

Solomon, P. and Draine, J. (1995a) The efficacy of a consumer case management team: 2-year outcomes of a randomized trial. *Journal of Mental Health Administration*, **22**(2), 135–46.

Solomon, P. and Draine, J. (1995b) One-year outcomes of a randomized trial of case management with seriously mentally ill clients leaving jail. *Evaluation Review*, **19**, 256–73.

Soni Raleigh, V. and Balarajan, R. (1992) Suicide and self-burning among Indians and West Indians in England and Wales. *British Journal of Psychiatry*, **161**, 365–8.

Steadman, H.J., Mulvey, E.P., Monahan, J., Robbins, P.C., Appelbaum, P.S., Grisso, T., et al. (1998) Violence by people discharged from acute psychiatric inpatient facilities and by others in the same neighbourhoods. *Archives of General Psychiatry*, **55**(5), 393–401.

Stefansson, C.G. and Cullberg, J. (1986) Introducing community mental health services. The effects on a suburban patient population. *Acta Psychiatrica Scandinavica*, **74**(4), 368–78.

Stein, L.I. and Santos, A.B. (1998) *Assertive community treatment of persons with severe mental illness*, W.W. Norton, New York.

Stein, L.I. and Test, M.A. (1978) An alternative to mental hospital treatment. In: *Alternatives to mental health hospital treatment* (ed. L.I. Stein and M.A. Test), Plenum Press, New York.

Stein, L.I. and Test, M.A. (1980) Alternative to mental hospital treatment. I. Conceptual model, treatment program, and clinical evaluation. *Archives of General Psychiatry*, **37**(4), 392–7.

Steinwachs, D.M., Kasper, J.D., and Skinner, E.A. (1992) *Family perspectives on meeting the needs for care of severely mentally ill relatives: a national survey. Final report*. Center of the Organisation and Financing of Care for the Severely Mentally Ill, John Hopkins University, Baltimore.

Stergiopoulos, V., Hwang, S., Gozdzik, A., Nisenbaum, R., Latimer, E., Rabouin, D., et al. (2015) Effect of scattered-site housing using rent supplements and intensive case management on housing stability among homeless adults with mental illness: a randomized trial. *JAMA*, **313**, 905–15.

Stiefel, M. and Nolan, K. (2012) *A guide to measuring the triple aim: population health, experience of care, and per capita cost*. IHI Innovation Series white paper. Cambridge, MA: Institute for Healthcare Improvement (available www.IHI.org).

Substance Abuse and Mental Health Services Administration. (2008) Assertive community treatment. DHHS Pub. No. SMA-08-4344, Rockville, MD: Center for Mental Health Services, Substance Abuse and Mental Health Services Administration, U.S. Department of Health and Human Services.

Swartz, M.S., Wagner, H.R., Swanson, J.W., Stroup, T.S., McEvoy, J.P., Canive, J.M., et al. (2006) Substance use in persons with schizophrenia: baseline prevalence and correlates from the NIMH CATIE study. *Journal of Nervous and Mental Disease*, **194**(3), 164–72. 10.1097/01.nmd.0000202575.79453.6e

Szmukler, G. and Appelbaum, P.S. (2008) Treatment pressures, leverage, coercion, and compulsion in mental health care. *Journal of Mental Health*, **17**, 233–44.

Talbott, J.A., Clark, G.H.J., Sharfstein, S.S., and Klein, J. (1987) Issues in developing standards governing psychiatric practice in community mental health centers. *Hospital & Community Psychiatry*, **38**(11), 1198–1202.

Tarrier, N., Barrowclough, C., Vaughn, C., Bamrah, J.S., Porceddu, K., Watts, S., et al. (1989) Community management of schizophrenia: a two-year follow-up of a behavioural intervention with families. *British Journal of Psychiatry*, **154**, 625–8.

Tarrier, N., Yusupoff, L., Kinney, C., McCarthy, E., Gledhill, A., Haddock, G., et al. (1998) Randomised controlled trial of intensive cognitive behaviour therapy for patients with chronic schizophrenia. *BMJ*, **317**(7154), 303–7.

Taylor, D. (1997) Pharmacokinetic interactions involving clozapine. *British Journal of Psychiatry*, **171**, 109–12.

Taylor, P.J. and Gunn, J. (1999) Homicides by people with mental illness: myth and reality. *British Journal of Psychiatry*, **174**, 9–14.

Teague, G.B., Bond, G.R. and Drake, R.E. (1998) Program fidelity in assertive community treatment: development and use of a measure. *American Journal of Orthopsychiatry*, **68**(2), 216–32.

Teague, G.B., Bond, G.R., and Drake, R.E. (1998) Program fidelity in assertive community treatment: development and use of a measure. *American Journal of Orthopsychiatry*, **68**(2), 216–32.

Test, M.A. (1992) Training in community living. In: *Handbook of Psychiatric Rehabilitation* (ed. R.P. Lieberman), Macmillan, New York.

Test, M.A. and Stein, L.I. (1980) Alternative to mental hospital treatment. III: social cost. *Archives of General Psychiatry*, **37**(4), 409–12.

The National Confidential Inquiry into Suicide and Homicide by People with Mental Illness. Annual Report 2015: England, Northern Ireland, Scotland and Wales (July 2015) University of Manchester.

Thornicroft, G. (2011) Physical health disparities and mental illness: the scandal of premature mortality. *British Journal of Psychiatry*, **199**(6), 441–2.

Thornicroft, G. and Tansella, M. (1999) *The mental health matrix: a manual to improve services*, Cambridge University Press, Cambridge.

Thornicroft, G., Strathdee, G., Phelan, M., Holloway, F., Wykes, T., Dunn, G., et al. (1998a) Rationale and design. PRiSM Psychosis Study 1. *British Journal of Psychiatry*, **173**, 363–70.

Thornicroft, G., Wykes, T., Holloway, F., Johnson, S., and Szmukler, G. (1998b) From efficacy to effectiveness in community mental health services. PRiSM Psychosis Study 10. *British Journal of Psychiatry*, **173**, 423–7.

Thornley, B. and Adams, C. (1998) Content and quality of 2000 controlled trials in schizophrenia over 50 years. *BMJ*, **317**, 1181–4.

Tsemberis, S. (2010) *Housing first: the pathways model to end homelessness for people with mental illness and addiction manual*. Hazelden, Minnesota.

Tsuda, Y., Saruwatari, J., and Yasui-Furukori, N. (2014) Meta-analysis: the effects of smoking on the disposition of two commonly used antipsychotic agents, olanzapine and clozapine. *BMJ Open*, doi:10.1136/bmjopen-2013-004216.

Tuckett, D., Boulton, M., Olson, C., and Williams, A. (1985) *Meetings between experts—an approach to sharing ideas in medical consultations*, Tavistock Publications, London.

Turkington, D., Kingdon, D., and Weiden, P.J. (2014) Cognitive behavior therapy for schizophrenia. *American Journal of Psychiatry*, **163**(3), 365–73.

Tyrer, P. (2000a) The future of the community mental health team. *International Review of Psychiatry*, **12**, 219–25.

Tyrer, P. (2000b) Effectiveness of intensive treatment in severe mental illness. *British Journal of Psychiatry*, **176**, 492–3.

Tyrer, P. (2013) A solution to the ossification of community psychiatry. *The Psychiatrist*, doi: 10.1192/pb.bp.113.042937.

Tyrer, P., Reed, G.M., and Crawford, M.J. (2015) Classification, assessment, prevalence, and effect of personality disorder. *The Lancet*, **385**, 717–26.

Tyrer, P., Coid, J., Simmonds, S., Joseph, P., and Marriott, S. (1999) Community mental health team management for those with severe mental illnesses and disordered personality. In: *Schizophrenia module of the Cochrane database systematic reviews* (ed. C.G. Adams, L. Duggan, and J. de Jesus Mari), Update Software, Oxford.

Tyrer, P., Morgan, J., Van Horn, E., Jayakody, M., Evans, K., Brummell, R., et al. (1995) A randomised controlled study of close monitoring of vulnerable psychiatric patients. *Lancet*, **345**(8952), 756–9.

Tyrer, P., Reed, G.M., and Crawford, M.J. (2015) Classification, assessment, prevalence, and effect of personality disorder. *The Lancet*, **385**(9969), 717–26.

UK700 Group: Burns, T., Creed, F., Fahy, T., Thompson, S., Tyrer, P., and White, I. (1999b) Intensive versus standard case management for severe psychotic illness: a randomised trial. *Lancet*, **353**, 2185–9.

UK700 Group: Burns, T., Fahy, T., Thompson, S., Tyrer, P., and White, I. (1999a) Intensive case management for severe psychotic illness [authors' reply]. *Lancet*, **354**, 1384–6.

UK700 Group: Byford, S., Fiander, M., Torgerson, D.J., Barber, J.A., Thompson, S.G., Burns, T., et al. (2000) Cost-effectiveness of intensive versus standard case management for severe psychotic illness. *British Journal of Psychiatry*, **176**, 537–43.

UK700 Group: Creed, F., Burns, T., Butler, T., Byford, S., Murray, R., Thompson, S., et al. (1999) Comparison of intensive and standard case management for patients with psychosis: rationale of the trial. *British Journal of Psychiatry*, **174**, 74–8.

UK700 Group: Tyrer, P., Hassiotis, A., Ukoumunne, O., Piachaud, J., and Harvey, K. (1999) Intensive case management for psychotic patients with borderline intelligence. *Lancet*, **354**(9183), 999–1000.

UNHCR (2014) *World at war global trends report: forced displacement in 2014.* Geneva: UNHCR.

Van Os, J. and Kapur, S. (2009) Schizophrenia. *Lancet*, **374**, 635–45.

Van Veldhuizen, J.R. (2007) FACT: a Dutch Version of ACT. *Community Mental Health Journal*, **43**(4), 421–33.

Van Veldhuizen, J.R. and Bähler, M. (2013) *Manual flexible assertive community treatment. FACT manual.* www.factfacts.nl, Groningen, The Netherlands.

Van Veldhuizen, J.R., Bähler, M., Mulder, N., Kroon, H., et al. (2015) *Handboek (Flexible) ACT.* De Tijdstroom, Utrecht.

Vaughan, K., Doyle, M., McConaghy, N., Blaszczynski, A., Fox, A., and Tarrier, N. (1992) The Sydney intervention trial: a controlled trial of relatives' counselling to reduce schizophrenic relapse. *Social Psychiatry & Psychiatric Epidemiology*, **27**(1), 16–21.

Vaughn, C. and Leff J. (1976) The measurement of expressed emotion in the families of psychiatric patients. *British Journal of Social Clinical Psychology*, **15**(2), 157–65.

Vocci, F.J. and Montoya, I.D. (2009) Psychological treatments for stimulant misuse, comparing and contrasting those for amphetamine dependence and those for cocaine dependence. *Current Opinion in Psychiatry*, **22**(3), 263–8.

Weisbrod, B.A., Test, M.A., and Stein, L.I. (1980) Alternative to mental hospital treatment. II: economic benefit-cost analysis. *Archives of General Psychiatry*, **37**(4), 400–5.

Weissman, M.M., Bland, R.C., Canino, G.J., Faravelli, C., Greenwald, S., Hwu, H.G., et al. (1996) Cross-national epidemiology of major depression and bipolar disorder. *Journal of the American Medical Association*, **276**(4), 293–9.

White, E. (1991) *The 3rd quinquennial national community psychiatric nursing survey*, University of Manchester, Department of Nursing, Manchester.

White, E. (1999) The 4th quinquennial national community mental health nursing census of England and Wales. *Australian & New Zealand Journal of Mental Health Nursing*, **8**(3), 86–92.

White, R., Tata, P., and Burns, T. (1996) Mood, learned resourcefulness and perceptions of control in Type 1 diabetes mellitus. *Journal of Psychosomatic Research*, **40**(2), 205–12.

Wig, N.N., Menon, D.K., Bedi, H., Leff, J., Kuipers, L., Ghosh, A., et al. (1987) Expressed emotion and schizophrenia in north India. II: Distribution of expressed emotion components among relatives of schizophrenic patients in Aarhus and Chandigarh. *British Journal of Psychiatry*, **151**, 160–5.

Wilkinson, G. (1994) Can suicide be prevented? Better treatment of mental illness is more appropriate aim. *BMJ*, **309**(6958), 860–1.

Williams, H., Clarke, R., Fashola, Y., and Holt, G. (1998) Diogenes' syndrome in patients with intellectual disability: 'a rose by any other name'? *Journal of Intellectual Disability Research*, **42**(4), 316–20.

Wing, J.K. (1968) Social treatments of mental illness. In: *Studies of psychiatry* (ed. M. Shepherd and D.L. Davies), Oxford University Press, London.

Wing, J.K., Cooper, J.E., and Sartorius, N. (1974) *The measurement and classification of psychiatric symptoms: an instruction manual for the PSE and the Catego Program*, Cambridge University Press, Cambridge.

Wing, J., Curtis, R.H., and Beevor, A. (1999) Health of the Nation Outcome Scales (HoNOS). Glossary for HoNOS score sheet. *British Journal of Psychiatry*, **174**, 432–4.

Witt, K., van Dorn, R., and Fazel, S. (2013) Risk factors for violence in psychosis: systematic review and meta-regression analysis of 110 studies. *PLoS ONE* **8**(2), e55942. doi:10.1371/journal.pone.0055942.

World Health Organisation (1992) *The ICD-10 classification of mental and behavioural disorders*, World Health Organisation, Geneva.

Wright, C., Catty, J., Watt, H., and Burns, T. (2004) A systematic review of home treatment services. Classification and sustainability. *Social Psychiatry and Psychiatric Epidemiology*, **39**, 789–96.

Yerkes, R.M. and Dodson, J.D. (1908) Relation of strength and stimulus to rapidity of habit-formation. *Journal of Comparative Neurology & Psychology*.

Zawilska, J.B. (2011) 'Legal highs'—new players in the old drama. *Current Drug Abuse Reviews*, **4**, 122–30.

Zigmond, A.S. and Snaith, R.P. (1983) The hospital anxiety and depression scale. *Acta Psychiatrica Scandinavica*, **67**(6), 361–70.

Zisook, S., McAdams, L.A., Kuck, J., Harris, M.J., Bailey, A., Patterson, T.L., et al. (1999) Depressive symptoms in schizophrenia. *American Journal of Psychiatry*, **156**(11), 1736–43.

Zubin, J. and Spring, B. (1977) Vulnerability—a new view of schizophrenia. *Journal of Abnormal Psychology*, **86**(2), 103–26.

Index

abuse, racial 98–103
abuse of power 89–90
access 8, 62, 68
accountability 306
ACT, *see* assertive community
    treatment (ACT)
active case load management 9
activity 260–9
activity analysis 274
adherence 122
affect dysregulation 177, 181
African-Caribbean patients
    schizophrenia 93
    suitability for outreach 28
Africans, schizophrenia 93
aftercare under supervision 301
aggression, *see* hostility
agoraphobia 211
akathisia 73
alcohol, safe limits 222
alcohol abuse 31, 222
    detoxification 226
    see also substance abuse
Alcoholics Anonymous 22–5
alienation 77, 79
amphetamine abuse, pharmacological
    treatment 226
anger 142
annual medical 251
antabuse 226
anticholinergics 73, 212
antidepressants 16, 72, 74, 126–7, 190, 210
antihypertensives 122, 253, 255
antipsychotics 175–7
    atypical 16, 71–2, 176
    maintenance 70–1
    side-effects 71, 72–3, 75, 190, 253
antisocial personality disorder 200
anxiety disorders 211–12
appetite 252
appointeeship 117, 239–41
appraisal 317
assaults 144–5
    prosecution following 148–9
assertive community treatment
    (ACT) 3, 10–11
    homelessness 246
    measures 11, 42
assertive outreach
    acceptance criteria 33–4, 39–40
    ACT model 11, 42–3, 52

alternative methods 52–4
    components 43–9
    compulsion in, *see* compulsion
    core competencies 314–16
    discharge 36–9
    dual diagnosis 31–2, 222–4
    fidelity to the model 20, 41, 42–3, 50,
        55, 331
    integrated model 322
    model of assertive outreach 11, 41–3, 54–5
    origins 4–11
    patient suitability 27–32
    patients' views of 114
    personal characteristics relevant to 310–11
    physical health care 254–8
    psychosocial intervention
        support 281–2, 289–90
    referral 20
    research 20
    UK and Europe 4–9
    vocationally focused 264–5
    weekly schedules 297–303
    what is it for? 25–6
    whole system 322–3
assessment skills training 315
attachment theory 58
atypical antipsychotics 16, 71–2
audit 291, 296, 304, 315, 316, 318, 319,
    328, 331–3
autonomy 77, 86

backing off 46
bank accounts 237
Beck Depression Inventory 153, 208
bed and breakfast accommodation 246
behavioural family management 18, 284–5
benefits 48, 231–6
    for carers 235–6
    fraud 238–9
    work and 260
benzodiazepines 73, 74–5, 189, 212
    alcohol detoxification 226
bereavement 214–15
beta-blockers 73
bias 336–8
bipolar affective disorder 182–95
    causes 183–4
    changes over time 32
    clinical picture 184–5
    community treatment 185–7
    depression 190, 210–11

bipolar affective disorder (*Cont.*)
early intervention 186–7
hypomanic episodes 187–9, 210–11
mood stabilizers 16, 73–4, 189–90
psychosocial interventions 190–4
relapse signatures 186–7, 191
sleep problems 186–7, 188–9
suitability for outreach 28
therapeutic alliance 185–6
black African-Caribbean patients
schizophrenia 93
suitability for outreach 28
black mental health services 96
Bleuler, Eugen 169, 172
borderline personality disorder 200, 204, 205
Boston method 53
brain disorders 79
breakaway 144
briefing 299, 300
Brief Psychiatric Rating Scale 153
brokerage case management 9, 52–3
budgeting 237–8
bulimia nervosa 216
business meetings 303

cannabis 31, 219, 220, 221, 222
carbamazepine 16, 74, 189
cardiovascular deaths 250
care, routine monitoring 329–31
care management 9
as ACT 11
Care Programme Approach (CPA) 56,
299, 301
carers
benefits for 235–6
information for 283
psychosocial interventions 282–6
use of term 15
working with 279–91
case control studies 18, 342
case histories 342
case load 45–6
case management 9–11, 52
case managers 9, 10
case notes 329
patient access 14
case studies 35, 36, 38, 45, 47, 60–1, 94, 95, 98,
105–6, 114, 116, 117, 129–30, 145, 155–6,
159, 165–6, 178–80, 184–5, 186, 190–1,
192–3, 194, 206, 209, 213–14, 215, 217,
227–9, 247–8, 257, 264–5, 268, 276–7,
323, 325–6, 331
CAT, *see* cognitive analytical therapy (CAT)
catatonic schizophrenia 170, 171
catchment areas 7
CBT, *see* cognitive behaviour therapy (CBT)
cigarettes 253
cleaning 164

client, use of term 15–16
clinical audit 328, 331–3
clinical case management 10
clinical effectiveness 280, 342
clinical governance 17–19
clinical opinion 26–7
clinical psychologists 21, 50, 51
clinical significance 340
clinical supervision 308–10
clozapine 16, 18, 52, 71, 72, 73, 130, 177, 316
clozaril 71
clubhouse model 265–6
CMHTs, *see* community mental health
teams (CMHTs)
cocaine abuse, pharmacological treatment 226
Cochrane Collaboration 343
cognitive analytical therapy (CAT) 17
cognitive behaviour therapy (CBT) 17,
280, 286
bipolar affective disorder 191
delusions and hallucinations 18, 287–8
depression 209
dropout 281
cognitive deficits 271–2
cognitive flexibility 272
cohort studies 18, 341–2
collaborative empiricism 286
colour blindness/sensitivity 95, 97
community care 19
community care grants 248
Community Mental Health Center
Movement 9
community mental health teams
(CMHTs) 5–6, 7–8
culture 8–9
discharge back to 36–9
community outreach, *see* assertive outreach
community psychiatric nurses (CPNs) 4–5
community psychiatry, evolution of 3–4
community treatment
bipolar affective disorder 185–7
schizophrenia 175–7
community treatment orders 87–9
comorbidity 218, 254
competencies 314–16, 324
compliance 28, 121–35
adherence/concordance 122
aids 131
improving 127–31
monitoring 131
suicide risk 152
therapy 134
see also non-compliance
comprehensive care 47–8
compulsion 79–80
abuse of power 89–90
community treatment orders 87–9
contingency management 85–7

early intervention 80
ethical issues 86, 257–8
financial incentives 85–7
honesty and 81–3
hospital admission 27, 81, 82, 83
inducements and threats 84, 85
leverage 84, 85–7
persuasion 83–5
power relationships 83
risks and benefits 83
therapeutic relationship and 81
compulsions 216
compulsory treatment orders (CTOs) 80, 328
computer training 267
concordance 122
concrete thinking 43
Confidential Inquiry into Suicide and
	Homicide 137, 138, 151, 152, 156
confidentiality 145
bipolar affective disorder 188
personality disorder 203–4
physical illness 256–7
confrontation 82
constructive approach 112–14
consultant psychiatrist 296–7
consumerism 14–16
consumer workers 311
contact frequencies 46–7
contingency management/
	planning 65–6, 85–7
cooking 275
coping strategies 155–6, 191, 287
co-production 14–15
Core Skills Training Framework 316–17
costed care 48
counselling 230, 290
vocational 267
Court of Protection 240–1
CPA *see* Care Programme Approach (CPA)
crack cocaine 220, 222
creative artists 184
criminal behaviour 13, 30–1
crisis access/response 46–7, 62–3
crisis teams 322, 333
critical incident analysis 148
cross-disciplinary supervision 307
cultural sensitivity 92–107; *see also* ethnicity

daily living skills 43, 51, 164, 270–8
assessment 272–3
cognitive deficits and 271–2
interventions 274–7
dangerous severe personality disorder
	(DSPD) 198
Dartmouth ACT scale 11, 42, 58, 119
data 330–1
day centres, work groups 267
debt 238

deception 81
deep cleans 164
de-escalation 140–4
deinstitutionalization 6–7, 9, 13, 19
delinquency 202
delirium tremens 226, 254
delusional disorders 78, 80, 169–81
cognitive behaviour therapy 287
treatment improvements 16–17
dementia praecox 169, 182
democratic therapeutic communities 200
denial and compliance 126
dental health 252, 254
dependency 39, 90–1
pathological 57
depot medication 133–4, 176–7
depression 74, 208–11
antidepressants 16, 72, 74, 126–7, 190, 210
assessment 153, 208–9
bipolar affective disorder 190, 210–11
cognitive behaviour therapy 209
psychotic symptoms 74, 209
rating scales 208–9
support 209–10
desensitization 211
detoxification 226
development meetings 304
diabetes 72, 73, 117, 118, 122, 161, 168, 253
diagnosis 35
Diagnostic and Statistical Manual, see
	DSM-III; DSM-IV; DSM-V
dialectical behaviour therapy 201
dialysis 163
diaries 154
diet 216–17, 253, 255
Dingleton Hospital 6
Diogenes' syndrome 160
direct access 8
disability employment advisers 267
discharge 36–9
supervised 302
disinhibition 185, 189
disorganization and compliance 44, 123
dissocial personality disorder 200, 202–4
disulfiram 226
diversion studies 337
doctors 50, 255–6; *see also* general
	practitioners
domestic commitments 308
dosette boxes 131, 255
double bind 173
double blind trials 18, 340
drug abuse 31–2; *see also* substance abuse
drug history 223
drug rehabilitation programmes 220
drug trials 18
dry mouth 252, 253
DSM-III 170

DSM-IV 198
DSM-V 170, 171, 198–200
dual diagnosis 218–30
    assertive outreach 31–2, 222–4
    assessment 221–2
    harm minimization 227–9
    incidence 220
    medication 226
    motivational interviewing 224–5
    relapse prevention 226–7
    service response 218–20
duty to warn 145
dynamic psychotherapy 201

early intervention 80, 288–9
    bipolar affective disorder 186–7
    schizophrenia 177–8
eating disorders 216–17
education
    family members 129
    patients, medication compliance 128–30
    public 32, 127
efficacy/effectiveness 280, 291, 342
emergency accommodation 245–6
employability 269
Employment Support Allowance (ESA) 232
engagement 27, 45, 86, 111–20
    classification 112, 113
    constructive approach 112–14
    failure 38, 117–18
    measuring and defining 118–19
    minimum period 36
    monitoring approach 115–16
    restrictive approach 116–17
equality and diversity training 94–5
ethics 86, 89, 257–8
ethnicity 92–3
    community engagement 103
    equality and diversity training 94–5
    local demographics 93–4
    'political correctness' 103–4, 106
    staff members 95, 96
    stereotypes 103–4
    suitability for outreach 28
    treatment uptake 93
ethnic representation/matching 96–8
evidence-based practice 3, 4, 17–19, 26–7, 40
experiments 345
expert opinion 42
expressed emotion 71, 174–5, 178, 284
extended hours 66–7
eye contact 143, 276

facilitators 304, 309, 310
families
    education 129
    impending loss 214
    information for 283
    medication compliance 126–7

psychosocial interventions 282–6
    racial harassment by/of 100, 102–3
    schizophrenia and 172–5, 283
    working with 279–91
family commitments 308
fidelity 20, 41, 42–3, 50, 55, 331
financial crises 231
financial incentives 85–7
first names 104
first onset (break) patients 32
flexible assertive community treatment
    (FACT) 53–4
flexible contact 46–7
flexi-time working 67
focus groups 324–5
folie circulaire 182
forensic patients 13, 30–1
Fountain House 265
franchising 320
fraud 238–9
frequent contact 46–7
Fromm-Reichmann, Frieda 174
full support 10
fun 105–6
furniture schemes 236, 247

general practitioners
    appointment keeping 256
    attendances 257
    non-registration 251–2
generic interventions 8
genetic factors 172–3, 183, 279
Goffman, Erving 7
'gold standard' in research 339
government intervention 22–3
graded exposure 211–12
graduate long-stay 13
grief 208, 215
group clinical supervision 309–10
group training 304
guardianship 113
guilt 156, 174, 175, 284

hallucinations 78, 80
    CBT for 287
hallucinogen abuse 32
Hamilton depression scale 208
handing back 33
handover 299, 300
harassment, racial 98–103
harm minimization 224
Hawthorne effect 338
health belief systems 124
health care apartheid 97
health services research 19–22
hebephrenic schizophrenia 170, 171
help-seeking behaviour 93, 250–2
heroin 32
hierarchy of evidence 17, 343–4

holism 290
home care 164, 275
homelessness 220, 242–9
  GP registration 251–2
  night shelters 245, 246
  prevalence 242–3
  service approaches 246–8
  see also housing
home visiting 4, 5, 6, 43–4
homework 212, 276
homicide 136–7, 138
honesty 81–3, 105
Hospital Anxiety Depression Scale 209
hospitals
  appointment keeping 255
  compulsory admission 27, 81, 82, 83
hostels 244–5
hostility 136–49
  incidence 136–7
  individual approaches 140–5
  risk assessment 139–40
  risk factors 137–8
  team approaches 145–9
housing 242–9
  crises 245–6
  furnishing 247
  repairs and faults 247
  types of 243–6
housing associations 244
housing benefit 232, 233
Housing First 246
human nature 123
humour 105–6
hybrid models 53
hypomania 99, 182, 184
  management 187–9, 210–11
hypothesis generation 27, 345–6

ICD-10 170, 171, 197, 198, 199,
  202, 203, 205
ICD-11 197, 200
Income-Related Employment and Support
  Allowance (ESA-IR) 233–4
income support 232, 233
independent accommodation 244
individual approaches
  hostility 140–5
  self-neglect 162–4
  suicide risk 153–6
individual placement and support (IPS)
  program 261–4
induction 296, 316
infectious disease 251, 252
information processing 27, 272
information sheets 283
informed patients 14
innovation 328, 333, 334, 335
inputs 328–9
insight 44, 77–9, 124–6

components 78, 125
scales 124
institutionalization 37, 57
institutional neurosis 6
insulin coma therapy 338
insurance-based systems 33, 329
intensive case management 11
International Classification of Diseases,
  see ICD-10; ICD-11
Internet 14
interpersonal therapy 17
interpreters 94, 95
interventions, generic/specific 8
intoxication 140, 141, 147, 224, 254
in vivo daily living skills 270, 271, 277
in vivo practice 43–5
IPS, *see* individual placement and
  support (IPS)
isolation 208, 211

Job Seeker's Allowance 233, 234
job shadowing 261
judgement 19
  in bipolar affective disorder 184, 185

KASI, *see* knowledge about schizophrenia
  interview (KASI)
key workers 56, 59, 60, 61, 82
  assumptions and responses 97
  competencies 316
  matching 96, 97
Klein, M. 183
knowledge about schizophrenia interview
  (KASI) 283
Kraepelin, E. 169, 170

Laing, R. D. 174
language 103–4
Lasting Power of Attorney 240
leadership 295, 297, 306
leaflets 283
learning disability 29
leave on Section 89, 302
leverage 84, 85–7, 117
life expectancy 250
lithium 16, 18, 73–4, 189
  side effects 254
liver enzymes 222
local needs profile 325
local sources of income and help 236
long-stay population 13

mainstreaming 49
maintenance medication 70–3
management approaches 306
management supervision 306–8, 317
mania 182
manic defence 183
manic-depressive psychosis 182

meals on wheels 166, 227, 235
means-tested benefits 232
medication 69–76
  compliance, *see* compliance
  depot 133–4, 176–7
  maintenance in psychoses 70–3
  reviews 75
  scepticism towards 126–7
  side-effects 71, 72–3, 75, 123–4,
    190, 253–4
  supervised 132–3
meetings
  business meeting 303
  development meetings 304
  duration 297
  weekly reviews 299–303
Mental Health Act (1959) 5–6, 197
mental health care, consumerism in 14–16
mental health nursing
  changes in 22
  training 22, 313
Mental Health Policy Implementation Guide
    (DoH) 52, 94
mental health services
  evaluation activities 328
  modernization 13–14
mental health support workers 8, 51–2
mental health work, fun of 105–6
mental hospitals 6–7
meta-analysis 18, 343
methadone 226
Milgram experiments 89
mind disorders 79
mindfulness-based cognitive therapy 17
mobile phones 312
mobile support teams 63
model fidelity 20, 41, 42–3, 50, 55, 331
modernization 13–14
money management 236–8, 239–41
monitoring
  care 329–33
  medication compliance 131
  mental health services 328
  training 317–18
mood matching 143–4
mood stabilizers 16, 73–4, 189–90
mortality 250
motivational interviewing 224–5, 275
mouth dryness 252, 253
multidisciplinary working 5, 49–54
multiprofessional teams 5, 6, 8

Nacka project 65
names, use of 104
Narcotics Anonymous 225
National Service Framework 52, 63
nature-nurture 92, 172, 183
needs, changing 313–14

needs profile 325
negative symptoms 30
neighbours, racial harassment by/of 100
neurocognitive factors 271
neurotic disorders 215–17
neurotic symptoms 208, 215
neurotransmitters 183
'New Deal for the Mentally Ill' 9
New Hampshire Model 224
new long-stay 38
new technologies 311–12
NHS Plan (DoH) 52, 320
night shelters 245, 246
non-compliance
  causes 122–7
  covert/overt 121
  extent of 122
  relapse risk 121
  suicide and 151
non-experimental studies 341–2
non-verbal techniques 143
normality 79
notes 329
  patient access to 14
nuisance crimes 31
nurses 50
  training 22
nursing homes 245

obesity 252–3
'observed meds' 132
obsessions 216
obsessive compulsive disorders, behavioural
    therapies for 17
occupational therapists 21, 50, 51, 273
offenders 13, 30–1
olanzapine 176, 190
open access 8
Open Dialogue 285
operational policy 304–5
operational training 316–17
opiate abuse 32
  methadone for 226
opportunity costs 64
outcomes 315, 327–8
overdose 151
over-treatment 221

panic disorders 211
paperwork 302
paranoid schizophrenia 170, 171
parasuicide 150, 152
pathological dependency 57
patients
  education 128–30
  informed 14
  matching 96–8
  racial harassment by/of 100–1

suitability for outreach 27–32
use of term 15–16
peer review/support 146–7
persistent delusional disorders 172
personal alarms 148
Personal and Social Performance
  Scale 272–3, 274
personal finance 231–4
Personal Independence Payment (PIP) 232,
  234–5, 236
personality disorders 196–207
  assertive outreach 201–2
  borderline 200, 204, 205
  clusters 199–200
  confidentiality and risk 203–4
  definitions 198–200
  diagnosis 197–8
  dissocial 200, 202–4
  suitability for outreach 29–30
  team approach and reviews 205–6
  therapeutic approach 204–6
  treatability 198, 200–1
personal narrative 196
personal space 143
persuasion 83–5
phobic disorders 211
physical assaults 144–5
  prosecution following 148–9
physical examination 161
physical health care 250–9
  confidentiality 256–7
  delivery by mental health staff 255–6,
    257, 258
  neglect of 163, 252–3
  outreach worker role 254–8
physical illness
  increased, causes of 252–4
  suicide risk 152
  toleration of 250–1
  treatment monitoring and supporting 255
pilot schemes 333
PIP, *see* Personal Independence Payment (PIP)
planning process 323–6
political correctness 103–4, 106
politicians 22
population matching 96
positive symptoms 169, 171
post-psychotic depression 208
post-review time 302
post-traumatic stress disorder 213–14
Powell, F. 7
power, statistical 341
power calculation 340
power relationships 83
  abuse of power 89–90
powers of attorney 240
pragmatic trials 342
pre-post studies 337

primary care, withdrawal of support by 257
prison 220
problem solving 143
process evaluation 328
professional developments 21
professionalism 330
programme in assertive community treatment
  (PACT) 11, 44, 270
prompting 130–1
prosecutions 148–9
psychiatrists 51, 244, 296–7
psychiatry 79
psychoanalysis 290
psychodynamic approaches 290
psycho-education 283–4
psychological treatments 21, 191
psychosis
  acute and transient 172
  CBT treatment 287–8
  first onset 32
  maintenance medication 70–3
  suitability for outreach 27, 28, 29, 30
psychosocial interventions 279–91
  bipolar affective disorder 190–4
  carers 282–6
  early intervention 288–9
  families 282–6
  patient-focused 286–9
  resistance 280–1
  schizophrenia 178–80
  supporting in community
    outreach 281–2, 289–90
  training 318
psychotherapy 17, 21, 57, 201, 280, 281
public
  education of 32, 127
  racial harassment by/of 100–1

qualitative research 344–6
quantitative research 344
quasi-experimental studies 335, 341

racial discrimination 97
racial harassment 98–103
racial sterotypes 103–4
randomized controlled trial (RCT) 17–18, 339
Rapp, C. 46
RCT, *see* randomized controlled trial (RCT)
realistic interdependence 275
reciprocal inhibition 211
records, *see* case notes
Recovery Approach 33, 53, 119, 136, 237, 271,
  268, 285
recovery goals 49, 53
recruitment 310–11
referral 32–6
rehabilitation-orientated case management 53
reinstitutionalization 13

relapse
  employment and 269
  management 162–3
  medication non-compliance 121
  severe 28
  substance abuse 226–7
relapse signatures 288–9
  bipolar affective disorder 186–7, 191
  schizophrenia 177–8
relationships 12, 77, 83, 105
Remploy 266
renal failure 255
renal problems 254
representative payeeship 239–40
research 9, 10, 19–22, 327, 335–6
  assessing studies 20, 23
  bias 336–8
  gulf between theory and practice 280
  methods 336, 338–42
residential provision 216–19
resistance 280–1, 324, 330
resource files 236
respiratory deaths 250
responsibility 306
restrictive approach 116–17
review for discharge 37
reviews 50, 72, 75
risk factors and risk assessment
  dissocial personality disorder 203–4
  hostility 137–40
  self-neglect 160–2
  suicide 151–3
risk management plans 140
risk reduction 207
role play 276
roles, changing 313–14
Royal College of Physicians 87

safety systems 147–8
sampling bias 337–8
SBAR 299
schism and skew 174
schizoaffective disorder 172
schizophrenia 169–81
  Africans/Afro-Caribbeans 93
  antipsychotics for 70, 175–7
  behavioural family management 284–5
  behavioural therapies 17, 18
  bordering disorders 172
  CBT treatment 18
  change over time 32
  classifications 170–1
  community treatments 175–7
  depression and 74, 209
  discharge follow-up, historical aspects 4
  early intervention 177–8
  family factors 172–5, 283
  family treatments 18

first description of 169
first-rank symptoms 169
four 'A's 169
genetic factors 172–3
institutional neurosis 6
life expectancy 73
positive symptoms 169
post-traumatic stress disorder 213–14
psychosocial interventions 178–80
relapse 177–8
substance abuse 31
treatment improvements 16–17
schizophreniform disorders 172
schizophrenogenic mother 174
schizotypal disorders 172
Schneider, K. 169
secteur approach 4
Section 17 leave 89, 302
sedation 253
self-disclosure 310–11
self-harm 152–3; *see also* suicide/suicidality
self-neglect 160–8
  ill health 163, 252–3
  incidence 160
  individual interventions 162–4
  risk factors and risk assessment 160–2
  team approaches 164–7
self-referral 8–9
service agents 9
service change 325–6
service development 328, 333–5
service examples 322
service planning 320–6
service proposal 325
service users 15
seven-day working 67–8
sexually transmitted disease 251
shame 264
sheltered accommodation 245
sheltered workshops 266
sick role 210
simple schizophrenia 170, 171
single point of entry 326
situational disorders 213–14
skill
  acquisition 271, 272
  maintenance 258
sleep problems 186–7, 188–9
smartphones 312
smoking 253
social drift 248
social enterprises 266
Social Functioning Scale 272, 273
social housing 244
social influences 6
social linking 163–4
social networks 155, 163–4, 272
social skills 269, 275–6

social stressors 6
social support 6, 194
social systems 285–6
social workers 48–9, 50, 58, 307
societal attitudes 127
Socratic dialogue 286
sodium valproate 74
specialist one-to-one work programmes 261
specific interventions 8
staff
 backgrounds 95
 personal issues 308
 racial harassment of 95, 96
 recruitment 310–11
 selection 310–11
 turnover 37
stakeholder conferences 324–5
standards 314
standing orders 240
staring 143
state benefits, see benefits
statistics 331, 340–1
steering group 324
Stein, L. L. 10, 19, 21, 41, 43, 57, 270, 323
step-down 37, 38–9
stereotypes 104–5
stigma 104, 127, 134, 137
strengths model 53, 113, 268
stress reduction, bipolar affective disorder 193
stress-vulnerability model 181, 248, 286–7
structured assessment tools 153, 209
 group training 315
structuring 130, 131
substance abuse 31–2, 118, 218–30
 acknowledged 221–2
 associated findings 220–1
 community outreach 222–4
 harm minimization 227–9
 incidence 150–1, 220
 motivational interviewing 224–5
 pharmacological intervention 226
 physical illness 254
 relapse prevention 226–7
 service response 218–20
 structured assessment 221–2
 violence risk 137, 138
suicide/suicidality 18, 150–9
 attempted 150
 incidence 150–1
 individual interventions 153–6
 post-suicide procedure 156, 158
 removing means 154–5
 risk factors and risk assessment 151–3, 157–8
 suicidal thoughts 152
supervised medication 132–3
supervision 306–10, 318, 330, 331
support 130–1, 209–10, 289–90
support workers 8, 51–2

survivors 15
symptom management 144
systematic care programme reviews 9
systematic reviews 343

take-away food 275
tardive dyskinesia 72
task-centred approach 59
team approach 49–54, 56, 57–8, 61
 drawbacks 58–9
 hostility 145–9
 personality disorder 205–6
 self-neglect 164–7
team building 303
team days 303–4
team doctors 255–6
team leaders 34, 295–6, 306
team management 295–312
team supervision 331
team targets 331
technology 311–12
telepsychiatry 312
terminology 15
Test, M. A. 3, 10, 19, 21, 41, 43, 270, 323
therapeutic alliance 128
 bipolar affective disorder 185–6
 compliance and 128
 compulsion and 81
 ethnic matching 96–7
 honesty 81–3
 knowing 'too much' 80–1
therapeutic communities 200
therapeutic efficacy 280, 291, 342
Thorn courses 280, 281
throughput 36–7
thyroid problems 254
Time Budget Measure 273
timetabling 297, 298
total institutions 7
traditional healing 103
training 313–19
 competencies 314–16, 317–18
 equality and diversity 94–5
 intervention skills 316
 monitoring 317–18
 operational 316–17
 outcomes 318
 structured assessment tool use 315
 work-related 267
training in community
 living 10, 43, 57, 262
trauma 254
treatment
 efficacy and effectiveness 280, 291, 342
 improvements 16–17
 societal attitudes 127
 uptake and ethnicity 93
 24-hour service 16, 62

treatment (*Cont.*)
  costs/benefits 64–5, 68
  need for 63–4
  sustaining the service 65

UC, *see* Universal Credit (UC)
UK700 study 20, 29, 42, 119, 247, 339
United States, case management 9–11
Universal Credit (UC) 233
unstable patients 27
urine drug screens 222
users 15
user workers 130, 133
utilities, paying for 238

venepuncture training 316
videoconference 312
videos 134, 283, 317
violence, *see* hostility
vocational counselling 267
vocationally focused
     outreach 264–5
vocational programmes 260
vocational training 267

voluntary sector teams 52
voluntary work 266–7

waiting lists 35
Warlingham Park Hospital 4
'Water Tower' speech 7
weekend working 67
weekly review meeting 299–303
weekly schedules 297–303
welfare benefits, *see* benefits
'when I am gone' (WIAG) 214
whole team approach, *see* team approach
WIAG, *see* 'when I am gone' (WIAG)
work assessment 268–9
work groups 267
working alliance 128; *see also* therapeutic alliance
working tax credit 233
work preparation 267
work-related activity 261–8
work training 267

Yerkes-Dodson curve 128, 129

zero tolerance 98–9, 148